W 18 BER £40

Lessons from Problem-based Learning

Lessons from Problem-based Learning

Edited by
Henk van Berkel
Albert Scherpbier
Harry Hillen
Cees van der Vleuten

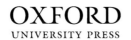

OXFORD
UNIVERSITY PRESS

OXFORD

UNIVERSITY PRESS

Great Clarendon Street, Oxford OX2 6DP

Oxford University Press is a department of the University of Oxford.
It furthers the University's objective of excellence in research, scholarship,
and education by publishing worldwide in

Oxford New York

Auckland Cape Town Dar es Salaam Hong Kong Karachi
Kuala Lumpur Madrid Melbourne Mexico City Nairobi
New Delhi Shanghai Taipei Toronto

With offices in

Argentina Austria Brazil Chile Czech Republic France Greece
Guatemala Hungary Italy Japan Poland Portugal Singapore
South Korea Switzerland Thailand Turkey Ukraine Vietnam

Oxford is a registered trade mark of Oxford University Press
in the UK and in certain other countries

Published in the United States
by Oxford University Press Inc., New York

British Library Cataloguing in Publication Data
Data available

Library of Congress Cataloging in Publication Data
Data available

Typeset in Minion by Glyph International, Bangalore, India
Printed in Great Britain
on acid-free paper by
the MPG Books Group, Bodmin and King's Lynn

ISBN 978-0-19-958344-7

10 9 8 7 6 5 4 3

Oxford University Press makes no representation, express or implied, that the drug dosages in this book
are correct. Readers must therefore always check the product information and clinical procedures with
the most up-to-date published product information and data sheets provided by the manufacturers and
the most recent codes of conduct and safety regulations. The authors and the publishers do not accept
responsibility or legal liability for any errors in the text or for the misuse or misapplication of material
in this work. Except where otherwise stated, drug dosages and recommendations are for the non-pregnant
adult who is not breastfeeding.

Contents

Preface

Problem-based learning has excited interest among educators around the world. Among the most notable applications of problem-based learning is the approach taken at the Faculty of Health, Medicine and Life Sciences (FHML) at Maastricht University, the Netherlands. The intention of the book is to inform an international audience on the situation of the Maastricht FHML, at that moment more than thirty-five years after its founding. Starting in 1974 as a medical school, the faculty embarked on the innovative pathway of problem-based learning, trying to establish a medical training programme. This programme applied recent insights of education which would be better adapted to the needs of the modern physician. The medical school, currently part of the FHML, can be considered an 'established' school, where original innovations and educational changes have become part of a routine. As an innovative school we believe there is an obligation to document our findings, and to share our experiences with others. This is our intention in producing this book.

We believe that this book supplies the reader with information which is not otherwise available from any one source, and hope that it proves useful and gives rise to further debate and refinement of problem-based learning in specific applications elsewhere and in general education discussion and thought.

The editors thank Mereke Gorsira for her excellent editorial work.

On behalf of the authors, the editors:

Henk van Berkel
Albert Scherpbier
Harry Hillen
Cees van der Vleuten
Maastricht, The Netherlands
January 2010

Contributors

Han Aarts
Mundo, Maastricht University,
The Netherlands

Marre Andrée Wiltens
Student at Maastricht University,
The Netherlands

Pie Bartholomeus
Maastricht University,
Faculty of Health, Medicine and
Life Sciences,
Skillslab,
The Netherlands

Esther Bergman
Maastricht University,
Faculty of Health, Medicine and
Life Sciences, Department of
Anatomy/Embryology,
The Netherlands

Henk van Berkel
Maastricht University, Faculty of Health,
Medicine and Life Sciences,
Department of Educational Development and
Educational Research,
The Netherlands

Lonneke Bokken
Pediatric Department,
UMC St. Radboud, Nijmegen,
The Netherlands

Emmaline Brouwer
Maastricht University,
Faculty of Health, Medicine and
Life Sciences,
Skillslab,
The Netherlands

Jan van Dalen
Maastricht University,
Faculty of Health, Medicine and
Life Sciences,
Skillslab,
The Netherlands

Agnes Diemers
Maastricht University,
Faculty of Health, Medicine and
Life Sciences,
Skillslab,
The Netherlands

Diana Dolmans
Maastricht University,
Faculty of Health, Medicine and
Life Sciences, Department of Educational
Development and Educational Research,
The Netherlands

Jeroen Donkers
Maastricht University,
Faculty of Health, Medicine and
Life Sciences, Department of Educational
Development and Educational Research,
The Netherlands

Robbert Duvivier
Maastricht University,
Faculty of Health, Medicine and Life Sciences,
Skillslab,
The Netherlands

Fons van den Eeckhout
Maastricht University Library,
The Netherlands

Anton 'Ton' de Goeij
Maastricht University,
Faculty of Health, Medicine and
Life Sciences, Department of Pathology and
Institute for Education,
The Netherlands

Willem de Grave
Maastricht University,
Faculty of Health, Medicine and
Life Sciences, Department of Educational
Development and Educational Research,
The Netherlands

Jeroen ten Haaf
Maastricht University Library,
The Netherlands

Erik Heineman
University Medical Center Groningen,
Department of Surgery, Groningen,
The Netherlands

Harry Hillen
Maastricht University,
Faculty of Health, Medicine and
Life Sciences,
The Netherlands

Nynke de Jong
Maastricht University,
Faculty of Health, Medicine and
Life Sciences,
School for Public Health and Primary Care,
Department of Health Care and
Nursing Science,
The Netherlands

Krista Koetsenruijter
Maastricht University,
Faculty of Health, Medicine and
Life Sciences,
The Netherlands

Marijke Kruithof
Maastricht University,
Faculty of Health, Medicine and
Life Sciences,
Skillslab,
The Netherlands

Bas de Leng
Maastricht University,
Faculty of Health, Medicine and
Life Sciences, Department of Educational
Development and Educational Research,
The Netherlands

Gaby Lutgens
Maastricht University Library,
The Netherlands

Gerard Majoor
Maastricht University,
Faculty of Health, Medicine and
Life Sciences,
Institute for Education,
The Netherlands

Stewart Mennin
Professor Emeritus,
Department of Cell Biology and Physiology,
University of New Mexico School of
Medicine,
Albuquerque,
New Mexico, USA;
Mennin Consulting and Associates Inc,
Sao Paulo, Brazil

Jeroen van Merriënboer
Maastricht University,
Faculty of Health, Medicine and
Life Sciences, Department of Educational
Development and Educational Research,
The Netherlands

Jos Moust
Maastricht University,
Faculty of Health, Medicine and Life
Sciences, Department of Educational
Development and Educational Research,
The Netherlands

Arno Muijtjens
Maastricht University,
Faculty of Health, Medicine and
Life Sciences, Department of Educational
Development and Educational Research,
The Netherlands

Susan Niemantsverdriet
University of Applied Sciences Leiden,
Department Policy Support and Strategic
Advice, Leiden,
The Netherlands

Martin Paul
Maastrucht University,
Faculty of Health, Medicine and
Life Science,
Dean's Office
The Netherlands

Jan-Joost Rethans
Maastricht University,
Faculty of Health, Medicine and
Life Sciences,
Skill lab,
The Netherlands

Herma Roebertsen
Maastricht University,
Faculty of Health, Medicine and
Life Sciences, Department of Educational
Development and Educational Research,
The Netherlands

Albert Scherpbier
Maastricht University,
Faculty of Health, Medicine and Life Sciences,
Institute for Education,
The Netherlands

Henk Schmidt
Erasmus University,
Department of Psychology,
Rotterdam,
The Netherlands

Marie-Louise Schreurs
Maastricht University,
Faculty of Health, Medicine and
Life Sciences, Department of Educational
Development and Educational Research,
The Netherlands

Lambert Schuwirth
Maastricht University,
Faculty of Health, Medicine and
Life Sciences, Department of Educational
Development and Research,
The Netherlands

Hetty Snellen-Balendong
Maastricht University,
Faculty of Health, Medicine and
Life Sciences, Department of Educational
Development and Educational Research,
The Netherlands

Renée Stalmeijer
Maastricht University,
Faculty of Health, Medicine and
Life Sciences, Department of Educational
Development and Educational Research,
The Netherlands

Fred Stevens
Maastricht University,
Faculty of Health, Medicine and
Life Sciences, Department of Educational
Development and Educational Research,
The Netherlands

Mascha Verheggen
Maastricht University,
Faculty of Health, Medicine and
Life Sciences, Department of Educational
Development and Educational Research,
The Netherlands

Daniëlle Verstegen
Maastricht University,
Faculty of Health, Medicine and
Life Sciences, Department of Educational
Development and Educational Research,
The Netherlands

Maarten Verwijnen
Maastricht University,
Faculty of Health, Medicine and
Life Sciences,
Skillslab,
The Netherlands

Cees van der Vleuten
Maastricht University,
Faculty of Health, Medicine and
Life Sciences, Department of Educational
Development and Educational Research,
The Netherlands

Wynand Wijnen
Maastricht University,
Faculty of Health, Medicine and
Life Sciences, Department of Educational
Development and Educational Research,
The Netherlands

Hubertina 'Incke' Wolfhagen
Maastricht University,
Faculty of Health, Medicine and
Life Sciences, Department of Educational
Development and Research,
The Netherlands

Chapter 1

Introduction: Sustainability of PBL and innovation in medical education at Maastricht University

Stewart Mennin

What PBL contributes

The development and spread of problem-based learning (PBL) is significant for contributing to the transformation of educational experiences for students and teachers in health professions institutions worldwide. In the latter part of the twentieth and beginning of the twenty-first century, learning has come to be understood more as an interactive situated and social process than one in which the teacher as knower transmits information to the student as knowee (Bleakley, 2006; Doll Jr, 1993). Problem-based learning has promoted explanation and questioning at the frontiers of understanding and propelled learners into self-directed, inquiry-based learning in authentic contexts relevant to the priority health needs of society. Learning has been reframed as a social interaction in which the quality of exchange and mindfulness of questioning has become the currency and source of understanding and knowing. Students develop the skills necessary to work and learn in teams early in their medical education. The sciences basic to medicine are more integrated and complementary with the clinical sciences and less frequently encountered as disarticulated and fragmented disciplines. Assessment of understanding as doing is more sophisticated than ever and is coming to be embedded with how and where learning occurs.

PBL: still relevant and practical?

Still, some may ask, 'Is PBL still relevant and practical for today's medical education?' What is relevant is learning and PBL is about transformative and enduring learning that emerges from interactive experiences, continuity, and variable iterations over time in a recursive social process of reflection and feedback (Dewey, 1938; Doll Jr, 1993; Mennin, 2007). Is PBL still practical? It depends. The practicalities of PBL present challenges for students, as well as teachers that shape the governance and organization of a curriculum. Do we need a new, exciting, more fashionable, cheaper, and easier approach to learning? A cheaper, easier health professions education is an oxymoron. Problem-based learning, when done well, continues to be necessary and relevant for the health professions as an interactive and humanistic approach to learning. Where there has been difficulty with PBL, in my experience, it has been when it is applied robotically as a formula, a technique, a tool, and an instrument. Problem-based learning requires continuous attention to faculty development (Dolmans et al., 2005a). Sustaining a quality PBL program is more difficult than starting one (Chapter 17).

The authors in this book make clear how they adapted and modified their approach to PBL as circumstances evolved, maintaining the relevance of their curriculum for more than three decades.

Central to this process was the extent to which small-group PBL was understood and applied by teachers and students (Chapters 12 and 19). Staff development (Chapter 18) is fundamental to Maastricht's story of sustainability.

Staff development and sustainability of PBL

From the beginning, Maastricht recognized the essential nature of informed teaching skills for a different concept of learning. Deliberate practice (Ericsson, 2004) based on well-established principles of staff development applied consistently formed the basis of the approach. The emphasis was on learning rather than teaching, on making connections, knowing in action through collaborative dialogue, promoting discovery and clarification, and, most important of all, formulating questions at the frontiers of understanding. Learning to question at the frontier of understanding meaningfully informs self-directed learning. The systematic development of teachers' pedagogic abilities is an essential part of the job and cannot be viewed as an add-on to the work and time required of a teacher/facilitator. Faculty development is mandatory at Maastricht, whereas at most of the world' schools it is voluntary. Staff development in resource-limited countries is a major challenge to effective and sustainable PBL programs.

Marie-Louis Schreurs and Willem de Grave (Chapter 18) describe how staff development for PBL has grown and remained relevant by developing new approaches as different needs arose. Similarly, Chapter 6 by Jos Moust provides a multidimensional framework for the abilities required of effective tutors. The work of Dolmans and Schmidt colleagues has shown that the well-formed cases and problems are essential for effective PBL (Dolmans, et al., 2005b) (Chapter 3). Maastricht has focused on the process of learning, making it complementary with what is to be learned. These are essential lessons that emerge from what is written in these pages.

Fundamental to the sustainability of Maastricht's curriculum has been the consistent high-quality, in-depth, research-based scholarship and abundant publications about how PBL works. The review of evidence about PBL at Maastricht by Henk Schmidt (Chapter 24) is a fine example of scholarship and research that has served to advance understanding of learning in a PBL setting. Debates about the efficacy of PBL (Colliver, 2000; Kirschner et al., 2006; Norman & Schmidt, 2000; Schmidt et al., 2006; Schmidt et al., 2009a; Schmidt et al., 2009b) continue to serve as a stimulus for further dialogue and study. Maastricht developed a series of scholarly programmes that include post-graduate study and degree programs in health professions education, a contribution with global impact.

Sustainability of innovation requires continuous reflection about supportive infrastructure (Chapter 20) and regular attention to quality indicators in the curriculum (Chapter 17). In addition, sustainability requires a thoughtful institutional response to reflection and quality evaluation. At Maastricht this has resulted in alternative adaptations of PBL (Chapter 14), which will be studied and refined over time.

Are there other ways to achieve what PBL has to offer? Probably, however, most modifications and variations of PBL seem, to this author, to be more teaching-centred than learning- and relationship-centred. The choice is made by each institution based on its practical realities, history, and understanding of the principles of learning and curriculum development (Mennin & Krackov, 1998). In the final analysis, bad PBL is worse than no PBL at all.

Lessons in sustainability

What deepens the value of this book are insights derived from reflection and descriptions of how Maastricht adapted and modified its approachs to PBL over the years while strengthening their basic philosophy and core principles. Readers will find a systematic, longitudinal, scholarly and research-based approach that created and sustained a culture of learning at Maastricht's Faculty of Health, Medicine and Life Sciences. It is a powerful and much needed message for other institutions involved with PBL and curriculum innovation. Wherever health professions education institutions are challenged to provide educational programmes relevant to society's priority healthcare needs, one finds issues of sustainability.

How did Maastricht do it? They began the medical school with PBL. They didn't have to deal with the challenges of changing from an existing traditional curriculum. They had resources and effective leadership; they were well organized; and they were situated in Western Europe with a culture supportive of collaborative work (Chapter 2). They had a meritocracy in which following the rules was part of the culture. They valued faculty development, scholarship, and research to understand and improve learning at the level of the individual, group, and institution. In many parts of the world, weak regulatory systems substitute power, longevity, politics, and position in the organizational hierarchy for merit, making sustainable change difficult.

Teaching mindfully is a powerful source of learning. Maastricht has been fortunate to have a significant role in encouraging and supporting innovation and change for individuals and institutions around the world and in so doing they have learned what works and how that experience helps to improve what they do at home (Chapter 25). What could other schools be doing to benchmark with Maastricht? They can strengthen their resolve to promote integration and learning relevant to the priority health needs of society as their most important activity. They can engage in scholarly studies of learning at their institution that go beyond reports of student satisfaction and unit grades and study the deeper issues of clarification and explanation of what is observed (Cook et al., 2008). Maastricht has been doing this consistently for the past 35 years.

Other powerful lessons in sustainability are derived from assessment where Lambert Schuwirth and Cees van der Vleuten discuss what led them to develop a comprehensive programme for assessment (Chapter 21). Their focus is on understanding how assessment is part of the learning process rather than a narrow perspective of the tools and instrumentality of PBL and assessment.

A postmodern curriculum

A curriculum for today's complex world, in the words of William Doll Jr., needs to be 'rich, recursive, relational and robust' (Doll Jr, 1993). Richness refers to the depth of the curriculum, its layers of meaning, and its different possible interpretations. Curriculum needs to be 'provocatively generative without losing form or shape . . . it needs disturbing qualities, perturbations, to provide richness'. Richness comes from negotiating passages between various interpretations of situations, data, and experiences. Recursion is about looping thoughts on thoughts in reflective interaction with the environment and with culture as an essential part of transformation. Formative assessment exemplifies this. In recursion, 'there is both stability and change; . . . in an orderly but often unpredictable manner', the educational structure is stable as the learner changes. Complex curricula are spiral, recursive, developmental, and comprehensive with tests, practicals, portfolios, and other completions that become the beginning of the next part of the learning process. Reflection conceived as recursion is helpful in developing competence and promoting inquiry. 'Without reflection engendered by dialogue, recursion becomes shallow not transformative; it is not reflective recursion, it is only repetition.' Relations are constantly changing and it becomes important to seek the connections between different things. An integrated learning experience values human relationships as an essential aspect of explanations about interactions. 'What becomes important are the connections with people, with the environment and the culture . . . our local perspectives integrate into a larger cultural, ecological, cosmic matrix.'

Rigor is important in a transformational curriculum. It means 'purposely looking for different alternatives, relations, connections', looking for and uncovering the assumptions that underlie our understanding. In the rapidly changing world of health professions education, it refers to the capability of learners to frame new questions, define problems, and seek understanding in new situations. This is what Maastricht has accomplished by sustaining its innovative PBL curriculum for 35 years, co-evolving, learning, and studying what it does to make it better for all concerned.

Reading this book was like coming home. It reminded me of my experiences between 1979 and 1993 with New Mexico's problem-based, community-oriented Primary Care Curriculum (Kaufman et al., 1989). Like Maastricht we had a coherent curriculum with an integrated and collaborative approach to learning. This book refreshed my love for learning, exploration, discovery, and understanding.

References

Bleakley, A. (2006). Broadening conceptions of learning in medical education: the message from team working. *Medical Education* **40**, 150–7.

Colliver, J. A. (2000). Effectiveness of problem-based learning curricula: research and theory. *Academic Medicine* **75**, 259–66.

Cook, D. A., Bordage, G., and Schmidt, H. G. (2008). Description, justification, and clarification: a framework for classifying the purposes of research in medical education. *Medical Education* **42**, 128–33.

Dewey, J. (1938). *Experience and education*. New York: Touchstone.

Doll Jr, W. E. (1993). *A post-modern perspective on curriculum*. New York: Teachers College Press.

Dolmans, D. H., de Grave, W., Wolfhagen, I. H., and van der Vleuten, C. P. (2005a). Problem-based learning: future challenges for educational practice and research. *Meical Edcuation* **39**, 732–41.

Dolmans, D. J. H. M., de Grave, W., Wolfhagen, I. H., van der Vleuten, C. P. M., and Wijnen, W. H. F. W. (2005b). Problem effectiveness in a course using problem-based learning. *Academic Medicine* **68**, 207–13.

Ericsson, A. K. (2004). Deliberate practice and the acquisition and maintenance of expert performance in medicine and related domains. *Academic Medicine* **79**(10 Supplement), s70–s81.

Kaufman, A., Mennin, S., Waterman, R., Duban, S., Hansbarger, C., Silverblatt, H., et al. (1989). The New Mexico Experiment: Educational innovation and institutional change. *Academic Medicine* **64**, 285–94.

Kirschner, P. A., Sweller, J., and Clark, R. E. (2006). Why minimal guidance during instruction does not work: an analysis of the failure of constructivist, discovery, problem-based, experiential, and inquiry-based teaching. *Educational Psychologist* **41**, 75–86.

Mennin, S. P. (2007). Small-group problem-based learning as a complex adaptive system. *Teaching and Teacher Education* **23**, 303–13.

Mennin, S. P., and Krackov, S. K. (1998). Reflections on relevance, resistance, and reform in medical education. *Academic Medicine* **73**, S60–S64.

Norman, G., and Schmidt, H. G. (2000). Effectiveness of problem-based learning curricula: theory, practice and paper darts. *Medical Education* **34**, 721–8.

Schmidt, H. G., Cohen-Schotanus, J., and Arends, L. (2009). Impact of problem-based, active, learning on graduation rates of 10 generations Dutch medical students. *Medical Education* **43**(3), 211–18.

Schmidt, H. G., van der Molen, H. T., te Winkel, W. W. R., and Wijnen, W. H. F. W. (2009). Constructivist, problem-based learning does work: a meta-analysis of curricular comparisons involving a single medical school. *Educational Psychologist* **44**, 227–49.

Schmidt, H. G., Vermeulen, L., and van der Molen, H. T. (2006). Long-term effects of problem-based learning: a comparison of competencies acquired by graduates of a problem-based and a conventional medical school. *Medical Education* **40**, 562–7.

Chapter 2

History of problem-based learning in medical education

Harry Hillen, Albert Scherpbier, and Wynand Wijnen

The Faculty of Medicine was founded in 1974, as the first faculty of the new University of Maastricht. From the outset, problem-based learning (PBL) has been the trademark of the university and the Faculty of Medicine. Other faculties were established later (from 1977 onwards) and followed suit by adopting PBL as their primary method of learning. This chapter concentrates on the history of PBL within the (former) Faculty of Medicine, which today has merged with the Faculty of Health Sciences into the Faculty of Health, Medicine and Life Sciences.

Introduction

PBL was introduced in medical faculties across Canada and Australia at approximately the same time that it was first introduced in Maastricht. The historical context of this international (PBL) development will be discussed. Was it a coincidence that PBL was exported overseas to Maastricht of all places? During the early years of the medical faculty, PBL was beset by a host of problems. What were the strategies employed by the faculty to meet these challenges? What were the decisive factors in the successful introduction of PBL in Maastricht? The early obstacles as well as the factors that have contributed to the success of PBL, not only in Maastricht, but in general, will be discussed.

The international context

Education, including PBL, is embedded in a social context. Educational innovation, PBL in particular, was part of the context of change that characterized the 1960s and 1970s. The post-war era with its sober, law-abiding social climate and conservative leadership was over and done with. Society as a whole was ready for change and innovation. In education, passive learning and the reward principles of behaviourism were replaced by active, student-centred learning, in accordance with the (new) principles of cognitive psychology. Authority and deductive learning lost their primacy, while independence, freedom, and personal growth gained increasing popularity. Educational innovation was the unmistakeable result of that societal context.

Based on the apprenticeship model of the professional guilds, medicine has long been a bastion of traditional learning. However, somewhere between 1960 and 1970, several developments occurred in medicine that would eventually lead to change and innovation in the training of medical doctors. With the advancement of biomedical technology and the rapid growth in the numbers of specialists and hospitals, medicine became very expensive, industrial, and indifferent. The French philosopher Michel Foucault (1963) published a critical review of the compulsory system of clinical medicine entitled *Naissance de la Clinique*. According to Foucault, many aspects of modern society were under the control of powerful medical institutions and the population was medicalized as a result of the primacy of hospital medicine. The English epidemiologist Thomas McKeown (1979) published influential and highly critical papers on the results and successes of medicine under the revealing title *The Role of Medicine: Dream, Mirage or Nemesis?* The improved health of the British people and the decline of infectious diseases were attributed not to the achievements of medicine or the good care of doctors, but to the introduction of toilets and sanitary systems and improved nutrition. In fact, the situation was even worse: medical interventions could be harmful. The doctor and the hospital had to change!

After the Second World War, together with increasing social criticism of medicine, a wealth of medical knowledge became available. As a result, two important developments emerged: new techniques, such as intensive care, haemodialysis, and cardiac catheterization, were the apparent and eminent signs of medical progress. But around 1970, progress came to a standstill. Societal factors, more than medical factors, played an important role in the emergence of new, poorly understood diseases, such as irritable bowel and chronic fatigue syndrome. The upsurge in complaints from many of the 'worried well' was blamed on the undesirable and costly medicalization of society. This process is convincingly analyzed in *The Rise and Fall of Modern Medicine* by the writer/columnist Le Fanu (1999). It was not only the voice of these authors that questioned modern medicine; experienced teachers and physicians also became convinced that, in lieu of these developments, more emphasis on the societal aspects of healthcare was called for both in medicine and in the education of future medical doctors.

In addition to social criticism and the rise and fall of clinical medicine, there was a third cause for serious concern with regard to medical education: the volume and changeability of medical knowledge. It was no longer feasible to master medical knowledge in its entirety. Not only had the volume of knowledge increased dramatically; it was also obvious that medical knowledge continued to evolve at a daunting pace. Thus, memorizing existing knowledge, the long-time mainstay of medical education, was no longer an attainable goal. Medical educators were forced to come up with a solution. This was, in a nutshell, the international context in which PBL came into being. At least this was the case in Hamilton, Canada, and Maastricht, the Netherlands.

History of PBL

PBL has its origins at McMaster University, Canada. In 1966, a small but influential group of educational innovators put together a new curriculum. The leading members of this group included Jim Anderson, Howard Barrows, and (founding) dean John Evans.

Jim Anderson, a professor of anatomy and physical anthropology, is considered the creator of PBL with learning in small groups of students. The idea of presenting real-life patient problems and the use of simulated patients for educational purposes was the brainchild of the neurologist Howard Barrows. Dean Evans was responsible for the central organization of education within the faculty. The (new) medical curriculum, based on PBL, was launched in 1969. The programme attracted broad international attention, especially from universities just starting out. Aside from the work at McMaster University, pioneer work was also being carried out at Newcastle University (Australia), Michigan State University (USA), and Maastricht University (the Netherlands).

The history of problem-based learning in Maastricht

In September 1969, the Dutch government decided that a new university was to be established in the City of Maastricht, Province of Limburg. The university began with one faculty, 'Medicine', the eighth medical faculty in the Netherlands. Maastricht was selected for several reasons: a policy decision to distribute higher education more evenly over the country; Maastricht's geographically attractive location in Europe; and compensation for the massive job losses caused by the closure of the coal mines in the region. The creation of an eighth medical faculty was initially justified by the general shortage of physicians in the Netherlands. Eventually, however, the political arguments were superseded by a call for the revitalization of medical education and the modernization of medical care as the primary task of the faculty.

The Netherlands now found itself in a period of transformation. Students took an active stance against the authoritarian university system and the *provo* movement in Amsterdam became a daily news item. Another determining factor was the excessive increases in scale and costs of 'specialist and technical healthcare' in the Netherlands. More attention was needed for primary healthcare and the education of family physicians. The government became increasingly keen to improve the efficiency of what had become a very costly medical education programme.

Dropout rates in medical education were high and many students ran into difficulties when the predominantly theoretical programme was transformed into a programme with a stronger clinical orientation. Traditionally, medical education was largely focused on the final exam. Many, including the students, felt that the education of doctors was poorly aligned with professional medical practice. This situation was fertile ground for the introduction of change and renewal.

The transformation of medical education can be traced back to the basic philosophy of Maastricht University. In line with international developments, the university board developed a four-point basic strategy:

♦ Extra attention given to the education of primary care physicians to counteract the highly specialized healthcare in hospitals;

♦ Educational revitalization by applying PBL to develop attitudes that will bridge the gap between education and professional practice and that will improve the communication skills of physicians;

♦ Research in multidisciplinary teams to counteract the autonomous and narrow scope of research in separate disciplines; and

♦ Transformation of all areas of healthcare to knock down the walls that separated the different chains of the healthcare system.

Discussions were held about distributing academic positions throughout academic regions that did not have an academic hospital. Within this basic philosophy the transformation of education played a major role.

The philosophy of education was based on the following principles:

♦ Problem orientation—to halt the division of disciplines;

♦ Attitude development—to pay more attention to the interpersonal and emotional components of healthcare;

♦ Involvement to increase student participation in the courses; and

♦ Progress evaluation—as an alternative to the year-end final exams.

At Maastricht, as at McMaster University, a small group of innovators laid the foundations for PBL. This group included Harm Tiddens, paediatrician; Wynand Wijnen, education psychologist; and the politician Jean (Sjeng) Tans, the first Chairman of the University Board.

Harm Tiddens visited the Michigan State and McMaster universities in 1969. Particularly inspired by John Evans, Tiddens was greatly impressed by the PBL method. Back in the Netherlands, he strongly advocated PBL in education circles and during informal meetings at the Ministry of Health. In 1970 he assumed the position of advisor to the preparatory committee of the new university at Maastricht. Together with Wijnen, Tiddens was invited to revitalize the Maastricht medical curriculum. As an education expert, Wijnen had previously conducted research on examinations for medical students in Groningen. Together with Tiddens, he assumed the position of education advisor to the faculty and was later appointed as *Rector Magnificus*.

In 1974, a large delegation from Maastricht, led by Tiddens, visited McMaster University. The delegation included not only core staff members, but also civil servants from the Ministries of Education and Health Care. It was during this visit that the commitment and content basis was created for the Introduction of PBL—agreed to be the most appropriate means for education renewal in the eighth faculty of medicine.

Meanwhile chairman Tans concentrated on securing commitment from the political and public sectors throughout the country and the region. Clearly, the introduction of PBL in Maastricht was not a coincidence. The circumstances made the revitalization of education not only desirable, but realizable. The Maastricht founding fathers created a university that wanted to be different by introducing education innovations, appointing a small, but highly motivated staff of education innovators, and building governmental and political commitment. These same factors had been present at McMaster University, exemplary conditions for the introduction of PBL.

Problems during the first years of PBL in Maastricht, and solutions

The first fifty medical students were welcomed at Maastricht University in September 1974 by Tiddens, the first dean of the new faculty. The Minister of Education had granted special permission for the initiation of the curriculum before the official opening of the university. During the early years, there were many internal and external problems, problems related to the renewal of university organizations. From the beginning, tensions between preclinical and clinical disciplines were evident. PBL called for faculty-led central management of education.

Education subjects are, almost without exception, multidisciplinary. When a student-centred programme is put in place, medical disciplines have to surrender some of their autonomy. Some professors were concerned that academic freedom was at stake. Some disciplines, which felt they were not properly recognized, were dissatisfied with their representation in the education programmes or the number of education hours allocated to 'their share' of the programme. The number of detectable hours of education is often interpreted as an indication of the relevance of a subject and the status of a discipline. From the very beginning, new staff members were asked to adopt the principles of the PBL programme. Nevertheless, a small but intriguing number of new staff members proved later on to be opposed to PBL.

The central education organization played a major role in achieving some stability in the organization. Structural feedback and annual meetings about the quantity and quality of education, with performance standards for the disciplines, have been successful in resolving many problems over the years. In many instances, feedback from disciplines led to changes in the curriculum. The faculty board has played a major role in securing maximum support for the principles of PBL and the thematic, multidisciplinary approach that has characterized the educational programme.

In every faculty, whether they use PBL or not, there is tension between education and research. In this respect PBL poses a special challenge, not only because it is felt to be labour intensive, but even more so because excellent teachers are needed if the faculty is to succeed in delivering a high-quality programme. For this reason the division of tasks for education, research, and patient care must be very clear and distinct.

If the faculty does not ensure a balanced allocation of tasks for education, research, and service and does not offer equal career prospects to staff members heavily involved in education, education will remain under constant threat. Resolving this situation has never been an easy task for the faculty board. Too often, in internal and external evaluations, the focus is on scientific research and development. Maastricht organized both education and research into multidisciplinary themes. Besides its role in education, central management has also been present in the thematic research institutes. The coordination between education and research institutes has achieved a very effective division of tasks in Maastricht.

During the early years the new faculty was closely watched by the other Dutch medical faculties. The public was doubtful about the quality of education and the quality of the physicians educated in Maastricht. Just as at McMaster, the method of the examinations at Maastricht, especially the formative examinations, came under critical scrutiny. In the early years the faculty teachers were not well prepared for the new assessment methods in the PBL programme. The first Maastricht students too were very critical of this aspect of the curriculum.

The faculty was very vulnerable in this respect in the early stages. During the first years, owing to the vulnerability of PBL, professors from other medical faculties were invited to observe examinations. From the outset, the faculty conducted investigations into the quality of the exams and the best methods for assessment. The progress test, developed by Wijnen (see Chapter 22), appeared to be an excellent instrument, not only for evaluating students' study progress but also for comparing the results of Maastricht students to those of students from other universities. Time and again it has been shown that the knowledge of Maastricht students is equal or superior to that of their colleagues from traditional schools.

Henk Schmidt, who until 2000 was Professor of Psychology in Maastricht, investigated the effects and outcomes of PBL early on (Norman & Schmidt, 1992; Schmidt et al., 1987; Schmidt & van der Molen, 2001). From the beginning, a comparison of the knowledge, skills, and attitudes of Maastricht students showed positive results. As a result, external criticism of PBL changed to interest and, at times, appreciation. Today, all medical faculties in the Netherlands include essential elements of PBL in their curricula.

During the difficult starting period, the faculty was supported by the World Health Organization (WHO). There was a great deal of unexpected interest in the development of PBL at Maastricht University, with many delegations visiting the school. International interest was not only welcomed; it also had a stimulating effect on the education staff, who embraced and expanded the WHO initiative of an international PBL Network: TUFH (Towards Unity for Health; see Chapters 25 and 26). The faculty organized an annual PBL summer course to build a widespread international network of friendly relations and cooperation.

In the beginning there were internal and external problems with the implementation of PBL, which demanded much attention from the central education organization. To resolve these problems, it was important that the faculty constantly safeguarded the basic principles of PBL. Developing commitment from the different medical disciplines was essential. And it was also essential in the early stages to eliminate the doubts about education quality by introducing transparent examinations and research of examinations.

Why is PBL in Maastricht successful?

The fact that Maastricht was a new faculty with a completely new education organization was very advantageous. Implementing PBL in a new faculty is undoubtedly easier than doing so in an existing faculty, where the education programme must be overhauled completely (see Chapter 15).

The establishment of a central education organization has been crucial for the success of PBL. Education experts have been on the staff from the beginning, when the mixture of education experts and staff with medical, psychological, and/or social science backgrounds appeared to be a propitious constellation. It also meant that education formats in PBL continued to develop, promoting variety and new approaches. An important pioneering effort was the establishment of the Skillslab, which has been the driving force for the development of new teaching models for clinical and communication skills in Maastricht.

The following chapters will delve deeper into these aspects.

Since 1999, the education organization has professionalized further by the establishment of an Institute of Education, responsible for the organization and quality improvement of education. Because of the fast growth of the faculty (from a yearly intake of fifty students at the start, to 250 students in 2002, and 340 students today), it was considered especially important to incorporate funds allocated for education, including the salaries of teachers, in the Institute's budget. The faculty sets great store by its own development. The Institute offers a programme to teach the essentials of PBL to staff members (staff development for PBL is discussed in detail in Chapter 18). Quality of education features prominently in the promotion decisions for all staff members. Currently, there is a separate career track for staff members whose main tasks and responsibilities are in education (see also Chapter 18).

From the beginning, the medical faculty has had a strong programme of educational research (Ten Cate, 2007). The ongoing research into assessment and the influence of the learning environment has met with strong international acclaim, as described by Cees van der Vleuten et al. in Chapter 23. At the same time the faculty has achieved compelling developments in biomedical research. Setting up thematic research in multidisciplinary institutes, in accordance with the basic philosophy of the faculty, has turned out to be a positive and stimulating factor which has probably been of significant importance for the success of PBL in Maastricht. The critical input of students during the start-up phase of the curriculum has led to improvements of many other aspects of PBL, and continues to make a valueable and vital contribution to the curriculum. Furthermore, the advice of alumni is sought on a regular basis in a longitudinal research project to evaluate the programme. The positive feedback of students and alumni has also heightened conviction within the faculty that PBL is not only a challenging and interesting method of learning but also a method that delivers well-qualified doctors who are ready for today's healthcare. Since 1996, Elsevier Magazine has published an annual survey of students about the quality and the infrastructure of university teaching programmes in the Netherlands. The leading position of the Maastricht Faculty of Medicine in the Elsevier rankings has continued without interruption for the past twelve years.

What does the future hold in store for PBL?

PBL has gained worldwide acceptance as an innovative teaching and learning method, not only in medicine, but in almost every other curriculum. Meanwhile ICT, the electronic library, and e-learning have gained an important place in PBL. This development is bound to continue as the role of distance learning and blended learning increases. Broader differentiation will develop within education. Honours programmes and special education programmes, such as the physician-clinical researcher curriculum, are the first indicators. Competency-based learning is gaining ground, a trend that will continue to develop.

Education research of PBL is a prerequisite to ensure future development of curricula and new learning methods. In addition to ideology, PBL must be underpinned by evidence. Further innovation of education will have to be driven and supported by research. Research will not only be directed at the methodology of PBL and the introduction of multimedia, but also at the physiology of human learning itself. Insights into learning from the neurosciences and molecular biology will open up new vistas with new methods of learning.

Epilogue

Since the start of the university, PBL has remained the hallmark of Maastricht University. The new faculty started out with a basic philosophy which has been translated into productive multidisciplinary research and academic patient care, and especially into the success of PBL. All the starting points in the basic philosophy with regard to education have become reality. One element has not been realized, however. This concerns the planning of an academic health region, fully focused on primary care, outside the academic hospital, and has proven to be out of reach and, in the end, not very practical for clinical teaching. Nevertheless strong emphasis on primary care remains a key characteristic of the Maastricht curriculum. Additionally, the concept of multidisciplinary care, the new chain model of healthcare, and teaching and learning of specialist and hospital medicine are likewise important to the PBL curriculum.

The evolving history of Maastricht University is founded on PBL, and this is, without question, the inspiration for the Maastricht University motto: Leading in Learning.

References

Foucault, M. (1963). *Naissance de la Clinique*. Paris: Presses Universitaire de France; *The birth of the clinic: an archaeology of medical perception*, trans. A. Sheridan (1973). London: Routledge.

Le Fanu, J. (1999). *The rise and fall of modern medicine*. London: Little, Brown.

McKeown, Th. (1979). *The role of medicine: dream, mirage or nemesis?* Oxford: Blackwell.

Norman, R. N., and Schmidt, H. G. (1992). The psychological basis of problem-based learning: a review of the evidence. *Academic Medicine* 67, 557–65.

Schmidt, H. G., Dauphinée, W. D., and Patel, V. L. (1987). Comparing the effects of problem-based and conventional curricula in an international sample. *Medical Education* 62, 305–15.

Schmidt, H. G., and van der Molen, H. T. (2001). Self-reported competency ratings of graduates of a problem-based medical curriculum. *Academic Medicine* 76, 466–8.

Ten Cate, O. (2007). Medical education in the Netherlands. *Medical Teacher* 29, 752–7.

Van der Vleuten, C. P. M., and Wijnen, W. H. F. W. (eds). (1990). *Problem-based learning: the Maastricht experience*. Amsterdam: Thesis.

Chapter 3

The problem-based learning process

Diana Dolmans and Henk Schmidt

Problem-based learning (PBL) works! Problems, tutors, and small groups are all important components of PBL. PBL is strongly based on contemporary insights on human learning: learning should be constructive, self-directed, collaborative, and contextual.

Description of PBL

PBL represents a major, complex, and widespread change in educational practice in higher education, professional education in particular. PBL was first implemented at McMaster University in Canada. According to Barrows and Tamblyn (1980), PBL's founding fathers, too much emphasis was placed in medical education on memorizing facts. They thought it would be better for students to learn how to solve patient problems rather than memorize facts that might or might not be relevant to medical practice. The upshot of this notion was that students were given (paper) patient problems to resolve instead of lectures to listen to. The patient problems were intended as a stimulus for students' learning activities. This approach is aimed at achieving two educational objectives: the acquisition of an integrated body of knowledge related to problems and the development or application of problem-solving skills (Barrows & Tamblyn, 1980).

Today, many medical schools all over the world have implemented PBL. Students in PBL groups discuss problems that generally consist of a description of certain phenomena that require explanation. The small groups of students are facilitated by a tutor, who does not convey expert knowledge but stimulates and monitors the group process and discussions. At the end of a session, several issues relevant to the problem remain to be clarified, because students do not have all the necessary knowledge. These issues are later studied by students during individual self-study. A few days later, the group reconvenes and students report the results of their self-study, sharing and discussing the insights they have gained. Basically, the problems, the tutors, and the small groups are the active ingredients of a PBL curriculum.

Problems

Problems are the driving force behind students' learning in PBL, both challenging them to actively engage in learning and stimulating them to construct new knowledge that is firmly linked to their existing knowledge. The problem is at the centre of knowledge acquisition and fosters flexible thinking (Hmelo-Silver, 2004). Problems used in PBL are often realistic and presented in the context of a patient scenario.

Problem: Ellen

The past few years, Ellen has grown taller very quickly. She has always been a tall girl, but at the age of 11 years and a height of five feet, four inches, she is head and shoulders above her age group. People always take her to be older, which can be quite wearisome.

In PBL students use an approach that involves *seven steps* to tackle a problem (Schmidt, 1983). In step 1 any terms that are new or not well understood by the group are explained. In step 2 the group identifies the problem (or problems). For example, problems related to the case of Ellen might be: Why is Ellen so tall? What are growth curves? Step 3 consists of brainstorming, during which students might for instance talk about what they know about hormones and their effects on height. In step 4 students generate a list of possible explanations, such as genetics or hormones. In step 5 students formulate learning issues and determine which issues are to be pursued during self-study, such as: Which factors influence growth and how? What are normal and abnormal growth rates? What are possible psychological effects of being too tall? Step 6 consists of self-study. Students search literature resources for information relevant to the learning issues. In step 7 the students meet and report the results of their self-study. They discuss, scrutinize, and synthesize the new information and determine how it affects their interpretation of the problem. For instance, how do students view Ellen's problem after having acquired more knowledge; is she really too tall?

Tutors

In PBL, tutors act as facilitators of student learning. Their task is to keep the learning process going, to probe the students' knowledge deeply, to ensure that all students are involved in the process, to monitor the education progress of each student, and to modulate the challenge of the problem (Barrows, 1988). They stimulate students to engage in elaboration and interactions by asking questions and inviting clarification (de Grave et al., 1999). Tutors are not expected to transmit their expert knowledge to students, but to probe students' knowledge and reasoning by encouraging specific kinds of cognitive activity.

Small groups

Students are stimulated to learn from interacting with each other when they discuss problems in small groups. For example, they explain concepts and phenomena, they ask each other questions, and they discuss the problem at hand. In PBL groups, students work together to construct collaborative explanations. This has the additional positive effect that not only students acquire knowledge and skills but they also learn to work together, which may help them become better collaborators (Hmelo-Silver, 2004).

Theoretical considerations

Modern insights into learning emphasize that learning should be a constructive, self-directed or self-regulated, collaborative, and contextual process (Dolmans et al., 2005). These four key principles are explained below. PBL is in keeping with these principles.

Constructive learning

The concept of constructive learning is closely related to constructivism, which views learning as the active construction of knowledge by learners who are active agents who build their own personal knowledge (Loyens & Gijbels, 2008). Mayer (2004) pointed to two important criteria for active learning. The first is activating or constructing knowledge essessential to making sense of new incoming information. The second criterion is the integration of new incoming information with an appropriate knowledge base. Learners use the knowledge they already possess to interpret new information. Activation of prior knowledge is thus essential for the acquisition and understanding of new information (Schmidt, 1993). Connecting new information with existing knowledge can be stimulated by activities like elaboration. Elaboration can take several forms, such as discussion, taking notes, or answering questions. During elaboration, new information and old information are being connected, a process that can generate new ideas. Elaboration creates rich knowledge structures, because it increases the number of connections between concepts and facilitates the activation of knowledge (Schmidt, 1993). Explaining is another activity that promotes elaboration, as well as the structuring and restructuring of knowledge (Chi et al., 1994). In other words, it is important for learners to be stimulated to actively construct their knowledge and engage in deep elaborations and explanations since this generates a deeper and richer understanding and better use of knowledge (Harris & Alexander, 1998). In PBL, students are encouraged to discuss and hence elaborate problems in small groups.

Self-regulated learning

Self-regulated learning, or self-directed learning, as it is also called, is an umbrella term covering various aspects, such as goal setting, self-observation, self-assessment, and self-reinforcement, all of which are believed to influence learning (Loyens & Gijbels, 2008). According to Ertmer and Newby (1996), self-regulated learning implies that learners play an active role in planning, monitoring, and evaluating their learning process. Planning implies that a learner first considers a variety of ways to approach a task, then sets a clear goal, selects appropriate strategies, and identifies potential obstacles to the successful attainment of the goal. Monitoring implies that learners are aware of what they are doing and anticipate what is to be done next by looking backward and forward. After completion of the learning process, the process itself and the results are evaluated. Reflection is critical to self-regulation (Ertmer & Newby, 1996). According to Boekaerts (1997), self-regulated learning can be defined as a complex interactive process involving not only cognitive but also motivational self-regulation. An increasing body of knowledge attests that cognitive self-regulation can be taught and that students who use self-regulatory skills have better grades in the content domain to which they apply these skills. Self-regulated learning can be a complex, demanding, and deliberate activity, but also an activity that is simple, habitual, and automatic (Boekaerts, 1997). Pintrich (1999) has demonstrated that motivational beliefs, such as task beliefs and self-efficacy, play an important role in self-regulated learning. In other words, learners should be stimulated to regulate their learning from both a motivational and a cognitive perspective. In PBL, students are encouraged to identify issues that require further study, an activity assumed to stimulate self-regulated learning. Furthermore, discussions and elaborations in PBL groups are assumed to stimulate students' intrinsic interest in the subject matter as well as their motivation to engage in self-study (Schmidt, 1993).

Collaborative learning

Collaboration is a social structure in which two or more people are interacting and which, in some circumstances, can produce interactions that have a positive effect on learning (Dillenbourg et al., 1996). At the heart of collaborative learning efforts is positive interdependence, which creates a situation in which students work together in groups to maximize the learning of all group members and stimulate each other to interact and share knowledge and information resources (Johnson et al., 2007). According to Johnson et al. (2007), collaborative learning is the instructional approach of choice to maximize student learning and retention in long-term memory, especially when the subjects or materials are complex. Collaborative learning is considered superior to individual learning when the learning task is complex (Kirschner et al., 2009). Factors within the collaborative learning situation that have the potential to enhance learning are elaboration, verbalization, co-construction, mutual support, criticism, and tuning in cognitively and socially (van der Linden et al., 2000). In other words, learners should be stimulated to collaborate and interact with each other because this has a positive impact on their learning. In PBL, students are stimulated to work together in small groups.

Contextual learning

The context or situation in which knowledge is acquired determines whether and how it is used. All too often it is difficult for students to transfer what they have learned in one context to new situations or different contexts. The reason for this is that students fail to discern that a similar deep structure underlies situations that, on the surface, may appear to be very dissimilar. As a consequence, knowledge transfers less easily across different types of situations (Billet, 1996).Transfer can be defined as applying what one has learned in different situations (Mayer, 2004). It can be facilitated by anchoring learning in meaningful contexts, revisiting content at different times, in rearranged contexts, for different purposes, and from different perspectives (Ertmer & Newby, 1993). Furthermore, when students are encouraged to view problem environments from multiple perspectives, they learn to recognize the critical features of the cases presented to them (Bransford & Schwartz, 1999). In conclusion, learners are preferably exposed to a professionally relevant context and confronted with cases or problems from multiple perspectives and in multiple contexts, because this stimulates the transfer of knowledge. In PBL, students are confronted with problems often highly relevant for their future professional practice (Dolmans et al., 1997).

Discussion: experiences and reflection

Changes in the PBL process over the years

The PBL process as described above was implemented at the Faculty of Health, Medicine and Life Sciences (FHML) some thirty years ago. The content and the structure of the medical curriculum have changed during these years and the numbers of new students entering medical school have increased dramatically. However, the basic characteristics of the PBL process continue to be present, especially in the first two years of the curriculum. In the third year, real patients have replaced the paper ones in the PBL group sessions. Chapter 8 describes this PBL format more extensively. Other changes are related to the role of the tutor and literature resources. Research in the past thirty years on the effectiveness of tutors has consistently demonstrated that it is preferable for tutors to be experts in the subject under discussion, although they should also know how to stimulate student learning, for example by asking critical questions (Dolmans, et al., 2002). In line with current insights into effective tutoring, tutor selection today is also guided by content expertise, whereas thirty years ago it was based exclusively on competence as a facilitator of group processes. Furthermore, our practical experiences have taught us that students need more guidance in selecting literature resources. Whereas thirty years ago students were merely told to search literature resources for relevant information, today students are given suggestions for which literature resources they might use. Another change of the past few years is the increased complexity of the problems. Students nowadays are also encouraged to collaborate on assignments, such as preparing presentations to a group or writing essays.

The difference between a PBL curriculum and hybrid curriculum

Many schools have introduced PBL in their curricula. Some schools use a hybrid model in which PBL is mixed with a traditional lecture-based approach. This raises the question of the distinction between a PBL curriculum and a hybrid curriculum. Firstly, it is important to consider that PBL is not a single unique instructional format. PBL can be implemented in different ways in various curricula.

Secondly, the PBL approach has several essential characteristics. Within PBL, student learning is organized around problems discussed by a group of students. The student group is facilitated by a tutor, who is not expected to transmit knowledge but to help students engage in constructive interactions and deep learning. Thus, the problems discussed in the group sessions are the central and main component of the curriculum. They drive the learning of students. All other educational activities within the curriculum are aimed at supporting these processes. The discussions around the problems drive students' learning and self-study activities.

The evidence for PBL

Several reviews of studies examining the effects of PBL have been published (Albanese & Mitchell, 1993; Berkson, 1993; Colliver, 2000; Dochy et al., 2003; Newman, 2003; Norman & Schmidt, 2000; Vernon & Blake, 1993). A consistent finding is that PBL students are highly satisfied with the PBL approach and that teachers find PBL a satisfying way to teach. Studies on the cognitive and motivational effects of small-group problem-based learning appear to demonstrate that several cognitive activities occur that are assumed to enhance student learning, such as activation of prior knowledge, elaboration, and interactions, and also that group discussion positively influences students' intrinsic interest in the subject matter under discussion (Dolmans & Schmidt, 2006). Although several studies have reported positive effects of group learning in PBL, much more research is needed to collect more evidence and insight into the mechanisms or active ingredients of small-group learning in PBL. Capon and Kuhn (2004) demonstrated in an experimental study in which they compared PBL with lecturing that PBL leads to superior explanations. This supports the hypothesis that the integration of new information with existing knowledge is the effective ingredient of PBL. In a more recent study, van Blankenstein et al. (2009) also concluded that being actively engaged in explaining phenomena during PBL small-group discussions has a positive impact on long-term memory. However, as yet there is no evidence that PBL leads to better learning outcomes in terms of academic achievement, problem solving, and transfer of knowledge. Nevertheless, a study conducted by Schmidt and van der Molen (2001) demonstrated that PBL graduates considered themselves to be better prepared than their colleagues from traditional curricula with regard to collaboration skills, problem-solving skills, skills to run meetings, and the ability to work independently. Prince et al. (2005) also demonstrated that, compared with non-PBL graduates, PBL graduates gave higher ratings for the alignment of school and work, their medical training, preparation for practice, and communication skills. In other words, PBL seems to stimulate the development of generic competencies that are very important for a successful career after graduation (Semeijn et al., 2005). Another chapter of this book (Chapter 24) will go into the evidence supporting PBL.

Future developments

PBL and work-based learning

Contextual learning and work-based learning have gained prominence in recent years. This has inspired changes in many medical curricula, such as the early introduction of real patient contacts. At FHML, a few years ago, instead of paper-based problems, real patients were introduced in the third year of the curriculum as a stimulus for student learning. This change has had a positive impact on students' motivation. In the future it could well be worthwhile to conduct experiments with PBL sessions around real patients during clinical rotations. But other innovative instructional approaches should be introduced as well, such as methods to stimulate collaboration among students during self-study.

PBL and information and communication technology

The use of information and communication technology continues to increase at a fast pace and it has come to play a dominant role in our day-to-day lives. Information and communication technologies also offer opportunities for PBL approaches. At FHML digital projectors are used to share the learning issues formulated in the group (see Chapter 20). Communication technologies are also used to exchange documents or literature resources and most curricular materials are available electronically. Curricular content is available via Blackboard, FHML's electronic learning environment. Additionally, experiments with blended PBL approaches have been conducted during clinical rotations. Use of an electronic discussion board enabled synchronous or asynchronous group discussions among students at different clerkship locations on issues they encountered during their clinical rotations and which required further study or on a video vignette of a patient case (de Leng, et al., 2007). This is one way to promote collaborative learning experiences during clinical clerkships. In the future, information and communication technology are expected to create opportunities for further innovations in PBL.

Annotated literature

Albanese, M. A., and Mitchell, S. (1993). Problem-based learning: A review of literature on its outcomes and implementation issues. *Academic Medicine* **68**, 52–81.

In this paper the authors report studies conducted between 1972 and 1992. It was concluded that PBL students are highly satisfied with the PBL approach and that teachers find PBL a satisfying way to teach.

Barrows, H. S., and Tamblyn, R. M. (1980). *Problem-based learning: an approach to medical education.* Springer: New York.

This book describes the process of PBL as it has been developed at McMaster University in Canada as well as the rationale behind problem-based learning.

Colliver, J. A. (2000). Effectiveness of problem-based learning curricula: Research and theory. *Academic Medicine* **75(3)**, 259–66.

In this paper eight studies that compared curricula are reviewed. It is concluded that PBL does not improve knowledge and clinical performance.

Dochy, F. Segers, M., van den Bossche, P., and Gijbels, D. (2003). Effects of PBL: a meta-analysis. *Learning and Instruction* **13(5)**, 533–68.

In this paper, 43 articles are reviewed. It is concluded that PBL has positive effects on skills and knowledge application, but not on knowledge.

Dolmans, D. H. J. M., de Grave, W., Wolfhagen, I. H. A. P., and van der Vleuten, C. P. M. (2005). Problem-based learning: future challenges for educational practice and research. *Medical Education* **39**, 732–41.

In this paper it is explained how PBL fits with current learning principles. Furthermore, problems experienced with PBL in practice are explained, as well as their solutions and suggestions for future research are summarized.

Schmidt, H.G. (1993). Foundations of problem-based learning: some explanatory notes. *Medical Education* **27**, 422–32.

In this paper the cognitive effects of PBL are explained. It is argued that PBL promotes activation of prior knowledge and elaborations.

References

Albanese, M. A., and Mitchell, S. (1993). Problem-based learning: A review of literature on its outcomes and implementation issues. *Academic Medicine* **68**, 52–81.

Barrows, H. S., and Tamblyn, R. M. (1980). *Problem-based learning: an approach to medical education.* Springer: New York.

Barrows, H.S. (1988). *The tutorial process*. Carbondatle, IL: Southern Illinois University School of Medicine.

Berkson, L. (1993). Problem-based learning: Have the expectations been met? *Academic Medicine* **68**, S79–S88.

Billet, S. (1996). Situated learning: Bridging sociocultural and cognitive theorising. *Learning and Instruction* **6**, 263–80.

Van Blankenstein, F. M., Dolmans, D. H. J. M., van der Vleuten, C. P. M., and Schmidt, H. G. (2009). Which cognitive processes support learning during small-group discussion? The role of providing explanations and listening to others. *Instructional Science*, doi 10.1007/s11251–009–9124–7.

Boekaerts, M. (1997). Self-regulated learning: A new concept embraced by researchers, policy makers, educators, teachers and students. *Learning and Instruction* **7**, 161–86.

Bransford, J. D., and Schwartz, D.L. (1999). Rethinking transfer: a simple proposal with multiple implications. *Review of Research in Education* **24**, 61–100.

Capon, N., and Kuhn, D. (2004). What's so good about problem-based learning? *Cognition and Instruction* **22**, 61–79.

Chi, M. T. H., DeLeeuw, N., Chiu, M. H., and LaVancher, C. (1994). Eliciting self-explanations improves understanding. *Cognitive Science* **18**, 439–77.

Colliver, J. A. (2000). Effectiveness of problem-based learning curricula: research and theory. *Academic Medicine* **75**, 259–66.

Dillenbourg, P., Baker, M., Blaye, A., and O'Malley, C. (1996). The evolution of research on collaborative learning. In: E. Spada & P. Reiman (eds), *Learning in humans and machine: towards an interdisciplinary learning science*. Oxford: Elsevier. Pp. 189–211.

Dochy, F., Segers, M., van den Bossche, P., and Gijbels D. (2003). Effects of PBL: a meta-analysis. *Learning and Instruction* **13**, 533–68.

Dolmans, D. H. J. M., Snellen-Balendong, H., Wolfhagen, H. A. P., and van der Vleuten C. P. M. (1997). Seven principles of effective design for a problem-based curriculum. *Medical Teacher* **19**, 185–9.

Dolmans, D. H. J. M., Gijselaers, W. H., Moust, J. H. C., de Grave, W. S., Wolfhagen, H. A. P., and van der Vleuten, C. P. M. (2002). Trends in research on the tutor in PBL: conclusions and implications for educational practice and research. *Medical Teacher* **24**, 173–80.

Dolmans, D. H. J. M., de Grave, W., Wolfhagen, I. H. A. P., and van der Vleuten, C. P. M. (2005). Problem-based learning: future challenges for educational practice and research. *Medical Education* **39**, 732–41.

Dolmans, D.H.J.M. & Schmidt, H.G. (2006). What do we know about cognitive and motivational effects of small group tutorials in problem-based Learning? *Advances in health Sciences Education* **11**, 321–36.

Ertmer, P. A., and Newby, T. J. (1993). Behaviorism, cognitivism, constructivism: Comparing critical features from an instructional design perspective. *Performance Improvement Quarterly* **6**, 50–72.

Ertmer, P. A., and Newby, T. J. (1996). The expert learner: Strategic, self-regulated, and reflective. *Instructional Science* **24**, 1–24.

De Grave, W. S., Dolmans, D. H. J. M., and van der Vleuten, C. (1999). Profiles of effective tutors in PBL: scaffolding student learning. *Medical Education* **33**, 901–6.

Harris, K. R., and Alexander, P. A. (1998). Integrated, constructivist education: Challenge and reality. *Educational Psychology Review* **10**, 115–27.

Hmelo-Silver, C. E. (2004). Problem-based learning: What and how students learn. *Educational Psychology Review* **16**, 235–66.

Johnson, D., Johnson, R., and Smith, K. (2007). The state of cooperative learning in postsecondary and professional settings. *Educational Psychology Review* **19**, 15–29.

Kirschner, F., Paas, F., and Kirschner, P. A. (2009). A cognitive load approach to collaborative learning: United brains for complex tasks. *Educational Psychology Review* **21**, 31–42.

De Leng, B. A., Dolmans, D. H. J. M., van der Wiel, M., Muijtjens, A. M. M., and van der Vleuten, C. P. M. (2007). How video cases should be used as authentic stimuli in problem-based medical education. *Medical Education* **41**, 181–8.

Loyens, M. M., and Gijbels, D. (2008). Understanding the effects of constructivist learning environments: introducing a multi-directional approach. *Instructional Science* **36**, 351–7.

Mayer, R. E. (2004). Should here be a three-strikes rule against pure discovery learning? The case for guided methods of instruction. *American Psychologist* **59**, 14–19.

Newman, M. (2003). *A pilot systematic review and meta-analysis on the effectiveness of problem based learning*. On behalf of the Campbell Collaboration Systematic Review Group on the effectiveness of problem based learning. University of Newcastle, Learning and Teaching Support Network LTSN-01. Newcastle, UK.

Norman, G. R., and Schmidt, H. G. (2000). Effectiveness of problem-based learning curricula: theory, practice and paper darts. *Medical Education* **34**, 721–8.

Pintrich, P. A. (1999). The role of motivation in promoting and sustaining self-regulated learning. *International Journal of Educational Research* **31**, 459–70.

Prince, K. J. A. H., van Eijs, P., Boshuizen, H. A. P., van der Vleuten, C. P. M., and Scherpbier, A. J. J. A. (2005). General competencies of problem-based learning (PBL) and non-PBL graduates. *Medical Education* **39**, 394–401.

Schmidt, H. G. (1983). Problem-based learning: rationale and description. *Medical Education* **17**, 11–16.

Schmidt, H. G. (1993). Foundations of problem-based learning: Some explanatory notes. *Medical Education* **27**, 422–32.

Schmidt, H. G., and van der Molen, H. T. (2001). Self-reported competency ratings of graduates of a problem-based curriculum. *Academic Medicine* **76**(5), 466–8.

Semeijn, J. H., van der Velden, R., Heijke, H., van der Vleuten, C. P. M., and Boshuizen, H. (2005). The role of education in selection and allocation in the labour market: An empirical study in the medical field. *Education Economics* **13**, 449–77.

Van der Linden, J., Erkens, G., Schmidt, H., and Renshaw, P. (2000) Collaborative learning. In: R.J. Simons, J. van der Linden, and T. Duffy (eds), *New learning*. Kluwer: Dordrecht. Pp. 37–54.

Vernon, D. T. A., and Blake, R. L. (1993). Does problem-based learning work? A meta-analysis of evaluative research. *Academic Medicine* **68**, 550–63.

Chapter 4

Designing a problem-based learning medical curriculum

Mascha Verheggen and Hetty Snellen-Balendong

Designing a problem-based learning (PBL) curriculum appears to be more complex than designing a traditional curriculum. This is partly due to the balance that must be struck between the central direction provided by the 'master' design and the responsibility delegated to those who develop the constituent elements of the curriculum, bearing in mind that small-scale educational formats and problem solving are the foundations of a PBL curriculum. Furthermore, the curriculum is to be orientated not primarily to the teachers but to the students and their learning needs, prior knowledge, and abilities.

In one sense the design of a curriculum for a Dutch medical school is relatively straightforward, because of the presence of Blueprint 2001, training of doctors in the Netherlands (Metz et al., 2001), a document that contains the statutory final objectives of undergraduate medical education which must be met by all medical schools.

Building a curriculum

There are a variety of definitions of the concept 'curriculum'. The older definitions emphasize curriculum content and how it is clustered around a central topic with all the related elements, and the sequencing of topics. Selection and arrangement of content is still important in the design of a curriculum, but nowadays the education goals of the various units and instruction and assessment tools are also essential elements.

The building bricks of a curriculum are units which:

+ Together cover the final objectives of the education programme in such a way that these objectives are achievable by the average student;

+ Offer content that, as regards volume and complexity, can be successfully mastered by students at that stage of the curriculum;

+ Together form a coherent curriculum in which preceding units prepare for the following ones; and

+ Are interesting and motivating to students.

The units of a PBL curriculum are typically not vertically arranged in time nor do they focus on one single discipline. Each unit lasts a certain number of weeks, is designed in a multidisciplinary way around a central theme, and requires full-time commitment from students. How much horizontal and vertical integration there is between basic and clinical sciences depends on the design of the curriculum. In a PBL curriculum there is a tendency for the distinction between basic and clinical sciences to become blurred, because basic sciences are frequently studied within the context of a clinical, pathophysiological, or social problem.

The first challenge to the designers of a PBL curriculum is to determine which themes are to be addressed during which year of the curriculum and during which units in that year. These themes should be covered in a meaningful way to ensure that the intended education goals are achieved, the study load is spread logically and evenly over the units, and the final objectives for each year are gained. When designers are considering options for themes to be included in a PBL curriculum, they should determine which related concept can serve as a suitable title for a certain period of the curriculum (a semester, a year). These overarching concepts must encompass the themes of the units of that period. Examples are acute complaints, chronic complaints, the course of life, body systems, body functions, etc. Once this has been done, it is less difficult to complete unit designs by determining more specific education goals, relevant teaching formats, assessment methods, and the sequence of the units. An early start of clinical skills training in the curriculum is an important factor to be considered in designing a PBL curriculum. Contacts with real patients as early as possible in the curriculum offer a strong motivator for students to study, facilitate the introduction of personal aspects of teaching goals, and help individual students to determine whether they really want to become a doctor.

Skills and clerkships

An early start with skills training is advisable, because it makes early clinical practice more meaningful. Even if it is not possible to introduce students to clinical practice at an early stage (e.g., because of the number of students and the (scarcity of) available accommodation and facilities in primary care settings and in hospitals) it is still important to offer early skills training, integrated with unit themes. Training skills stimulates the acquisition of theoretical knowledge and is highly appreciated by students.

In a PBL curriculum, as in most traditional curricula, clinical clerkships are scheduled in the last phase of the curriculum. Students spend this period in hospitals and primary care settings. Important conditions for a successful clerkship period include the following:

- Students see patients independently;
- Students are regularly observed during patient contacts;
- Students receive formative and summative feedback;
- Students are given dedicated time and facilities for self-study activities; and
- Students are not given routine tasks.

In essence, these considerations are not characteristic of a PBL curriculum, but over the past 35 years they have dominated the discussions about clerkships with hospital staff and primary care doctors. What is considered characteristic of a PBL curriculum is the integration of disciplines, also during clerkships. It is true that horizontal integration (between disciplines) is less important during clerkships, but what is important is vertical integration: refreshing and elaborating knowledge and insights from basic sciences and their relationship to clinical science. This can be pursued in short presentations, lab practicals, and assignments.

Planning group

Once the unit themes and the clerkships are determined, the next step is the attribution of education goals for each unit and clerkship. Units are composed from a multidisciplinary perspective. In other words, they deal with topics of various disciplines. The integration of different disciplines promotes integrative thinking in students, which is the keystone of medical expertise. In order to achieve integration, a unit should be designed, implemented, and evaluated by a multidisciplinary group of teachers, a planning group. Every planning group is headed by a coordinator, preferably a staff member who has had previous experience with the unit as a planning group member, to ensure the presence within the team of sufficient affinity and expertise with regard to the unit.

A planning group works within a framework determined by three factors. The first factor is the unit blueprint, designed by the Education Committee or a specially appointed curriculum committee. The second and third factors are the education and examination regulations, which are issued annually, and the guidelines for organization and implementation, issued by the central administration of the medical school. It is the task of the planning group to design (or revise, as the case may be) a unit, ensure appropriate delivery during the curricular period allocated to it, and evaluate it afterwards. Generally a year coordinator is appointed to ensure adequate coordination and organization of the different units in one curricular year. The developmental stage of a unit determines the planning group's main focus of attention. With a new unit, the emphasis will be on design; with an existing unit, the planning group's task is to revise and update the unit.

Planning group members should preferably be directly involved in the delivery of the unit. Tutoring one or two groups offers first-hand experience of student response to the unit. When planning group members together possess all the required expertise, it will be easier to achieve multidisciplinary and interdisciplinary collaboration. Planning groups are at their most effective when they comprise not only expertise in different areas but also different personalities. Students can play an important role with regard to implementation, and evaluation in particular. A prerequisite for effective student contribution is that student members communicate with their fellow students and with other students who have an official function in the education programme.

Blueprint

Unit blueprints are designed at faculty level by the Education Committee and incorporated in the final curriculum design (Snellen-Balendong, 1993). They are part of the overarching curriculum design and the main instrument for controlling curriculum content. There is an individual blueprint for each unit. A result of having blueprints is that individual departments are prevented from developing activities without consulting with other departments or setting requirements that may jeopardize the 'do-ability' of the curriculum. The Education Committee is responsible for ensuring coherence among the different blueprints.

The blueprint is particularly important when a new curriculum is being introduced and during the first years of its implementation. In order to develop a unit systematically a number of steps must be taken by the planning group. The first step involves analysing and discussing the blueprint and developing a broad outline of unit content. Next, relevant topics are determined and a list is made of the disciplines that are to participate in the unit. When topics and participating disciplines are known, a conceptual framework representing unit content and showing the interrelationships of the topics is developed. The final step is to formulate the learning objectives which define the knowledge and skills students are expected to have acquired at the end of the unit.

The construction of a unit

After the conceptual framework and the objectives have been generated, a start can be made with the actual construction of the unit. Four stages are distinguished: design, implementation, evaluation, and revision (Geerlings and Snellen-Balendong, 1995). During the design stage the planning group uses the formulated objectives and the conceptual framework as the starting point for selecting educational formats (problems, lab practicals, skills training, etc.), learning resources, and assessment tools. Problems play a central role in PBL. They drive students' learning activities and obviously must be of high quality. At the Maastricht Faculty of Health, Medicine and Life Sciences considerable experience in problem design has been gained over the years (see next chapter). The implementation stage is part of the design process, because it is only when a unit is being implemented that it can become clear whether the educational activities meet the goals set by the planning group. During the evaluation stage the planning group ascertains to what extent the objectives are actually being achieved and whether it is necessary to make changes in the original design or fill in any gaps. During the revision stage the planning group directs its efforts at improving the unit in line with the information from the evaluation. At that point the unit design process has come full circle.

Description of the implementation of different curricula

During the 35 years of its existence, Maastricht medical school has seen two full curriculum revisions.

Curriculum 1

The first edition of the curriculum, running from September 1974 to September 1988, showed all the signs of the haste that had characterized its implementation. This haste was due to political reasons. During the first years faculty staff was small and not all the disciplines were represented. More importantly, the notions related to PBL, how to design a unit, a problem, or a task had not yet fully crystallized. In these pioneering years unit books came from the copiers the weekend before the unit started. This implies that there was only a very global master plan. The curriculum was literally growing as more disciplines started to participate. Inevitably, this led to curriculum overload in the later years of the curriculum due to attempts to compensate gaps in the coverage of topics that emerged as the curriculum was developing. An analysis of curriculum content revealed an imbalance between the different components. Some topics were dealt with repeatedly, while other topics were not addressed at all or disappeared during the curriculum. A probable cause was that the planning groups were operating with too much autonomy. Despite several attempts to improve the curricular structure, the evaluation of several units consistently revealed negative appraisal. Another worrying phenomenon was that students enthusiastically tackled clinical problems during the first two years but progressing through the curriculum they began to experience a lack of basic science knowledge. More guidance from tutors did not effectively solve these problems.

Appendix 4.1 gives a global overview of the units in the first four years of this curriculum. Years 5 and 6 were completely taken up by traditional clerkships.

Curriculum 2

The second version of the curriculum ran from September 1988 till September 2001. The aim of this version was to remedy the detected flaws and shortcomings. The plan was based on the following didactic guidelines:

- Gradual integration of disciplines;
- A gradual shift from basic science knowledge to patient problems: in the first two years clinical problems were used to illustrate the relevance of basic science knowledge, which was an important factor that had to be taken into account in the construction of problems;

+ A gradual shift from normal functioning to pathology, with emphasis on the broad borderline area between normal and abnormal functioning; and

+ More systematic organization of content, with human functioning as the leading theme for the first two years and the main complaints in healthcare for the third and fourth year.

Traditional clerkships determined the outline of years 5 and 6.

The Curriculum Change Review Committee was installed to supervise and control the curriculum change. This committee was authorized to review the tasks and problems and oversee the work of the groups developing the new units. Appendix 4.2 gives an overview of curriculum 2.

A reorientation of the format and organization of the curriculum took place in the second half of the nineties. At that time senior students were complaining that the tutorial group process was becoming too much of a fixed routine. They felt that groups were becoming less productive. Another problem was that the growth in the number of students with each new cohort made it more and more difficult and sometimes impossible to offer all students clinical contacts or an introduction to healthcare in the first four years.

On top of that there was a growing demand for more scientific training and implementation of 'best available evidence medical education'. A renewal of the curriculum also facilitated the incorporation of the most advanced information and communication technology.

Curriculum 3

One of the opportunities that should be grasped by those designing a new curriculum is a reorientation of the old basic principles. Another opportunity is offered to faculty members who have experience with all sorts of educational roles in the curriculum but never had the chance to design a new unit. A new curriculum offers them the challenge of actually designing a new unit. Additionally, account can be taken of the latest developments in healthcare. In curriculum 3, the basic principles of curriculum design are, apart from problem orientation, patient and project orientation. The student remained the pivotal factor, but attention was also focused on 'how to learn' and 'working together'. Working in small groups, a multidisciplinary approach, and alignment of teaching and the learning process remained important factors.

The leading theme in the first year of curriculum 3 is regulating systems and emergency medicine. The aim is to facilitate learning and retention in memory. The leading theme in the second year is the life cycle together with the diagnostic process. Important topics in this year are normal human development from conception to old age, the borderline between normal and abnormal, and the main complaints and diseases in certain stages of life. Clinical reasoning during the diagnostic process is an important focus of attention.

The programme of the first two years is aimed at preparing students to take a history and do a physical examination in real patients in the third year. The skill training programme in the first two years is attuned to this goal. The central theme of the third year is chronic diseases. Students take part in weekly (or more) consultations with real patients. In view of the large number of students, this requires optimal use of the available facilities with regard to patients, accommodation, and supervision. In order to achieve that, the student cohort is divided into four groups, who follow the units, or clusters as they are named in the third year, in different sequences. This means that each cluster is delivered four times a year. During the clusters tutorial groups meet once a week for at least three hours to discuss the patient contacts, compare experiences, learn from each other, and prepare for the next patient contact. Years 4 and 5 are completely devoted to clerkships. The difference with the previous two curricula is the introduction of a 'preceding week' and a 'concluding week' before and after traditional clerkship rotations in healthcare settings. The aim of the preceding week is to give students more time to prepare for the upcoming clerkship, make the introduction to the workplace less stressful, and promote integration of basic and clinical sciences. In the 'concluding week' there is time for assessment, remedial teaching, and evaluation of the clerkship. Some clerkships include a weekly 'return day' (to the medical school). The central theme for the sixth and final year is 'participation'. During one half of the year students stay in the same healthcare setting, either in a hospital or in primary care, where they have an active role in patient care with more responsibilities than was customary during the earlier clerkships. During the other half of year 6, students participate in a project of one of the research schools of the faculty and are responsible for their own research project. At the end of this period students must hand in a substantial essay or paper.

Experiences and reflection

The question to be answered now is: is everybody—students, staff, and management—satisfied with the latest version of the curriculum?

The answer is not a simple yes or no. There is a general satisfaction with the design of the third year with early patient contacts. This setup stimulates the motivation of students and the programme evaluation shows that they work very hard indeed. There is also general satisfaction with the way the plans for the sixth year have turned out and the increased attention for scientific research. Nevertheless, a committee has been installed to investigate the format and content of the scientific aspects of the curriculum. This committee will formulate a proposal with a broader spectrum, including philosophy of science.

A drawback recognized by the whole community of the medical school is the lack of contact with patients and healthcare in the first two years. However, this is a logistical problem that is not easy to resolve given that the regional healthcare system already accommodates large numbers of students in years 4 through 6. The 'preceding' week and 'concluding week' around the clerkships in years 4 and 5 have been the subject of prolonged and heated debate at all levels of the medical school. Most clinicians thought that these weeks would be spent more profitably in the clinical setting. Especially when these weeks were first introduced, criticism from students and staff was widespread. At the moment the discussion seems to have faded, probably because these weeks are now better structured and all parties are familiar with the goals, format, and content.

There is general dissatisfaction among students with life cycle as the theme of the second year and with the last two units of that year in particular. In these units the main emphasis is on the role of environmental factors in the development of disease. Apparently, at that stage of the curriculum these topics have no great urgency or relevance to the students. The fact is that they study fewer hours in these two units than in other ones. The planning groups of these units are inclined to increase the study load by putting more basic science or clinical content into the problems and tasks.

In the introduction to this chapter the ideal design and implementation of a PBL curriculum was described. One of the issues mentioned in this regard was the importance of a consistent and persistent focus on the final objectives of the curriculum. The designers of units, clerkships, and other formats to implement the curriculum master plan should be mindful of their responsibility to design a curriculum that offers students sufficient and adequate opportunities to meet the final objectives of undergraduate medical training. Nevertheless, while the third version of the curriculum was not yet fully implemented, a committee was installed to investigate suspicions of important gaps/omissions in the first two years. Indeed, the committee concluded that some repair was needed.

All this shows that it is difficult to strike a good balance between central directives from a board, dean, or special curriculum committee on the one hand and the need to allocate decentralized responsibility to specific (planning) groups.

References

Geerlings, T., and Snellen-Balendong, H. A. M. (1995). Cursusconstructie [Construction of learning modules]. In: J. C. M. Metz, A. J. J. A. Scherpbier, and C. P. M. van der Vleuten (eds), *Medisch Onderwijs in de Praktijk*. Assen: Van Gorcum. Pp. 283–98.

Metz, J. C. M., Verbeek-Weel, A. M. M., and Huisjes, H. J. (2001). *Raamplan 2001 Artsopleiding*. Nijmegen: Mediagroep Nijmegen. Translated into English as: Blueprint 2001: training of doctors in the Netherlands; adjusted objectives of undergraduate medical education in the Netherlands.

Snellen-Balendong, H. A. M. (1993). Rationale underlying the design of a problem-based curriculum. In: P. A. J. Bouhuijs, H. G. Schmidt, and H. J. M. van Berkel (eds), *Problem-Based Learning as an Educational Strategy*. Maastricht: Network Publications. Pp. 69–78.

Appendices

Appendix 4.1 The first four years of curriculum 1974–88

Year 1	Year 2
Unit 1.1 Study at the University of Limburg	Unit 2.1 From Cell to Human Being
Unit 1.2 Traumata	Unit 2.2 The Child
Unit 1.3 Infection and Inflammation	Unit 2.3 Electives
Unit 1.4 Psychosomatic Disorder	Unit 2.4 The Adolescent
Unit 1.5 Atherosclerosis	Unit 2.5 The Adult
Unit 1.6 Tumours	Unit 2.6 Elderly People
	Unit 2.7 Health, Healthcare, and Community
Year 3	**Year 4**
Unit 3.1 Fever, Infection, and Inflammation	Unit 4.1 Abdominal Pain
Unit 3.2 Fatigue	Unit 4.2 Gynaecological Problems and Reproduction
Unit 3.3 Chest Pain	Unit 4.3 Blood Loss
Unit 3.4 Life Style	Unit 4.4 Electives
Unit 3.5 Electives	Unit 4.5 Headache
Unit 3.6 Electives	Unit 4.6 Backache and Pain in the Extremities

Appendix 4.2 The first four years of curriculum 1988–2001

Year 1	Year 2
Unit 1.1 Introduction: 'Studying at the University of Limburg'	Unit 2.1 Perception, Consciousness, and Emotion
Unit 1.2 Metabolism	Unit 2.2 Locomotion
Unit 1.3 Interaction and Regulation	Unit 2.3 Electives
Unit 1.4 Attack and Defence	Unit 2.4 Basics of Scientific Research
Unit 1.5 Balance/Imbalance	Unit 2.5 Growth and Differentiation
Unit 1.6 Caring for Help	Unit 2.6 Born and Raised
	Unit 2.7 Ageing
Year 3	**Year 4**
Unit 3.1 Shortness of Breath and Chest Pain	Unit 4.1 Sexuality, Fertility, and Problems Related to Pregnancy
Unit 3.2 Mental and Behavioural Problems	Unit 4.2 Abdominal Complaints
Unit 3.3 Disturbances of the Nervous System and Special Senses	Unit 4.3 Fever, Infection, and Inflammation
Unit 3.4 Pain	Unit 4.4 Electives
Unit 3.5 Appearances and External Manifestations of Disease	Unit 4.5 Blood loss
Unit 3.6 Electives	Unit 4.6 Fatigue and Weight Loss
Unit 3.7 Electives	Unit 4.7 Emergencies

Appendix 4.3 The Maastricht medical curriculum from September 2001 till now

Bachelor programme		
Year 1	Year 2	Year 3
Unit 1.1 Emergencies Unit 1.2 Traumata Unit 1.3 Dyspnoea Unit 1.4 Shock Unit 1.5 Abdomen Unit 1.6 Unconsciousness	Unit 2.1 Cell growth Unit 2.2 Pregnancy, Birth, and Growth Unit 2.3 Puberty/Adolescence Unit 2.4 Adulthood and Health Unit 2.5 Ageing Unit 2.6 Electives	Cluster Abdomen Cluster Locomotor Apparatus Cluster Circulation and Lungs Cluster Psychomedical Problems and Mental Health
Master programme		
Year 4	Year 5	Year 6
Dermatology ENT Ophthalmology Internal medicine, Surgery Electives	Social Medicine Paediatrics Gynaecology Psychiatry Neurology General Practice	Research Participation Participation in Health Care

Chapter 5

Designing problems

Henk Schmidt and Jos Moust

At the heart of problem-based learning stands the problem. The analysis of a problem by students, based on their prior knowledge, is the starting point for their learning inside as well as outside the tutorial groups. The quality of a problem seems to influence the depth of the learning process as well as the quantity and quality of the interaction of the students. In the past quite a lot of research has been conducted, in particular at Maastricht University, into the characteristics of problems. Based on epistemological analysis, there are four kinds of distinguishable knowledge: explanatory knowledge (theories), descriptive knowledge (facts), procedural knowledge (knowledge of how to do things), and subjective knowledge (personal convictions or attitudes of the learner). These kinds of knowledge are addressed in problem-based curricula, respectively, by four types of problems: explanation problems, fact-finding problems, strategy problems, and moral dilemma resolution problems. The chapter also provides teachers with some rules about what to do and what to avoid in designing problems.

Introduction

This chapter reports on the development of a taxonomy of didactic problems used in problem-based learning (PBL) curricula. The study has three goals. The first is to make a transparent taxonomy available that would enable teachers to develop a repertoire of skills useful for designing materials for this type of education. Second is to help students, by using the taxonomy, to recognize the nature of the learning task and optimize their learning strategies, which are thought to be dependent on the type of problem they deal with. Third, such a taxonomy could help answer the question of what 'works' in PBL and why (see also Chapter 24). A further reason for this study was that until now the design of problems for PBL curricula has received only limited attention in the relevant literature. Barrows (1985) spends only a handful of pages on problem selection and preparation. A book describing the University of New Mexico experience with PBL (Kaufman, 1985) limits itself to giving a few examples. Boud and Feletti's (1992) treatment of the subject includes only a short descriptive chapter. No text currently available proposes rules for designing PBL problems.

This contribution is idiosyncratic in nature. It is based largely on informal observations made in PBL curricula all over the world. It is not that no previous attempts have been made to characterize problems for use in educational contexts. For instance, Krumm (1985) proposes no less than twenty possible attributes of such problems. In the social psychological literature, which is relevant because PBL relies heavily on small-group collaborative work, are classifications abound (see, for instance, Shaw, 1976). These previous attempts, however, have concentrated largely on the characteristics of problems, such as concreteness, complexity, ambiguity, or familiarity, which can be verified only empirically because they depend on the characteristics of the student population for which the problems were designed. What may be a familiar problem for one student group may be not a familiar problem for another group. This chapter offers an alternative approach. Problems are characterized in terms of the nature of the knowledge addressed by them.

Two assumptions guided this approach: (a) that teachers design problems with certain subject matter in mind, subject matter to be acquired by students through working on these problems; and (b) that the nature of this subject matter may be different, depending on the particular goals of the teacher. Social-work teachers, who wish their students to acquire skills in dealing with drug addicts, have a different goal than criminology professors who encourage students to study theories on the causes of drugs-related crime.

The importance of high-quality problems for students' learning

Gijselaers and Schmidt (1990), Schmidt and Gijselaers (1990), and van Berkel and Schmidt (2001) provide evidence for the impact of problems on students' learning. In line with the models-of-school-learning tradition, these researchers developed a theory of problem-based learning in which three categories of variables (input, throughput and output) played a role. They subjected this model to a series of tests in which they measured each of the variables involved and studied their relations. They analyzed data from units of the medical curriculum and additional data from the health sciences curriculum using the structural equations modeling technique. Figure 5.1 displays the results of one of their analyses.

The researchers found that the quality of problems does not only affect the functioning of the tutorial group, but also two other elements of the model as well; 'time spent' and 'interest in

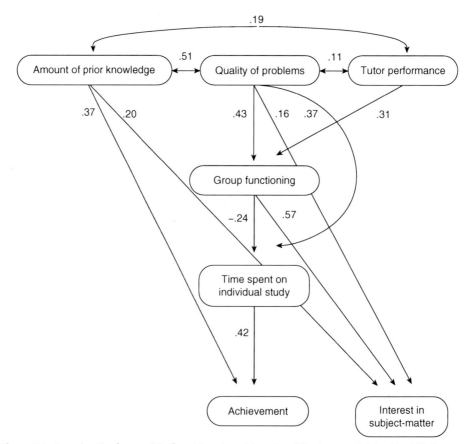

Figure 5.1 Causal paths for model of problem-based learning (Gijselaers and Schmidt, 1990).

subject-matter'. The higher the quality of problems used, the better students in the tutorial groups collaborate, the more time they spend on self-directed learning activities and the more interest is raised in the materials studied. Gijselaers and Schmidt (1990) concluded 'Problems are central to the learning in problem-based curricula.' (p. 110). In line with this conclusion the researchers suggested that poorly designed problems seems to be more of a hazard to student learning than the presence of a poor tutor, and that improving the quality of problems is bound to have a greater beneficial effects on learning than extending tutor training activities to improve tutor performance.

Previous attempts to taxonomize problems for PBL

As early as the 1970s, it was noticed that problems used in PBL curricula could be different in ways more fundamental than that suggested in the preceding section. These observations were called *a problem typology* (Schmidt & Bouhuijs, 1980). This work distinguished between five types of stimulus materials presented to students: (patient) problems, strategy tasks, action tasks, discussion tasks, and study tasks. A problem is defined as an explanation type of assignment, students are supposed to come up with explanations for the phenomena described in the story. A strategy task is defined as a 'what-if' task: 'What would you do if you were in the position of . . . (the physician, the lawyer, the engineer)?' While a strategy task is essentially geared towards the simulation of some kind of (professional) activity, an action task requires students to engage themselves in some kind of field activity, for instance, a visit to a community to undertake an epidemiological or demographic study, or to interview community leaders. Discussion tasks are described as those that focus on students' personal opinions rather than on the acquisition of book knowledge. Finally study tasks are those that do not require group discussion and can be accomplished through individual study.

Based on an analysis of the problems in use in a medical curriculum, Snellen-Balendong (1982) identified no less than thirteen types of stimulus materials. The distinctions made by Snellen-Balendong and by Schmidt and Bouhuijs (1980), together with attempts of others at Maastricht University (e.g., Dolmans & Snellen-Balendong, 1995; Moust & Beurskens, 1994), were not always clear-cut. In some cases, categories seemed to overlap. Sometimes, new variations would arise in the materials produced by teachers that turned out to be difficult to categorize with the existing approaches. After it was fully understood why these teachers needed these different formats, it was possible to come up with the solution that is presented in this chapter.

Different categories of knowledge and related problem types

The proposed taxonomy of PBL problems is based on two assumptions: (a) That during the course of their study, students acquire different kinds, or categories, of knowledge about relevant aspects of their domain of study; and (b) that the problem types to be distinguished are meant to guide learners towards these different knowledge categories. The example below may elucidate these assumptions.

Example 1: Gaining weight suddenly: a normal process when you are over forty?

A man in his forties comes to your office complaining that he has grown fat in a short time. His abdomen is swollen, and he finds it difficult to fasten his belt. His eyelids and the skin around his eyes appear to be swollen too. The percentage of plasma protein in his blood is lower than normal.
Instruction (a): What is the matter with this man?
Instruction (b): How would you manage his problem?

Instruction (a) requires students to offer explanations of the phenomena described in terms of underlying processes. It encourages students to acquire knowledge about the effects of kidney failure on the location of extracellular fluids. This kind of knowledge contributes to an understanding and explanation of the observed phenomena, which is referred to as explanatory or causal knowledge. It is knowledge that explains why a man in his forties may develop these symptoms. In instruction (b), the emphasis is not on explanation but on (simulated) action. What would you do if you were this patient's doctor? The problem designer apparently has assumed that students already understand the problem and are able to explain the signs and symptoms in terms of their underlying disease processes. The intention of the instruction is to guide students into learning how to act upon their understanding of this particular case, that is, to manage this case. The kind of knowledge being addressed is not explanatory or causal knowledge about why things are the way they are, but knowledge of how to act upon the situation in order to change it. This kind of knowledge is called procedural knowledge.

The distinction between explanatory and procedural knowledge is, however, not the only one made by philosophers of science. It is assumed that there are at least four different ways of knowing the world around us. These four ways of knowing are summarized in Figure 5.2.

To elucidate these four ways of knowing (or knowledge categories), some additional distinctions must be made. The first important distinction is that between knowledge in the public domain and normative, personal knowledge, a distinction made by, among others, the philosopher of science Karl Popper (1972). Public knowledge is available in libraries, books, journals, and research reports. It is accessible and can be criticized or improved upon. Therefore, Popper sometimes uses the term objective knowledge to refer to knowledge in the public domain. The knowledge produced and recorded by scientists, journalists, and other writers is considered objective—not because their points of view are objective in the sense of being 'true', but because these viewpoints can be critically discussed, tested, and improved upon. In contrast, personal, normative knowledge is that which exists in peoples' minds. It represents the whole of their

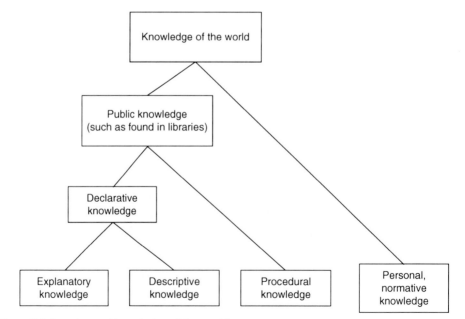

Figure 5.2 Four types of knowledge of the world.

attitudes and deeply felt convictions about the world. Personal knowledge can be considered normative knowledge, because it is not about what is 'true' or 'false', but about what is 'right' or 'wrong'. Personal knowledge is not as easily revealed because people may not want to disclose their convictions. It is also more difficult to criticize or improve upon than public knowledge because people tend to stick with their convictions despite facts or experience.

In many professional domains, normative ideas and convictions are important because they play a role in the way a future professional will conduct his or her profession. This is the case in particular with moral dilemmas, small and large, with which the professional may be confronted. Problems that lead into this kind of knowledge are called moral dilemma resolution problems or dilemma problems. The following situation comes from the medical profession.

Example 2: Blood transfusion for a child of Jehovah's Witnesses

A child is admitted to the First Aid Ward of a hospital. She has been knocked down by a motorcar and has lost a substantial amount of blood. The only way to save the child's life, in the judgment of the attending physician, is a blood transfusion. However, the child's parents are not likely to give their consent because their religion forbids the transmission of another person's blood into their child's body: 'She is in God's hands.'
Instruction: What do you think the physician should do?

Students have different ideas and different convictions of what should be done in situations such as these. Should the physician accept the ultimate responsibility of the parents with regard to the child's welfare? If so, would that not be at variance with his or her Hippocratic oath to save the life of a patient if s/he can? What about the will of the patient herself and her right to self-determination? These questions deal with personal ethics in the context of healthcare. It is important to the professional development of medical students that they confront personal values and norms with regard to the dilemma sketched. Hence, dilemma problems arise.

Ryle (1949) distinguishes between two forms of knowledge: knowing *that* and knowing *how*. Anderson (1983) makes a similar distinction, namely between declarative knowledge and procedural knowledge. Knowing that, or declarative knowledge, is knowledge of the world as it is, whereas knowing how, or procedural knowledge, is knowledge of how to act upon the world. Declarative knowledge is similar to explanatory knowledge discussed earlier. A distinction is necessary, however, because explanatory knowledge often is considered a subset of declarative knowledge that also includes descriptive knowledge (Bromage & Mayer, 1981). Descriptive knowledge consists only of empirical facts, whereas explanatory knowledge consists of causal theories. Put another way, descriptive knowledge describes the facts of life, whereas explanatory knowledge explains them. This distinction is useful, because we may know all kind of facts about the world but not be able to explain them. For instance, it is known that small amounts of aspirin or acetylsalicylic acid, taken on a daily basis, lower the chances of developing a myocard infarct (fact), but it is largely unknown why this is so (explanation). Sometimes, facts exist even without a (potential) explanation. For instance, we happen to remember that Sir Edmund Hillary was the first to climb Mount Everest in 1953, and that his Sherpah's name was Tenzing. These are statements of fact; they can be true or false, but they require no further explanation. They describe the world as it is. In some cases, students may have to acquire these facts even in the absence of scientific explanation, for instance, because these facts are professionally useful. Therefore, if facts and fact acquisition play a role in most curricula, then PBL curricula must use fact-finding problems. Here is an example.

Example 3: The legal map of the Netherlands

The Netherlands can be observed through many different glasses. A topographical map discloses the locations of roads, rivers, canals, and hills. A Roman-Catholic map distinguishes between parishes, dioceses, and an archdiocese. An administrative map has different colors for communities, cities, metropolitan areas, and provinces.

Instruction: What would a legal map look like?

This problem will lead students into finding out how the Dutch judicial system is organized; how many courts there are; and where they are located. These are facts, useful to know for law students that do not require further explanation in terms of some underlying principle or theory. They do not even require much discussion. Therefore, Example 3 is a fact-finding problem, because it encourages law students to acquire these facts.

In summary, four types of knowledge can be distinguished: explanatory knowledge, descriptive knowledge, procedural knowledge, and normative knowledge. Problems developed for problem-based guide students towards these knowledge types. Therefore, four types of problems exist in these curricula, no less and no more: explanation problems, fact-finding problems, strategy problems, and moral dilemma resolution problems. All other types found are either combinations of these four or can be reduced to one of these. Figure 5.3 displays the relationship between problem types and knowledge types and summarizes the examples provided in this chapter.

Some further examples of problems and some cautionary notes

In this paragraph some further examples of the four types of problems are presented. These examples will be offered in the format of prototypes to demonstrate in the most rudimentary way the differences between them.

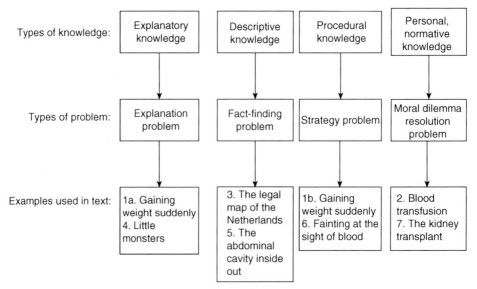

Figure 5.3 Taxonomy of problems, related to types of knowledge.

Explanation problems

An explanatory problem is a description of a set of phenomena or events in need of explanation in terms of an underlying process, mechanism, or principle. The following is an example.

Example 4: Little monsters!

Coming home from work, tired and in need of a hot bath, Peter, an account manager, discovers two spiders in his tub. He shrinks back, screams, and runs away. A neighbour saves him from his difficult situation by carrying the little insects in her hands outside. In the days and months to come Peter's behaviour changes. He insulates all windows of his house thoroughly. Often he asks his neighbour to inspect all his rooms before he enters them. Words such as Spiderman and Webmaster makes him very nervous.
Explain.

An explanation problem has several advantages. It stimulates students to study facts as well as the relations between facts. It also, invites students to activate their prior knowledge and to elaborate about possible hypotheses that can explain underlying processes, mechanisms, or principles. Explanation problems are closely related to the hypothetico-deductive processes PBL wants to support. A third advantage is that this type of a problem offers students, even in its most rudimentary format a professional context which support students' memory storage and retrieval processes.

Fact-finding problems

A fact-finding problem can be described as a problem that helps students to research facts which they should know in order to better understand a subject-matter studied within a certain discipline. Example 5 shows an example of a fact-finding problem.

Example 5: The abdominal cavity inside out

The digestive tract consists of a hollow pipe that is an extension of the outside world. Each part of the tract is distinguished by its relation to specific glands and organs. Study the parts of the digestive tract that can be distinguished macroscopically, the location of the parts in relation to each other, and their functions.

Fact-finding problems have a serious disadvantage. They do not stimulate students' previous knowledge and, consequently hinder students from elaborating on the subject matter to be studied. On the other hand, teachers may have difficulties designing another type of problem. In that case a fact-finding problem may be the solution for stimulating the students to work at the subject matter which needs to be studied.

Strategy problems

A strategy problem is a description of a set of phenomena or events where students learn how to *act* upon their understanding of a particular case, that is, how to manage the case. The instructional goal is to guide students into mastering all procedures appropriate to managing the problem. Example 6 offers an example of a strategy problem.

Example 6: Fainting at the sight of blood

In biology class, some blood is taken from several students. One of the bystanders faints. How would you manage his problem?

The format given above is not the only format a teacher can use to support student's understanding of how to act. A teacher can stimulate students by offering them a role play in which one of the group members acts as a general practitioner and the other as a patient. The patient has learned about a number of complaints, which he offers to the physician. The physician must work out a strategy to help the patient. The interview can be videotaped and be looked at after the play. The other members of the tutorial group can give feedback and suggestions. Students can also be stimulated to participate in a simulation game. In a health science curriculum students are divided in several parties (each party from a different country) who have to negotiate about limited resources in healthcare. Students are able to experience the dynamics of bargaining in a multicultural setting. Another example is an action problem. Students conduct interviews with laborers in a factory (e.g., chemical factory). Students must develop their own questionnaire (open and closed questions) about the way the healthcare system in and outside the factory is able to provide, care, and cure diseases related to working with advanced chemical products. Students must work out their data and create a report in which they deliver suggestions for improvement.

Moral dilemma problems

A moral dilemma problem is a description of a set of phenomena or events where students are invited to bring forward their own norms and values regarding this event. Example 7 presents such a problem.

Example 7: The kidney transplant

Two adolescents with a severe kidney disease are brought to your department last week. Research has shown that they will die soon without kidney transplant. At the moment there is only one possible donor. You know that one of these adolescents is a brilliant student who wants to become a surgeon. However, she is so sick now that there is only a 50% chance to survive the transplant. The chances she will have a healthy live will also be small. The other patient seems not to be very interested to have a successful career in life. He neglects a lot of school activities and only seems to be interested in being a merry-maker. There is a nearly 100% chance he will survive the transplant and live a healthy life.
To whom would you give the kidney?

As said before, these problems are prototypes to show the basic process teachers want to provoke of students: understanding, acting, and reflecting. Explanations and facts are particularly important for the scientific part of the programme, whereas procedural and normative knowledge are particularly important for the professional part. The various types of problems can be offered to students in one unit. Teachers involved in developing a unit book can start with explanation and fact-finding problems, stimulating students to understand the phenomena and events related to a specific topic. Later they can offer strategy problems that encourage students to think about how to handle problems like these. At the end of a unit book they can offer moral dilemma problems, which challenge students to reflect about ethical norms and values they have as well as those professionals should have concerning the subject matter offered. This schedule, however, is not obliged. Depending on the subject matter offered, teachers can start with strategy problems, go on to explanation problems and end with dilemma problems. The objectives of the planning group define the way a unit bock is designed and the order of the problems offered.

The problems distinguished here represent prototypical models. The problems offered are focusing on either the normal or abnormal functioning of phenomena at the cell, tissue, organ, personal, family or group, organization or community level. The problems are designed in a well-structured way, whereby students get all the information necessary to understand or solve the problem. In the reality of problem-based curricula these problems are to be found particularly in the first year of study. In more advanced years, problems should become longer, more complex, and real life. There are several ways to foster problem complexity. First, problems can be combined prototypes, e.g., an explanation problem combined with a strategy problem, or a strategy problem integrated with a dilemma problem. Students must deal with problems that require them to explore conceptual issues, while also focusing on patient management issues and/or moral dilemmas.

Second, offering students ill-defined problems can also foster complexity. As in real-life situations students must analyse problems which lack certain information or which contain false information. Clients (individual patients, groups, or even organizations) may purposefully, unaware, or uninformed give information that may set the physician or consultant on the wrong track. Students must recognize this lack or distortion of information, and look for additional information to clarify and solve the problem in one or more correct ways.

Until now the discussed problems have had a written format. The problems had a title and a problem text. This text was a description of some phenomena to be observed in the outside world or some events told in the format of a story. Problems in a written format can, however, also be graphics, cartoons, laboratory outcomes, etc. Students, however, may be offered other formats too: a videotape showing contact between a client or patient and a healthcare professional, a simulated patient contact, or a computer program offering various photos which must be analysed.

Some additional rules for problem design

Next a set of rules is presented. These rules are mainly based on common sense and knowledge of 'what works and what doesn't'. They are suggestions for good problem design and not universally applicable 'laws', so exceptions and alternatives may be thought of.

A well-formed problem consists of a title

A title is important because it provides a context for a problem. It often contains cues as to what the focus of the problem is; it frames the problem. It gives the students an idea of the approach they must take to clarify or solve the problem. Of course, in the broader context, the objectives of the particular unit book may influence the students' interpretation of the problem. A title can be intriguing or funny to raise student interest.

A well-formed problem consists of a concrete body text

The body text should contain a theoretically neutral description of the phenomena or events to be explained or solved, phrased in concrete terms and common language. When a problem text contains a lot of jargon, e.g., domain-related terminology, students will focus too much in particular directions. Another argument for being concrete is that most clients will not use medical or healthcare concepts while seeking help. They will use common sense terminology or even direct attention to the areas in their body where they feel pain. The advice not to use specific terminology applies in particular to problems written for first-year students who have not yet mastered the kind of concepts professionals or scientists use to denote certain phenomena. For more advanced students this may be less of a problem. The rule of thumb here is that the problem should always be framed in terms that are adapted to the students' prior knowledge and that can be understood immediately.

The problem text should also give students the opportunity to imagine the situation as clearly as described. Students should be able to build a mental model of the situation. A lively and concrete problem text helps students to 'visualize' what is going on, and stimulates their prior knowledge.

The body text should also only contain a limited number of cues and no distracters. This sub-rule regards especially problems presented to novice students. In the previous section it was said that in the later years of their study, students can be offered ill-defined problems to better understand the real life of their profession. However, 'messy' problems, which contain information irrelevant to its understanding must be used carefully. To experts, understanding messy, complex, real-life problems in terms of their underlying structure usually presents no difficulty because they discover, almost instantly, the pattern of cues in need of explanation. For experts, one could say, the pattern of the phenomena 'pops up' from the data and almost immediately triggers an explanation (in the form of a diagnosis or another kind of understanding). For students, who are novices by definition, the situation is quite different. They do not see a pattern and must reason from each of the cues actively, elaborately, and often laboriously (Schmidt & Boshuizen, 1993). If the number of cues presented in a problem increases, the complexity of their task increases substantially more. Students not only have to consider separate reasonable explanations for each of the cues but also for their combinations. This is a formidable task, often too difficult for novices to cope with. Students will deal with messy, complex, ill-structured problems by having endless and sometimes repetitive discussions and building a basically unrelated micro-theory for each cue, or they will come up with a fairly superficial analysis, leading to the formulation of learning goals largely in terms of the original cues. Subsequently their understanding of the phenomena will often be meaningless. Students will become surface-level learners. This kind of learning behavior is inefficient, laborious, and frustrating for students. Therefore, particularly when students are novices, problems should be short, should contain only a limited number of cues, and should not contain pitfalls. As students progress, the complexity of the problems may expand, until, after sufficient time has passed, real-life problems becomes the ones students can deal with. In other words, curricula and unit book designers should be careful in using complex and real-life problems. There should be an alignment between the increasing domain of knowledge of the students and the level of complexity of problems offered.

Each problem needs an instruction as to what to do with it

Among designers of problems there is some discussion about this rule. Some teachers say it is evident that students should explain the underlying phenomena, so this instruction can be skipped. Others warn that students tend to be more oriented towards solving the problem, i.e., to find strategies or solutions, than to look for explanations. Students seem to be more focused on the management of a problem. They put themselves vicariously in the position of a physician or another healthcare professional and act accordingly. They focus on the features of appropriate action rather than on explanations per se. Here, again the difference in thinking between experts and novices is important. For experts, understanding (the diagnosis of a problem) and action go hand in hand, because experts acquired the necessary knowledge previously. For novices this will not be the case. Management of a problem concentrates on how to confirm or refute a differential diagnosis, and how to treat a client provided a certain diagnosis is confirmed. Explanation, on the other hand, deals with understanding the diagnosis itself. For students (novices), understanding should always precede action if the action is to be rational.

There are two other arguments to instruct students on what to do with a problem. An explanation instruction will lead students to acquiring declarative knowledge, while a management instruction will engage students in the mastery of procedure. In line with this argument the nature of the learning activities of the students confronted with a management instruction will be quite different from those of students stimulated by an explanation instruction.

To avoid students neglecting explanation of the phenomena included within the problem text, instruction on how to approach the problem in the tutorial group would be wise.

A problem should be connected to the prior knowledge base students have

Starting from student's prior knowledge base is very important. As students must analyse the problem to understand underlying mechanisms and processes, students need their previous knowledge to take the first step. The connection with the prior knowledge base is very delicate. If students are able to explain or solve the problem with their existing knowledge the problem is too easy. Students are not challenged to study external resources. If the problem, on the other hand, is too far from students' prior knowledge the problem is too difficult. Students will experience an inability to bring forward their ideas, and their discussion and learning will come to an end.

A problem should raise students' curiosity

Curiosity supports motivation and interaction. There are several techniques to make students curious. The first is 'contrasting situations'. Two individuals experience a different situation: one is afraid of spiders, the other is not. Why? The skin of a dark-haired person and the skin of a blond person are exposed to bright sun for a period of two hours. In the evening, the skin of the blond person looks very red, the skin of the dark person less so. Why? You also can contrast an animal with a human being. For example, a rat can survive total starvation for 6–7 days while an average human can survive 3–4 months. Why? Or you can compare two blood cells: A red blood cell is put into pure water under a microscope. The blood cell swells rapidly and eventually bursts. Another red blood cell is added to a solution of salt in water and is observed to shrink. Why?

Another technique for raising student curiosity is 'counterintuitive situations'. In this case, the description in the problem text consists of phenomena that seem to be contradictory to the intuitive knowledge students have. Students get in a situation of cognitive dissonance. They feel an urgent need to underpin or reject explanations. A brief example follows:

> A man is traveling by foot in a snowy and frostbitten area for hours. He, however, seems to feel very happy. He has a good bottle of vodka in his pocket. Sometimes, when the cold sends too many shivers down his back, he stops and drinks a good few gulps of vodka to get warm. Suddenly, he falls to the ground. Within a short period of time he is dead.
>
> Explain.

Or another one:

> For more than 15 minutes an eight-year-old girl, Mary, has been lifelessly floating around in water colder than 60°F. Fortunately, a passer-by succeeds in bringing her out of the water. Mouth-to-mouth resuscitation is applied immediately. Everyone of the onlookers is astonished to notice that the girl is

still alive. Presently, Mary is on the intensive care ward of the local hospital and is out of danger. According to her doctor she is expected to recover completely.

Explain why this is possible.

In these problem texts students' expectations of how the outside world is functioning is disturbed. (Vodka keeps people warm!—People die quickly when immersed in cold water.) When your expectations are disturbed, your worldview may be undermined. Most people do not like that; they will look for information either to reduce their ruffled view of the world or to understand the new information and adapt to the new circumstances. (Some brief explanations to the above problems: Vodka opens your blood veins, so you become even colder. In cold water, the oxygen needs of the body may be reduced, and since a child has a smaller body surface, her body may not decrease in temperature to the same extent of an adult's.)

A problem should only introduce a limited number of issues for learning

People cannot handle too many topics at the same time. When they are forced to handle several subject matters their cognitive system becomes overloaded (Van Merriënboer, 1998). This rule applies even more for novices in a specific domain. Sometimes designers of a problem offer students large (several pages of information) problems. Students are expected not only to study in depth the biomedical, pathophysiological, and clinical aspects of the problem but also its psychological, social, and epidemiological aspects. In order to have students delve into those different domains, the problem designers must describe many different cues in the body text, each leading to a different discipline. This makes the learning (of novices) unnecessarily complicated and a burden. The reaction of students to these problems is typical; they engage frantically in all kinds of learning activities for long hours of study and end up feeling frustrated because they 'failed' to master the topics to a reasonable extent. There is, however, no reason to make the burden heavier by requiring (novice) students to deal with problems beyond their grasp. Within one problem, two or three major issues are sufficient to keep a student busy. As has been suggested already in this chapter, this rule applies particularly to novices in a domain. The rule demands that those responsible for the development of a PBL curriculum carefully consider the subjects that students subsequently must study. The members of a planning group should also meticulously research which aspects of students' prior knowledge is related to the subjects offered in a unit book. A precise investigation of what students have studied previously and what can be built upon gives the planning group members opportunities to offer students problems that have a different level of complexity.

A problem should not take too much self-directed study time to acquire a fair understanding of the issues at hand

As has been explained in Chapter 3, students meet twice a week, each session lasting for about two hours. They work on average two problems a week. Assume that the students of a tutorial group meet on Monday and Thursday. In that case they analyse a new problem and formulate learning issues related to that problem during the second hour of the Monday meeting. Considerable time is dedicated on Tuesday and Wednesday to self-directed learning and the students discuss their findings on Thursday, during the first hour of the tutorial group, the second hour being spent on the initial analysis of the week's second problem. On Friday and over the weekend self-study activities devoted to the second problem are undertaken. On Monday the first hour is used for information exchange with regard to the second problem, etc. This schedule implies that students can spend about two days of self-study for each problem. This rhythm is responsible for intensive and stimulating tutorial sessions because much work needs to be done in a relatively short period. There is no time to relax because the next problem is already around the corner. When members of a planning group offer students problems that require quite a lot more self-study time, students will not be able to study all the information. Many undesirable consequences can occur as a result. Students will not be able to discuss all the information from their learning resources; they might skip the analysis phase in order to have more time to synthesize the information. By skipping time to analyse the new problem students might formulate half-hearted learning issues, which influence the quality of their self-study. Doing this quite often will result in the students' learning process falling into a downward spiral. Students might also decide to stop the synthesis phase after about an hour of discussion. This can lead to feelings of frustration, with students not sure whether they've understood the information correctly, whether there are misconceptions, and whether they've applied the information well. So, members of a planning group should try to estimate the amount of study time students need in order to understand the subject matter accurately. Besides underestimating the amount of study hours, members of a planning group can also, of course, overestimate the amount of study time students need to grasp the information. In that case students will be students. They will spend their free time during the period of self-study on student-related activities. And they will suggest that the time for the tutorial meeting can be reduced in that unit.

After offering these 'do's' it is also useful to offer you some 'don't's'.

Do not offer students a problem which includes many questions in or under the problem text. Questions seem to trigger students' attention. Often it seems that students are drilled to answer questions. They seem not to be able to think for themselves and to ask themselves questions when a designer of a problem offers them questions. They often stick to the questions offered and do not look further.

Do not offer students a problem supplemented with keywords, either under the problem or somewhere in the unit book. Keywords have nearly the same effect as questions. They hinder the students brainstorming about the ideas that come to mind. As a result, the stimulating prior knowledge and elaborating on ideas do not, or do so very slowly, get off the ground. Students seem to think 'Oh that is what we have to study? I don't know very much about that topic! Let's come up with some learning issues!'

Do not provide one or two literature suggestions under a problem. Literature suggestions may, of course, be offered to the students. Somewhere in the unit book a list of numerous books and journals as well as other resources can be offered. Students must learn for themselves how to find, select, and read relevant resources. Literature suggestions provided under a problem text, however, kills students' self-directed learning. Most students will stick to the resources offered. Students will form the idea that these resources are the most relevant to understanding or solving the problem.

In general one may say that the core of these 'don'ts' is that they hinder the process of self-directed learning. At the end of this section a warning should be given. The rules offered so far may be interpreted as a number of prescriptions which should be followed strictly. That is not the case! In a unit there may be situations which impel a teacher, as a problem designer, to deviate from these rules. What should be kept in mind is to raise students' curiosity.

Concluding remarks

In this chapter, a distinction of four categories of knowledge acquired by students in the course of their PBL training was offered: explanatory, descriptive, procedural, and normative knowledge. Other authors have made similar distinctions (for instance, Farnham Diggory, 1994). In response to the need for students to acquire these kinds of knowledge relevant to their discipline, and because problems are the main instruments through the learning process is directed in PBL curricula, teachers develop any of four types of problems: explanation problems, fact-finding problems, strategy problems, and moral dilemma resolution problems. The purpose of the taxonomy is to describe sufficiently and exhaustively the variety of problems found in PBL curricula. Thus, each of these kinds of problems matches one type of knowledge. A taxonomy such as this may help teachers to design appropriate problems for PBL, and it may guide students in their choice of learning strategy.

A limitation of the proposed taxonomy is that it is descriptive rather than prescriptive. It describes the kind of problems used in PBL curricula and the reasons why these problems are used versus others. The taxonomy, however, does not provide explicit and detailed guidelines on how to design problems optimal for particular subject matter. Formulating such explicit guidelines may prove an impossible task, because the quality of a problem seems related not so much to its actual formulation as to the characteristics of the students, such as the nature of their prior knowledge through which they tackle the problem, or the students' interest in the subject to which the problem refers. Research has shown that neither subject matter experts nor educationalists are able to distinguish between poorly and well-formulated problems when asked to give such a judgement (Kokx & Schmidt, 1990).

A final remark on what is the purpose of the whole PBL exercise: The reader should be aware that the position taken in this chapter, namely, that using problems helps students to acquire different kinds of knowledge, is somewhat controversial. Other definitions of PBL emphasize helping students to learn to solve professional problems as its main goal, rather than acquiring different types of subject matter knowledge (Barrows and Tamblyn, 1980; Boud and Feletti, 1992). These definitions, in other words, emphasize procedural learning exclusively. It is believed, however, that the definition presented here is more generally applicable.

Annotated literature

Dolmans, D. H. J. M., Snellen-Balendong, H. A. M., Wolfhagen, I. H. A. P., and van der Vleuten, C. P. M. (1997). Seven principles of effective case design for a problem-based curriculum. *Medical Teacher* **19(3)**, 185–9.

This article described several principles for effective case design deduced from programme evaluation research. Several examples are offered.

Schmidt, H. G., and Moust, J. H. C. (2000). Towards a taxonomy of problems used in problem-based curricula. *Journal on Excellence in College Teaching* **11(2–3)**, 57–73.

This contribution contains the report of an attempt to develop a taxonomy of problems used in problem-based curricula in Maastricht.

Schmidt, H. G., van der Molen, H. T., te Winkel, W. W. R., and Wijnen, W. F. F. W. (2009). Constructivist, problem-based, learning does work: A meta-analysis of curricular comparisons involving a single medical school. *Educational Psychologist* **44**, 227–49.

This article describes in an elaborated way three types of PBL. It also compares the effects of PBL of one medical school with seven other medical schools in the Netherlands. The results suggest that students and graduates from the particular curriculum perform much better in the area of interpersonal skills and with regard to practical medical skills. In addition, students from this school consistently rate the quality of the curriculum higher. Moreover, fewer students drop out and those students surviving need less time to graduate. Differences with respect to medical knowledge and diagnostic reasoning were on average positive but small.

References

Anderson, J. R. (1983). *The architecture of cognition.* Cambridge, MA: Harvard University Press.

Barrows, H. S. (1985). *How to design a problem-based curriculum for the preclinical years.* New York: Springer.

Barrows, H. S., and Tamblyn, R. M. (1980). *Problem-based learning: an approach to medical education.* New York: Springer.

Van Berkel, H., and Schmidt, H. G. (2001). Motivation to commit oneself as a determinant of achievement in problem-based learning. *Higher Education* **40**, 231–42.

Boud, D., and Feletti, G. (eds). (1992). *Problem-based learning: an approach to medical education.* New York: Springer.

Bromage, B. K., and Mayer, R. E. (1981). Relationship between what is remembered and creative problem-solving performance in science learning. *Journal of Educational Psychology* **73**, 451–61.

Dolmans, D. H. J. M., and Snellen-Balendong, H. A. M. (1995). *Constructie van taken [Construction of tasks].* Maastricht, The Netherlands: Vakgroep Onderwijsontwikkeling en-research, Maastricht University.

Farnham Diggory, S. (1994). Paradigms of knowledge and instruction. *Review of Educational Research* **64**, 463–77.

Gijselaers, W. H., and Schmidt, H. G. (1990). Development and evaluation of a causal model of problem-based learning. In: Z. M. Nooman, H. G. Schmidt, and E. S. Ezzat (eds), *Innovation in medical education: an evaluation of its present status.* New York: Springer. Pp. 95–113.

Kaufman, A. (1985). *Implementing problem-based medical education: lessons from successful innovations.* New York: Springer.

Kokx, I. P. A., and Schmidt, H. G. (1990). *The quality of problems in problem-based learning: expert judgments.* Paper presented at the Second International Symposium on Problem-Based Learning, Yogyakarta, Indonesia.

Krumm, V. (1985). Anmerkungen zur rolle der aufgaben in didaktik, unterricht und unterrichtsforschung [Remarks on the role of assignments in didactics, education and educational research]. *Unterrichtswissenschaft* **2**, 102–15.

Moust, J. H. C., and Beurskens, W. (1994). *Ontwikkelen van leermateriaal voor probleemgestuurd leren [Development of learning materials for problem-based learning].* Maastricht, The Netherlands: Faculteit der Rechtsgeleerdheid, Maastricht University.

Popper, K. R. (1972). *Objective knowledge: an evolutionary approach.* London: Oxford University Press.

Ryle, G. (1949). *Collected papers, vol. II: Critical essays.* London: Hutchinson.

Schmidt, H. G., and Bouhuijs, P. A. J. (1980). *Onderwijs in taakgerichte groepen [Instruction in task-oriented groups].* Utrecht, The Netherlands: Het Spectrum.

Schmidt, H.G., and Boshuizen, H. P. A. (1993). On acquiring expertise in medicine. *Educational Psychology Review* **5**, 1–17.

Schmidt, H. G., and Gijselaers, W. H. (1990). *Causual Modelling of Problem-based Learning.* Paper presented at the Annual Meeting of the American Educational Research Association, Boston, MA, April 16–22.

Shaw, M. E. (1976). *Group dynamics.* New York: McGraw-Hill.

Snellen-Balendong, H. A. M. (1982). *Curriculumoverzicht fakulteit der geneeskunde jaar I t/m IV 1981/1982 [Curriculum overview faculty of medicine year 1 to 4 1981/1982 (19b)].* Maastricht, The Netherlands: Department of Educational Development and Research.

Van Merriënboer, J. J. G. (1998). Cognitive load theory and the design of problems in PBL. In: J. van Merriënboer and G. Moerkerke (eds), *Instructional design for problem-based learning.* Proceedings of the Third Workshop of the EARLI SIG Instructional Design. Maastricht: The Netherlands: Datawyse Publishing Maastricht.

Chapter 6

The role of the tutor

Jos Moust

Teachers perform various roles in problem-based learning (PBL): designer of problems, assessor of performance, trainer of skills, and facilitator of learning. The last role seems to have the highest importance because teachers in this role can observe students in action during individual and collaborative learning. Tutors see students struggling to acquire new knowledge. They observe how students use their prior knowledge, the pitfalls they encounter, and their motivation to engage with the subject matter. They also see how students collaborate within the group. Apart from observing students' behaviour, tutors also intervene: they can facilitate learning by asking questions, offering analogies and metaphors, and giving feedback about students' thinking and reasoning. Tutors fulfil an important role in guiding students to work together as a team and perform at a high level of self-directed learning. And last but not least, tutors act as intermediaries between students and teaching staff: they can offer feedback about the quality of the problems in unit books and they are the first-line 'officers' who observe what motivates students.

The responsibilities and tasks of a tutor

It goes without saying that the responsibilities of a tutor are in line with the activities students are expected to undertake inside and outside tutorial groups (Chapter 3). Students must acquire knowledge and insights concerning the domains in their field of study, they must collaborate efficiently and effectively, and they must become increasingly self-directed learners (Figure 6.1).

In order to promote these activities, tutors should facilitate the acquisition of knowledge, stimulate collaboration, and guide students to become independent learners. Figure 6.2 shows the various activities of a tutor. Figure 6.2 also shows another competency for tutors: relevant general pedagogical knowledge. In this chapter, the responsibilities of a tutor in the PBL programmes of the Maastricht Faculty of Health, Medicine and Life Sciences (FHML) as well as the main tasks tutors must perform to fulfil these responsibilities are discussed.

General pedagogical knowledge

As university teachers, tutors are expected to have some knowledge about educational subjects with relevance to higher education (left upper part of Figure 6.2). They should have some basic knowledge and skills with respect to the principles and theories of the learning and teaching of (young) adults. For instance, they should know about the key principles of adult education, as the students they guide are approximately eighteen years old or older (for example, Kaufman et al., 2000; Merriam & Caffarella,1999). They should also have some knowledge about curriculum and unit design, assessment, and various instructional methods (Dent & Harden, 2006) and they should be familiar with important modern educational concepts, like constructive, contextual, and collaborative learning. And, at a more specific education level, they should understand the

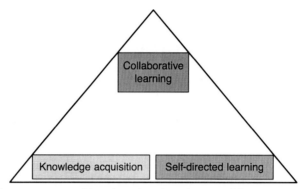

Figure 6.1 Three important areas of learning of students in a tutorial group.

learning processes underpinning PBL, such as the activation of prior knowledge to acquire new information, and the role of elaboration in storing and retrieving information, and questioning behaviour (Schmidt, 1983, 1993). General pedagogical knowledge helps tutors to understand the main teaching and learning processes promoted in a PBL environment.

Content and pedagogical content knowledge

In order to help students acquire knowledge and insights about the subject matter offered in unit books, tutors should, first of all, have be knowledgeable about the subject matter (Figure 6.2). A tutor who cannot follow the discussions in the tutorial group during the analysis and synthesis phases is unlikely to be able to determine whether the students are on the right track, have any misconceptions, do or do not grasp the main and side issues, and apply information correctly. Knowledge of subject matter is a prerequisite for effective performance as a tutor. Apart from content knowledge, a tutor should also possess pedagogical content knowledge: knowledge of content-specific instruction. This special form of knowledge is unique to teachers and develops through the repetitive experience of teaching specific content to specific groups of students. The resulting knowledge becomes organized in teaching scripts containing general goals of instruction, key teaching points, specific representations of content (explanations, analogies, examples), an understanding of learners' conceptions and misconceptions, and procedures for overcoming learning difficulties. The essence of content-specific instruction is that content knowledge is

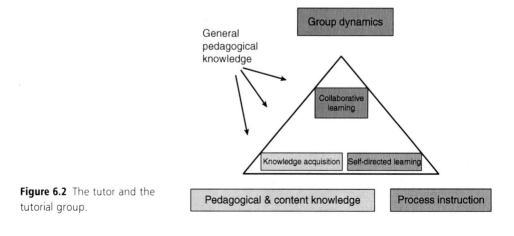

Figure 6.2 The tutor and the tutorial group.

organized for teaching purposes in such a way that it can be made comprehensible to learners (Irby, 1994).

An overview of the tutor's tasks in this area is presented in Box 6.1.

Facilitating collaboration in a tutorial group

Because students work in a group of some ten to twelve students for a considerable period of time, tutors should know how groups function and how to enhance collaboration inside and outside the tutorial group. Knowledge about group dynamics is essential for this (Figure 6.2). Tutors should know how to get a group started, how to agree on and adhere to a code of conduct, how groups develop over time, what groups should do at the task and maintenance level to function effectively, how to handle conflicts between group members, and how to give interpersonal feedback about group members' behaviour. Such knowledge and skills are essential for fostering a collaborative learning climate in which students can work together in an open and trustful way. Box 6.1 gives an overview of the tasks of a tutor as a facilitator of collaboration in tutorial groups.

Box 6.1 An overview of the tasks of a tutor in a problem-based context

A. A tutor plays an active and stimulating role in a tutorial group with respect to students' learning processes (Triangle point: content and pedagogical-content knowledge).

To this end a tutor:
- Prepares thoroughly before and during a unit;
- Establishes, in dialogue with the group members, a code of conduct to support a constructive learning environment;
- Facilitates students' knowledge construction process by 'reading' students' prior knowledge base;
- Listens actively to students' contributions with regard to both content and intentions;
- Stimulates students to formulate in-depth ideas on the subject matter under discussion;
- Helps students to organize the subject matter in meaningful structures;
- Diagnoses the intellectual processes going on within and between students;
- Stimulates students to reflect on what they bring up for discussion;
- Keeps himself informed of students' opinions concerning the group proceedings; and
- Prevents himself from dominating the discussion.

B. A tutor plays an active and stimulating role with respect to students' collaborative activities. (Triangle point: group dynamics)

To this end a tutor:
- Ensures that arrangements are made for working procedures, participation, group roles, etc., and sees to it that group members act accordingly;
- Improves the way students chair the tutorial group;
- Tries to anticipate problematic behaviour of group members and helps them to resolve problems;

Box 6.1 An overview of the tasks of a tutor in a problem-based context (continued)

- Evaluates group members' perceptions of the collaborative process and offers alternatives to improve collaboration; and
- Provides feedback on the behaviour of group members.

C. A tutor plays an active and facilitating role with respect to students' self-directed learning. (Triangle point: process instruction)

To this end a tutor:

- Helps students to reflect about their knowledge acquisition during tutorial group sessions. By offering students feedback about the way they discuss subject matter, e.g., how they structure, relate, apply, and concretize subject matter, the tutor can make students aware of how they are learning in a collaborative setting;
- Pays attention to the way students study outside tutorial group sessions. Tutors may bring up topics like planning, preparation for tests, and reflection on strengths and weaknesses in relation to independent learning;

D. A tutor serves as an intermediary between the faculty and the students.

To this end a tutor:

- Assists students in consulting experts as learning resources;
- Attends tutor meetings during the unit to remain well informed about the intentions of the planning group, the problems and progress of fellow tutors, and last-minute changes to the unit; and
- Provides feedback to the members of the planning group regarding the quality of the unit book and the assignments.

Stimulating students' self-directedness

An important goal in PBL is to foster students' growth in self-directedness. Self-directed learning can be defined as students' ability to assume control of their own learning process. PBL is a learning environment that fosters self-regulation of learning activities by students. It is important for students to develop cognitive skills for independent learning in order to be able to cope with the huge amounts of information in today's world. Students must be able to continue to learn after they have completed their training. In other words, they should become life-long learners. Regulating one's own learning process requires three essential activities: planning, monitoring, and evaluation. Planning involves goal setting and determining strategies for goal attainment. Monitoring and evaluation involve judgement of how well and to what degree a plan is executed successfully and require conscious reflection on determining the extent to which learning has taken place and the ability to recognize errors. Self-assessment, peer feedback, and tutor feedback can support students' reflective ability. Tutors can help students to become self-directed learners. Their interventions to support self-directed learning are summarized by the concept of 'process instruction', i.e., instruction focused on students' learning processes (Figure 6.2). Knowledge about process instruction is part of a teacher's general pedagogical knowledge. Since self-directed learning plays such a prominent role in PBL, tutors should acquire specific skills in this area of pedagogical knowledge. An overview of the tasks of a tutor in relation to self-directed learning is presented in Box 6.1.

Acting as an intermediary between the faculty and students

Tutors act as intermediaries between students and staff. As tutors are in daily contact with students for several months, they are able to observe how students perform in the PBL curriculum. They have first-hand knowledge of aspects like the activities of a year group, whether the problems offered are adequately connected to students' prior knowledge, students' motivation, and students' sense of well being. Tutors can offer information and feedback to unit coordinators during regular meetings. An overview of the tasks of a tutor as an intermediary can be found in Box 6.1.

The tasks of a tutor are not simple. It is quite a demanding teaching role. Some teachers prefer to focus on the content and pedagogical content knowledge part of the spectrum of tutor activities, while others tend to concentrate on group dynamics or process instructional dimensions. All in all, many tutors have difficulty attending to all the areas of the tutor role simultaneously. That is why faculty development activities are very important to help staff members optimize the tutor role (Chapter 18). Introductory tutor courses have an important role to play in this respect.

The preparation of teachers for the role of tutor

Since the founding of the Maastricht Faculty of Medicine in 1974, staff members have engaged in activities to prepare for the tutor role. Initially, staff members observed each other while guiding a tutorial group and discussed their experiences and the advantages and disadvantages of interventions in plenary sessions. With the rapid increase in the number of staff members, however, it gradually became quite difficult to share beliefs, experiences, and behaviour in this rather informal way. After several years it was decided to set up two courses for new staff members: a course offering newcomers insight into the backgrounds and design of PBL at FHML and a course offering new staff members basic training in the tutor role. Both courses last two days and are mandatory for staff members who take on the tutor role.

Topics of the first course are the educational background of PBL, important principles of learning, the seven-step approach as a method for analysing, studying, and synthesizing information, experiences of students in a PBL environment, the design of the FHML curricula, student assessment, and some specific topics related to programmes within FHML (e.g. the skills laboratory). The course is designed to invite the participants to be active learners. The second course relates more directly to the role of the tutor. Participants take turns in playing the roles of the tutor, chairperson, note taker, and group member in a tutorial group and tackle the same problems offered to students in tutorial sessions. Some participants are invited to observe the tutorial group process. At the end of each exercise the participants evaluate the process and give feedback to each other. Specific attention is given to topics like the start of a new tutorial group, developing a code of conduct, handling difficult situations in tutorial groups (such as silent or dominant students, free rider behaviour, superficial problem analysis, etc.), and dealing with poorly written problems.

An overview of the content of the two introductory courses for tutors is given in Table 6.1.

What aids are available to a tutor?

Before the start of a unit, tutors receive a tutor guide containing background information about the outline of the unit book, the subjects of the unit, and some pedagogical content information. It will be obvious that tutors read parts of the tutor guide carefully before every group session, because the guide informs them about the content and pedagogical content knowledge related to

Table 6.1 An overview of the introduction courses for tutors at FHML

Day	Topics	Formats
1	Getting acquainted. Goals of the course, design of the course.	Plenary session
	What do you mean by learning? Some positive and negative personal learning experiences you had in the past.	Individual, triads, plenary
	The tutorial group. Analysis of a non-FHML problem. Introduction to the seven-step procedure and the roles of the tutor, chair, note-taker, and group member.	Exercise, plenary
	Some important learning principles underlying the PBL environment.	Interactive lecture
	A tutorial group by students and a tutor. Experiences of students and staff members in a PBL environment.	Demonstration, observation, plenary discussion
	The role of assessment in a PBL environment.	Interactive lecture
	Evaluation of Day 1.	Plenary session
2	Designing a PBL unit.	Plenary, subgroups, plenary
	Designing a PBL problem.	Plenary, subgroups, plenary
	Students work with your problem; feedback about the quality of your problem.	Plenary discussions
	The role of ICT in PBL.	Plenary, individual exercises
	Specific issues in relation to the FHML programmes, e.g., skillslab, progress test, practicals.	Plenary
	Evaluation of Day 2.	Plenary
3	The tutorial group. Analysis of a FHML problem. More in-depth understanding of the seven-step procedure and the roles of the tutor, chair, note-taker, and group member. Special attention for the task and maintenance level in groups.	Exercise, observation, feedback, discussion
	How to start a new tutorial group? Brainstorming in dyads. Presenting your approach to other group members.	Individually, subgroups, simulations, discussion
	The tutorial group. Analysis of a problem relating to how memory works and how people acquire, store, retrieve, and forget information. Participants must formulate learning objectives and study resources at home.	Plenary
	Reflection exercise: what are the main responsibilities and tasks of a tutor?	Individually, subgroups, plenary
	The tutorial group. Analysis of a poorly designed problem. What can/should a tutor do?	Plenary

Table 6.1 (*continued*) An overview of the introduction courses for tutors at FHML

Day	Topics	Formats
4	Synthesis (integration and application) of the information studied at home. Special attention to important cognitive learning activities like structuring, relating, applying, and concretizing information.	Plenary
	Evaluation of tutorial group sessions. Evaluation procedures and skills in giving and receiving interpersonal feedback	Interactive lecture
	What do you look forward to with some apprehension? Participants discuss situations in tutorial groups that can potentially raise tensions.	Individually, subgroups, plenary
	Difficult situations in tutorial groups.	Role plays, video presentations, giving and receiving feedback
	Being a tutor within other educational formats in a PBL environment.	Interactive lecture
	Your educational future as a teacher in FHML. What do we have to offer to improve your teacher skills?	Presentation of written materials
	Evaluation of Day 4. Evaluation of the whole course.	Plenary session Answering a questionnaire

the individual problems. In addition to the tutor guide, most planning groups inform tutors about the unit in a meeting before the start of the unit, in which members of the planning group describe their overall goals, potential problems students may have with the subject matter (e.g., misconceptions), and other previous experiences with the unit.

Most planning groups also organize weekly one-hour meetings with all tutors in which the chair of planning group and the tutors exchange experiences about what is going on in the various tutorial groups, discuss difficulties encountered by tutors in relation to unit content, group dynamics, and students' independent behaviour, and look ahead to the problems of the upcoming week. Tutors who attend these meetings get a good idea of what is going on in parallel groups, how colleagues solve problems with respect to learning and collaboration, and become more aware of potential learning difficulties in the sessions ahead. The tutors are also informed of last-minute changes in the course. Because they are in a position to closely observe students' learning and collaboration processes, tutors are in an excellent position to make suggestions to planning groups about how they could adapt their unit to enhance students' performance.

A brief look at outcomes of research on the tutor role

Because of the high importance placed on it, the role of the tutor in PBL has been researched extensively at FHML. Within the space available in this chapter it is not possible to expatiate upon this research (for elaborate discussions on this topic see the References).

Three major trends can be observed: studies on the differential influence of content expert and non-content expert tutors on student achievement; studies on process variables; and studies on the relationship between tutor characteristics and differential contextual circumstances. What follows are the main outcomes of these issues. First, it is concluded that no firm conclusions can be drawn about the question of whether tutorial groups should be guided by content expert tutors. Non-expert tutors and peer students seem to be equally capable of guiding students, because of their ability to show cognitively and socially congruent behaviour. Second, studies on process variables show that content expert tutors tend to make more use of their content expertise to direct group discussions, e.g., by explaining topics that students do not understand, whereas non-content expert tutors tend to make more use of their expertise in process facilitation to guide groups. Third, tutor performance is not a stable characteristic but is partly situation specific. Contextual circumstances like differences in students' prior knowledge levels, the quality of the problems, the level of structure in the PBL unit, and the functioning of the students in the group influence the performance of the tutor. A conclusion from the research is that tutors should know how to deal with subject matter expertise and how to facilitate learning processes (van Berkel & Dolmans, 2006; Dolmans et al., 2002; Schmidt & Moust, 1995, 2000).

A look into the future

In general major changes in the role of the tutor are not expected in the near future. It will remain the task of the tutor to facilitate students' learning of subject matter, stimulate collaborative group processes, and encourage students' self-directed learning. PBL curricula will continue to need tutors with expertise in these domains. What will change in the near future is the context in which students learn. Two changes are anticipated. First, there will be less face-to-face contacts between students and between students and the tutor. Students will be offered more ICT opportunities and work at home to clarify and solve problems, in either asynchronous or synchronous learning situations. Tutors will be confronted with new ICT facilities for use during tutorial group sessions and in between group meetings. A wider range of learning resources is becoming available on the Internet. These resources are increasingly available for free and no longer limited to text and pictures but include videos, virtual patients, and other interactive packages. A virtual learning environment facilitates the sharing of resources, notes, and other information. Interactive whiteboards and laptops will be used during group sessions and impact on communication and group dynamics. In either case students will be guided by a tutor who needs new ICT skills to foster dialogue and collaboration among students.

A second development, somewhat diametrical to the previous one, is the need for more team development in tutorial groups. Society needs team players who are able to work in (sometimes quickly changing) interdisciplinary and multidisciplinary self-directed teams. Currently, the FHML curricula offer students scant preparation to meet these societal demands. In the present curriculum, students work in the same group for eight or four weeks. Sometimes groups work together quite well but often tutorial groups are loose groups of individuals who work together more or less accidentally. The focus is on effective and efficient problem solving rather than on the development of high-performance learning teams that can work independently. This results in high costs for tutors, who are needed to guide student groups. Two measures seem to offer promise to help students to become professional team players. First, the level of accountability of individual group members and the group could be raised. Second, tutorial groups are temporary groups working together for four to eight weeks and this period is too short to achieve a high level of group cohesiveness. This might be remedied by extending the period during which groups work together, for example to a semester. With higher levels of accountability and cohesiveness students will gradually learn to become members of effective learning teams. More information about other ways to foster students' self-directed learning behaviour in a PBL context is provided in Chapter 14, in which the authors advocate for more variation in group formats in a PBL curriculum.

Annotated literature

Moust, J. H. C., Bouhuijs, P. A. J., and Schmidt, H.G. (2007). *Introduction to problem-based learning: a guide for students*. Groningen: Wolters-Noordhoff.

In this book tutors can find the basic principles of problem-based learning as well as procedures for analysing different types of problems offered in unit books. The book also gives extensive information about collaborative learning, the skills students must perform during tutorial sessions, and the skills of the chair of a tutorial group to support his peers in engaging in efficient and effective discussion. Observation lists, checklists, and questionnaires which will be very helpful for tutors in facilitating students' knowledge acquisition, collaboration, and self-directed learning are provided.

Dolmans, D.H. J. M., Gijselaers, W. H., Moust, J. H. C., de Grave, W. S., Wolfhagen, H. A. P., and van der Vleuten, C. P. M. (2002). Trends in research on the tutor in problem-based learning: conclusions and implications for educational practice and research. *Medical Teacher* **24**, 173–80.

This article gives a good overview of the major trends in the research on the tutor role during the past ten years.

Dolmans, D. H. J. M., and Schmidt, H. G. (2006). What do we know about cognitive and motivational effects of small group tutorials in problem-based learning? *Advances in Health Sciences Education* **11**, 312–26.

This article summarizes research concerning the cognitive and motivational components of the tutor role. The studies in this article demonstrate that activation of prior knowledge, recall of information, causal reasoning or theory building, and cognitive conflicts foster conceptual change in students. Other studies have shown that an elaborate group discussion positively influences students' intrinsic interest in subject matter. Several studies have provided suggestions for optimizing group work in PBL.

Schmidt, H. G., and Moust, J. H. C. (2000). Factors affecting small-group tutorial learning: A review of research. In: D. H. Evensen and C. E. Hmelo (eds) *Problem-based learning: a research perspective on learning interactions*. Mahwah, NJ: Lawrence Erlbaum. Pp. 19–53.

This chapter presents four different aspects of problem-based instruction: (1) the role of problems used to stimulate the learning of students; (2) the cognitive processes elicited by small-group discussion and their effects on achievement; (3) motivational influences; and (4) the influence of the tutor on students' learning. The chapter discusses a large number of studies carried out at Maastricht on tutors' expertise and on differences between staff and peer tutors as well as evidence supporting a particular model of tutor functioning in problem-based contexts.

References

Van Berkel, H. J. M., and Dolmans, D. H. J. M. (2006). The influence of tutoring competencies on problems, group functioning and student achievement in problem-based learning. *Medical Education* **40**, 730–6.

Dent, J. A., and Harden, R. M. (eds) (2006). *A practical guide for medical teachers*, 2nd edn. Edinburgh: Elsevier Churchill Livingstone.

Dolmans, D. H. J. M., Gijselaers, W. H., Moust, J. H. C., de Grave, W. S., Wolfhagen, H. A. P., and van der Vleuten, C. P. M. (2002). Trends in research on the tutor in problem-based learning: conclusions and implications for educational practice and research. *Medical Teacher* **24**, 173–80.

Irby, D. (1994). What clinical teachers in medicine need to know. *Academic Medicine* **69**, 334.

Kaufman, D. M., Mann, K., and Jennett, P. A. (2000). *Teaching and learning in medical education: how theory can inform practice*. Edinburgh: Association for the Study of Medical Education Monograph.

Merriam, S. B., and Caffarella, R. S. (1999). *Learning in adulthood: a comprehensive guide*, 2nd edn. San Francisco: Jossey-Bass.

Schmidt, H. G. (1983). Problem-based learning: Rationale and description. *Medical Education* **17**, 11–16.

Schmidt, H. G. (1993). Foundations of problem-based learning; Some explanatory notes. *Medical Education* **27**, 422–32.

Schmidt, H. G., and Moust, J. H. C. (1995). What makes a tutor effective? A structural-equations modelling approach to learning in problem-based curricula. *Academic Medicine* **70**, 708–14.

Schmidt, H. G., and Moust, J. H. C. (2000). Factors affecting small-group tutorial learning: A review of research. In: D. H. Evensen and C. E. Hmelo (eds) *Problem-based learning: a research perspective on learning interactions*. Mahwah, NJ: Lawrence Erlbaum. Pp. 19–53.

Chapter 7

Basic sciences in problem-based learning

Esther Bergman and Ton de Goeij

Clinical reasoning, an essential cognitive element in medicine, needs to be built upon conceptual and factual knowledge of the basic sciences (Norman, 2000). Although this is widely accepted, it is less clear how this fundament of basic sciences is integrated with clinical knowledge and skills, and (ultimately) leads to good diagnostic and therapeutic practice of physicians (Woods et al., 2005). In parallel, the role and position of the basic sciences in medical education are under debate (Norman, 2000). Since the introduction of problem-based learning (PBL) in medical education, this discussion has intensified and is leading to significant changes in curricula worldwide. It is to be expected that the role of basic science knowledge will be one of the focal issues in further transformation of medical curricula in the near future (Kaufman et al., 2008).

The position and function of basic sciences in medical curricula

What are basic sciences?

Basic sciences are generally defined as the scientific foundation of clinical reasoning and medical practice (Kaufman et al., 2008). A 'narrow' definition of basic sciences includes the disciplines anatomy, biochemistry, and physiology. In this chapter the 'broad' definition is used, including anatomy, biochemistry, physiology, and (at least) epidemiology, statistics, microbiology, pharmacology, molecular biology, cell biology, immunology, pathology, psychology, sociology, and ethics. However, others might assign these disciplines to alternative categories like clinical sciences, behavioural sciences, social sciences, or human sciences (McCrorie, 2000; Verhoeven et al., 2002).

Basic sciences in traditional medical curricula

In a 'traditional' curriculum, basic sciences have a clear position and function, which is described here somewhat simplistically. The first years usually focus on basic sciences while subsequent years deal exclusively with clinical education and skills training. Learning is viewed as a simple accumulation of knowledge. A firm foundation of basic science knowledge is considered an absolute requirement for clinical reasoning, and knowledge of normal structure and function is thought necessary to understand abnormal structure and function. This fundament of basic science knowledge is concentrated in a 'preclinical phase', usually lasting four years. Every basic science is presented in an isolated course, which is strictly department based and there is little or no integration across disciplines. Courses consist mainly of lectures and teacher-centred instruction in laboratories. Assessment of student knowledge is predominantly based on written or oral tests. There is little deliberate instruction in the application of basic sciences to clinical problems and limited student–patient interaction (Dahle et al., 2002; Drake, 1998; Swanson & Case, 1997). Basic clinical skills, like taking a patient history, communicating with patients, and performing a structured physical examination, are taught in the 'clinical phase', at the beginning of clerkships, or not at all. The traditional curriculum exists 'primarily for its efficiency, not necessarily for its effectiveness' (Way et al., 2000, p. s118).

A changing role of basic sciences in medical education

Medical knowledge has expanded dramatically over recent decades, with an exponential growth in nearly all basic sciences. Since the early 1980s, it has been recognized that the amount of basic science information with potential relevance to medical practice is far too large for instructors to teach and for students to learn. In other words, attempts to include everything in the under-graduate curriculum have become a mission impossible (Swanson & Case, 1997). Furthermore, significant parts of what students learn today will be outdated soon: 'We can be certain that the doctors of tomorrow will be applying knowledge and deploying skills which are at present unforeseen' (General Medical Council, 1993; quoted in Monkhouse & Farrell, 1999, p. 131). Therefore, the development of more generic competencies, such as interpersonal skills and skills for lifelong learning, is receiving increasing attention in medical education. Nevertheless, basic science education is probably not less but even more important: 'future developments in medical practice [such as diagnostic technology or surgical approaches] will best be dealt with by those who have a sound knowledge of the structure and function of the human body' (Monkhouse & Farrell, 1999, pp. 131–2). Currently the focus is changing from rote learning and memorization of factual details for later recall at examinations to understanding key concepts and principles of medical problem solving (Drake, 1998; Swanson et al., 1996). In coherence with these changes, the variety of assessment tools for (basic science) knowledge has expanded (e.g., portfolio, progress test and OSCE).

Research on the psychology of learning has revealed findings relevant to the retention and application of basic science knowledge. Active learning, elaboration, and discussion build and strengthen connections between and within students' knowledge networks (Regehr & Norman, 1996). Therefore, many medical curricula have incorporated student-centred education focused on active, self-directed learning either individually or in groups (Dolmans et al., 2005). In addi-tion, knowledge retrieval is facilitated when knowledge is acquired in situations resembling the situation of its practical application (Smith & Vela, 2001). The transfer of knowledge from educational settings to clinical practice can be improved by matching the contexts. In a PBL setting, basic science learning is thus based on authentic patient problem scenarios or contacts with patients early in the curriculum, wherever possible (Dornan et al., 2006).

Furthermore, students and teachers became increasingly dissatisfied with the basic sciences being taught unrelated to each other and to the students' future practice. Together with several research findings, this has resulted in fundamental changes in medical curricula (Custers & Ten Cate, 2002; Drake, 1998). In 'innovative' curricula, basic sciences are taught simultaneously and in an interrelated manner—the so-called *horizontal integration*. Furthermore, clinical sciences are frequently introduced in the early years of the curriculum, integrated with basic sciences, the so-called *vertical integration* (Dahle et al., 2002). Consequently, traditional curricula can be represented by an *H-shape* and innovative curricula by a *Z-shape* (Figure 7.1).

Basic sciences in a PBL curriculum

In PBL horizontal and vertical integration are very important, since this is necessary to make full use of the advantages of PBL (Brynhildsen et al., 2002). PBL curricula should facilitate many aspects of learning: integration of knowledge, transfer of concepts to new problems, application of basic science concepts to clinical problems, intrinsic interest in the subject matter, the develop-ment of skills in problem solving, learning to learn, self-directed learning, and an interest in

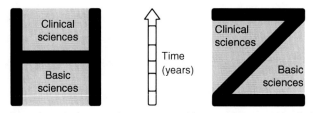

Figure 7.1 The traditional curriculum can be represented by an H-shape, with all clinical sciences later in the curriculum. The innovative curricula can be represented by a Z-shape, where students are introduced to clinical sciences at the beginning of the curriculum.

lifelong learning (Dahle et al., 2002; Norman & Schmidt, 1992). Whereas in traditional curricula students may have the impression that they are studying basic sciences because they must, PBL should stimulate them to learn basic sciences in order to understand clinical problems. Research suggests that if students recognize the relevance of basic sciences, their learning is enhanced (McCrorie, 2000; O'Neill, 2000; Prince et al., 2003). In addition, integrated teaching of basic and clinical sciences should facilitate the notoriously difficult transition from the preclinical phase to clerkships (Prince et al., 2000).

Issues concerning basic sciences in a PBL curriculum

In the literature on basic sciences in PBL curricula, the focus is mainly on perceptions and attitudes of students, teachers, and clinicians as well as on the level, retention, and growth of the knowledge of students. Studies by, for example, Kaufmann and Mann (1997), Way et al. (2000), Custers and Ten Cate (2002), Prince et al. (2000), and Brynhildsen et al. (2002) support the theory that horizontal and vertical integration contributes to a more positive attitude of students towards basic sciences and increases students' awareness of their relevance to clinical practice. On the other hand, innovative curricula seem to have a negative effect on the importance of basic sciences as perceived by the students. In other words: '[The] potential disadvantage [of PBL] is that students may become more interested in the clinical aspects of a problem and neglect the underlying basic science knowledge' (O'Neill, 2000, p. 608). Students have reported a tendency to skip the initial exploration of probable causes and underlying mechanisms of patient problems and not to bother formulating appropriate learning objectives related to basic sciences. Instead, they confined themselves to looking up a diagnosis and its associated symptoms and treatments (Prince et al., 2000).

Last but not least, it is claimed that the perceived and actual basic science knowledge of PBL students is reduced. Interestingly, studies assessing the level, retention, and growth of basic science knowledge of PBL versus non-PBL students have yielded conflicting and inconclusive evidence (for example, Albanese & Mitchell, 1993; Prince et al., 2003; Swanson et al., 1996; Verhoeven et al., 2002; Vernon & Blake, 1993) (see Chapter 24).

A historical perspective on basic sciences in the Maastricht PBL curricula

First experiences with basic sciences in PBL: curriculum 1974–1987

In 1972, before the establishment of the medical school in Maastricht, the so-called 'Basic Philosophy' was published, stating the position and aims of the new university as well as guidelines for the development of medical education, research, and patient care. The main objective

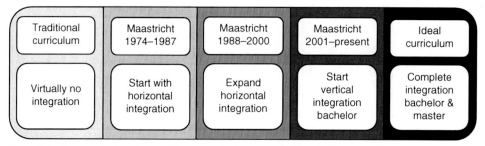

Figure 7.2 Characteristics of a traditional curriculum, an ideal curriculum and the past and present Maastricht curricula.

was to design a curriculum based on the healthcare desired by *society* and the role of the physician therein. To avoid traditional thinking and to promote a flexible attitude it was advised not to divide the curriculum into disciplines, but to arrange it into themes and put it into context (Table 7.1). Furthermore, it was strongly suggested that subject matter be uncoupled from a single discipline when appointing teaching staff, in order to promote integration. For example, elementary anatomy could be taught by a surgeon, a pathologist, or an anatomist, and learning physiology could be supported by an internist, pharmacologist, or physiologist.

The first curriculum started in 1974 (see Figure 7.2) with a new approach to medical education: learning in small groups based on patient problem scenarios, so-called 'tutorial sessions'. The focus was not on teaching but on the learning of students. The first two years dealt mainly with normal and abnormal human functioning. The first year was divided into thematic units, such as 'Traumata', 'Atherosclerosis', and 'Tumours', and the units in the second year were dedicated to the life cycle. The third and fourth year concentrated on the most prevalent clinical problems in thematic units like 'Fatigue', 'Shortness of breath', and 'Blood loss'. Here, basic sciences, such as anatomy, physiology, and biochemistry, had a minor role, whereas disciplines like epidemiology, pathology, and pharmacology were delivered mainly in this part of the curriculum.

Table 7.1 Organizing basic science content around themes and patient problems: an example of anatomy

Traditional	PBL		
Teaching according to organ systems	Theme	Patient problem scenario	Teaching according to patient problem scenario in theme
Digestive tract	Chronic disease	Boy with diabetes	Glands of digestive tract
Nervous system	Disturbed consciousness	Girl with epilepsy	Brain
Musculoskeletal system	Trauma	Woman with sprained ankle	Ankle and foot region (Skeleton, muscles, ligaments, nerves, blood vessels etc.)
	Life cycle	Man with osteoarthritis in hip	Hip region (Skeleton, muscles, ligaments, nerves, blood vessels, etc.)
Heart and circulation	Trauma	Man with heart attack	Heart and coronary arteries
Respiratory tract	Shortness of breath	Girl with asthma	Trachea and lungs
Urogenital tract	Life cycle	Woman trying to get pregnant	Female genital tract

Learning goals for the basic sciences formulated in the tutorial sessions served to explain the patient problems. In conclusion, the basic sciences were delivered in a medical context as much as possible, but horizontal and vertical integration was limited. Lectures were scarce in the first four years. Besides tutorial sessions, the main learning format with relevance to basic sciences was laboratory sessions, although computerized simulation programmes and direct consultations of basic scientists by tutorial groups occurred occasionally.

The knowledge of the students was assessed by formative end-of-unit tests, containing a large proportion of questions on basic sciences, particularly in the first two years. In 1976, an additional tool was developed for summative and formative purposes: the progress test (see Chapter 22). With roughly one-third of the approximately 250 questions in each test pertaining to the basic sciences, the progress test is a valuable tool for monitoring the acquired level of basic science knowledge.

Since 1974, the Maastricht medical faculty has emphasized the importance of quality assurance in education. Almost every activity in the curriculum is systematically evaluated by the students and by the medical faculty (Chapter 17). This has provided an understanding of the role of the basic sciences in a PBL curriculum and their impact on the learning of medical students. In fact this understanding played an important role in setting the stage for a series of curriculum reforms. Between 1983 and 1985 the Education Committee identified several major problems in the curriculum: too complicated problem scenarios in the first year, gaps and duplications in (basic science) topics, low student ratings for some units, the content and structure of the second year not meeting the requirements, and a significant overload in the fourth year. This led the Education Committee to propose 'The Read Thread', a concept of a new curriculum, in 1985. In 1986, students stirred up the faculty by presenting 'The Blue Spiral': a plan proposing the idea of a spiral in the curriculum, with an increasing level of complexity and integration of basic and clinical disciplines, regular revisiting of topics, and a logical, structured line in the first four years. Now it was felt that minor changes would not be sufficient to meet the demands of the next decade. In 1987 the medical faculty decided to design and implement a new curriculum.

More integration of basic sciences: curriculum 1988–2000

Proposals of the Education Committee and the students were combined in a programme on the theme 'human functioning' in the first two years and 'disturbed human functioning' in the third and fourth year. Psychosocial disciplines, such as psychology, sociology, and psychiatry, were no longer set apart but integrated with the biomedical sciences. The life cycle and its fundamental topics were reduced to three units at the end of the second year. All unit themes in the first two years focused on basic sciences in a medical context. Again, the themes in the next two years dealt with the major medical complaints. However, in contrast to the previous curriculum, the basic sciences were better distributed over the whole range of the first four years. As a result, the integration of basic and clinical sciences was significantly increased, but only in the first four, preclinical years. The clerkships in the fifth and sixth year remained unchanged. In other words, horizontal integration was improved, but vertical integration lagged behind.

Problems arose with respect to the assessment of basic sciences because the unit tests, which had been formative, were changed into strongly summative assessments. This caused student learning behaviour to become more test directed and less PBL orientated.

The current status in Maastricht: curriculum 2001–present

Reform of the complete medical programme, comprising all six years and aiming at full integration of basic and clinical sciences, was the logical next step. This approach has resulted in a Z-shaped curriculum (Figure 7.1), with an emphasis on theory and learning of fundamental aspects and basic sciences at the beginning, as well as a gradual shift of focus towards practice, application of knowledge, and clinical performance at the end.

The curriculum is now divided into a bachelor phase (years 1–3) and a master phase (years 4–6) (Figure 7.3). The first two years did not change profoundly as compared to the previous curriculum. Some extra lectures were introduced as they had proved to be indispensable for the explanation of difficult or key concepts, and the laboratory sessions became increasingly student centred as a result of the implementation of activating work forms. Major alterations with respect to the position and role of the basic sciences were made in the third and the sixth year.

The third year is divided into four clusters. Within these clusters, students learn fundamental aspects of disease in weekly small-group sessions coached by staff members, either clinicians or basic scientists. Patient contacts supervised by clinicians provide the problems tackled in these sessions. The basic science content of the first two years is repeated and expanded during the clusters.

After two years of clerkships combined with theoretical education at the medical school, students in the sixth year participate in patient care as well as in a research project for a more extensive period. The participation in research is made feasible by theoretical and practical training in the preceding years.

With respect to the assessment of basic sciences no major changes were made compared to the preceding curriculum. However, complaints are rising that the unit tests are not integrated and it seems to be increasingly difficult to construct relevant and novel test questions.

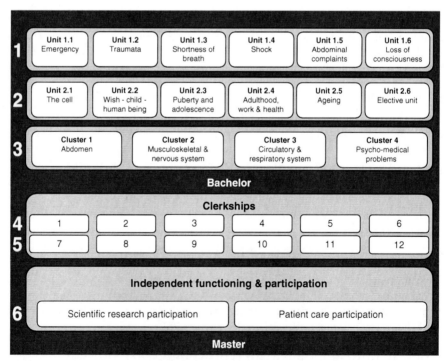

Figure 7.3 Maastricht University curriculum 2001–present. The first and second years are each divided into six thematic units, the third year is divided into four clusters. The fourth and fifth year are devoted to twelve different clerkships. Half of the sixth year is dedicated to participation in a research project; the other half is dedicated to patient care (extensive clerkship).

Lessons learned

Obviously, the role of basic sciences in medical education, encompassing the spectrum of disciplines building the fundament for good clinical practice, is changing dramatically. The explosion in biomedical knowledge means that choices must be made based on the impact of these developments on healthcare and cure. Parallel with this process, there are shifts in educational concepts, such as from monodisciplinary teaching to integrated learning, and from a focus on facts and details to the understanding of general principles, mechanisms, and concepts. Research on the psychology of learning, educational innovations, and quality assurance procedures, especially systematic programme evaluation by teachers *and* students, have been crucial in these developments.

Since the integration of basic sciences in PBL curricula is pivotal for the successful education of physicians and their later clinical practice, the collaboration between basic scientists and clinicians is a primary requirement. It has also become clear that comprehensive horizontal and vertical integration is very hard to achieve and may not even be strictly necessary. Crucial, however, is an interdisciplinary design of the curriculum (with respect to theory as well as practice) in which important topics are delivered in context and repeated with increasing complexity. In this respect coherence in curriculum structure and function can only be obtained by central governance of the programme and good collaboration between programme coordinators, clinicians, scientists, teachers, students, and patients, supported by organizational and financial staff.

An interesting finding is that the level, growth, and retention of basic science knowledge are limited when this knowledge is not applied by students. For example, when basic science issues are neglected in the discussion of patient problem scenarios during tutorial sessions, full understanding of the problems will not be achieved. This can result in low scores on student assessments. Therefore, student assessment should ideally be focused on evaluating basic science knowledge and its application in a medical context, using a variety of assessment formats, as often as possible, and integrated with learning wherever possible.

Future developments

Based on the lessons learned during 35 years of experience and research at the Maastricht Faculty of Medicine, several trends likely to have an impact on PBL worldwide can be identified.

Quality assurance is and will remain a significant issue. However, a more profound and detailed insight into the evaluation of educational programmes by students as well as teachers may lead to significant improvements. Consequently, the emphasis in gathering student and teacher feedback and opinions should (partly) shift from quantitative to qualitative data.

With respect to the early years of the curriculum, additional stimuli to apply basic science knowledge in solving patient problem scenarios in tutorial groups is likely to give students a better understanding of normal and abnormal human functioning. Later in the curriculum, possibilities for expanding the vertical integration of basic sciences by interdisciplinary collaboration between basic scientists and clinicians should be explored further and may well yield important progress. Coherent cooperation between management, researchers, and teachers as well as integration of theory and practice are prerequisite for success.

Furthermore, improvements in formative and summative assessment of medical competencies (e.g., by using electronic portfolios), integrated within educational programmes, is expected to increase the efficiency and effectiveness of the education of health professionals.

A crucial, but unfortunately poorly developed, area in most medical schools is human resource management and the rewarding of teaching accomplishments. For academic staff, there is a strong emphasis on research targets, whereas teaching in both basic and clinical sciences has low priority as it is less valued as an academic activity than research (Older, 2004). Selection for rewards (promotions, space, endowed chairs, etc.) is almost exclusively based on the number of publications and grant funding, and not on teaching and clinical competence (Cahill & Leonard, 1999; Fasel et al., 2005). Rewarding good teaching practice should be drastically changed and actively pursued. Why? Future developments and improvements can only be accomplished by rewarding excellent and enthusiastic teachers and educationalists willing to work hard to improve the quality of education in their institution.

Annoted literature

Prince, K. J., van Mameren, H., Hylkema, N., Drukker, J., Scherpbier, A. J., van der Vleuten, C. P. (2003). Does problem based learning lead to deficiencies in basic science knowledge? An empirical case on anatomy. *Medical Education* **37**(1), 15–21.

This study aimed to identify differences between PBL and non-PBL students in perceived and actual levels of knowledge of anatomy. Year 4 students of all eight medical schools in the Netherlands completed a questionnaire and took part in an anatomy test. Although no significant differences were found, interesting trends on the effects of teaching in context and repetition within the curriculum are identified.

Swanson, D. B., and Case, S. M. (1997). Assessment for basic science instruction: Directions for practice and research. *Advances in Health Science Education* **2**, 71–84.

In this essay, assessment of students' understanding of the basic sciences is discussed from the perspective that assessment should follow from, and be congruent with, course and curricular goals. A special section is devoted to assessment issues that arise in the context of PBL and discusses the merits and use of novel as well as traditional assessment approaches.

Woods, N. N., Brooks, L. R., and Norman, G. R. (2005). The value of basic science in clinical diagnosis, creating coherence among signs and symptoms. *Medical Education* **39**(1), 107–12.

This study is based on the theory that basic science may be useful for creating a coherent mental representation of diagnostic categories and their signs and symptoms, by providing a framework of meaning and hence aid retention and recall. The interesting results are discussed in light of other theories, like learning probability matrices and prototypes, and research results.

References

Albanese, M. A., and Mitchell, S. (1993). Problem-based learning: a review of literature on its outcomes and implementation issues. *Academic Medicine* **68**(1), 52–81.

Brynhildsen, J., Dahle, L. O., Behrbohm Fallsberg, M., Rundquist, I., and Hammar, M. (2002). Attitudes among students and teachers on vertical integration between clinical medicine and basic science within a problem-based undergraduate medical curriculum. *Medical Teacher* **24**(3), 286–8.

Cahill, D. R., and Leonard, R. J. (1999). Missteps and masquerade in American medical academe: clinical anatomists call for action. *Clinical Anatomy* **12**(3), 220–22.

Custers, E. J., and Ten Cate, O. T. (2002). Medical students' attitudes towards and perception of the basic sciences: a comparison between students in the old and the new curriculum at the University Medical Center Utrecht, The Netherlands. *Medical Education* **36**(12), 1142–50.

Dahle, L. O., Brynhildsen, J., Behrbohm Fallsberg, M., Rundquist, I., and Hammar, M. (2002). Pros and cons of vertical integration between clinical medicine and basic science within a problem-based undergraduate medical curriculum: examples and experiences from Linkoping, Sweden. *Medical Teacher* **24**(3), 280–5.

Dolmans, D. H., de Grave, W., Wolfhagen, I. H., and van der Vleuten, C. P. (2005). Problem-based learning: future challenges for educational practice and research. *Medical Education* **39**(7), 732–41.

Dornan, T., Littlewood, S., Margolis, S. A., Scherpbier, A., Spencer, J., and Ypinazar, V. (2006). How can experience in clinical and community settings contribute to early medical education? A BEME systematic review. *Medical Teacher* **28(1)**, 3–18.

Drake, R. L. (1998). Anatomy education in a changing medical curriculum. *Anatomical Record* **253(1)**, 28–31.

Fasel, J. H., Morel, P., and Gailloud, P. (2005). A survival strategy for anatomy. *Lancet* **365(9461)**, 754.

Kaufman, D. M., and Mann, K. V. (1997). Basic sciences in problem-based learning and conventional curricula: students' attitudes. *Medical Education* **31(3)**, 177–80.

Kaufman, D. R., Yoskowitz, N. A., and Patel, V. L. (2008). Clinical reasoning and biomedical knowledge: implications for teaching. In: J. Higgs, M. A. Jones, S. Loftus, and N. Christensen (eds), *Clinical reasoning in the health professions*, 3rd edn. Edinburgh: Elsevier, pp. 137–49.

McCrorie, P. (2000). The place of the basic sciences in medical curricula. *Medical Education* **34(8)**, 594–5.

Monkhouse, W. S., and Farrell, T. B. (1999). Tomorrow's doctors: today's mistakes? *Clinical Anatomy* **12(2)**, 131–4.

Norman, G. (2000). The essential role of basic science in medical education: the perspective from psychology. *Clinical and Investigative Medicine* **23(1)**, 47–51.

Norman, G. R., & Schmidt, H. G. (1992). The psychological basis of problem-based learning: a review of the evidence. *Academic Medicine* **67(9)**, 557–65.

O'Neill, P. A. (2000). The role of basic sciences in a problem-based learning clinical curriculum. *Medical Education* **34(8)**, 608–13.

Older, J. (2004). Anatomy: a must for teaching the next generation. *Surgeon* **2(2)**, 79–90.

Prince, K. J., van de Wiel, M., Scherpbier, A. J., van der Vleuten, C. P., and Boshuizen, H. P. (2000). A qualitative analysis of the transition from theory to practice in undergraduate training in a PBL-medical school. *Advances in Health Sciences Education: Theory and Practice* **5(2)**, 105–16.

Prince, K. J., van Mameren, H., Hylkema, N., Drukker, J., Scherpbier, A. J., and van der Vleuten, C. P. (2003). Does problem-based learning lead to deficiencies in basic science knowledge? An empirical case on anatomy. *Medical Education* **37(1)**, 15–21.

Regehr, G., and Norman, G. R. (1996). Issues in cognitive psychology: implications for professional education. *Academic Medicine* **71(9)**, 988–1001.

Smith, S. M., and Vela, E. (2001). Environmental context-dependent memory: a review and meta-analysis. *Psychonomic Bulletin and Review* **8(2)**, 203–20.

Swanson, D. B., and Case, S. M. (1997). Assessment in Basic Science Instruction: Directions for Practice and Research. *Advances in Health Sciences Education* **2**, 71–84.

Swanson, D. B., Case, S. M., Luecht, R. M., & Dillon, G. F. (1996). Retention of basic science information by fourth-year medical students. *Academic Medicine* **71(10 Suppl)**, S80–2.

Verhoeven, B. H., Verwijnen, G. M., Scherpbier, A. J. J. A., and van der Vleuten, C. P. M. (2002). Growth of medical knowledge. *Medical Education* **36(8)**, 711–17.

Vernon, D. T., and Blake, R. L. (1993). Does problem-based learning work? A meta-analysis of evaluative research. *Academic Medicine* **68(7)**, 550–63.

Way, D. P., Hudson, A., and Biagi, B. (2000). Comparison of three parallel, basic science pathways in the same medical college. *Academic Medicine* **75(10 Suppl)**, S118–20.

Woods, N. N., Brooks, L. R., and Norman, G. R. (2005). The value of basic science in clinical diagnosis: creating coherence among signs and symptoms. *Medical Education* **39(1)**, 107–12.

Chapter 8

The introduction of real (ambulatory) patients early in the curriculum

Agnes Diemers, Erik Heineman, and Diana Dolmans

Since the establishment of Maastricht University, PBL has been used as the educational approach of the Faculty of Health, Medicine and Life Sciences (FHML). Initially, students used only paper patient problems as the starting point for learning in the four preclinical years of the six-year curriculum. Although PBL is supposed to 'promote the transfer of knowledge concepts to new problems and the integration of basic science concepts into clinical problems' (Norman & Schmidt, 1992, p. 557), students reported difficulties in transitioning from the theoretical preclinical years to the mainly workplace-based, clerkship years(Prince et al., 2000, 2005), as they had no idea how to apply the knowledge they had acquired when confronted with real patients. As a result, real patient contacts during the preclinical phase were considered to resolve this so-called shock of practice (Prince et al., 2000, 2005).

Theoretical considerations

The literature reports several advantages of early real patient contacts. First of all, patient contacts are expected to ease the transition from the preclinical to the clinical phase (Prince et al., 2000; Seabrook, 2004). They are also assumed to motivate students to learn (Prince et al., 2000); make students feel more comfortable performing physical examinations (O'Brien-Gonzales et al., 2001); and increase students' awareness of the impact of disease on patients' lives (Cooper et al., 2001). Furthermore, real patient encounters are assumed to stimulate the process of professional socialization (Dornan et al., 2006; O'Brien-Gonzales et al., 2001). Finally, there is the presumed beneficial effect on student learning, because patient contacts are considered to enhance the acquisition and retention of knowledge (Prince et al., 2000; Seabrook, 2004). So patient contacts can promote meaningful and deep learning (Dornan & Bundy, 2004; Littlewood et al., 2005; Norman & Schmidt, 1992; Parsell & Bligh, 2001; Prince et al., 2000) as well as internalization of newly acquired knowledge (Prince et al., 2000).

The implementation and integration of patient contacts is not easy though, and success cannot be taken for granted. The main reported problems in the literature are matching patient problems to course themes and potential difficulties in selecting sufficient numbers of patients to ensure coverage of the core curriculum (Mainhard et al., 2004; O'Neill et al., 2000). Another problem is that students can have difficulty identifying meaningful links between theory and practice and across problems (Eva, 2005; van de Wiel et al., 1999) and as a result tend to jump straight to diagnosing without first trying to understand underlying pathophysiological mechanisms. Students should therefore be explicitly instructed to look for connections between patient problems and basic science knowledge and make comparisons across patient problems, strategies that have been reported to stimulate transfer of knowledge (Eva, 2005; van de Wiel et al., 1999).

From literature about expertise development it is known that expert physicians rarely use basic science knowledge during routine practice (Patel et al., 1989), but do turn to basic science knowledge when faced with complex patient problems (Joseph & Patel, 1990; Norman et al., 1994). Woods (2007) found additional beneficial effects of the use of biomedical knowledge by students. Making explanatory connections not only enhances students' recall and application of clinical knowledge, their diagnoses become more accurate as well, particularly after a time delay and under time constraints (Woods, 2007). This implies that medical education should be structured to explain and make students aware of the relationships between biomedical and clinical knowledge (Woods, 2007). These insights have prompted the recommendation to introduce clinical experience at an early stage of medical education. One way to do so is early patient contacts.

In order to realize the combined educational potential of early patient encounters and PBL, FHML developed a new curriculum in 2001 in which real patient encounters are offered in the third year. The next section of this chapter describes how PBL with real patients is organized at FHML.

Description

The 'old' Maastricht PBL Curriculum was H-shaped with a clear divide between the first (pre-clinical) four, primarily theory-based years and the final two clinical, mainly practice-based years. In the 'new' Maastricht curriculum, implemented in 2001, the amount of practice-based activities gradually increases from year 1 to 6, while simultaneously the amount of theory-based activities gradually decreases, a so-called Z-shaped curriculum. The first two years of this new curriculum consist of thematic units of about six to ten weeks, in which students in small tutorial groups are given paper patient problems as the starting point for learning. The tutorial groups are supported by lectures, practicals, and a longitudinal skills training programme. In the skills laboratory, students practise skills (including communication skills) with models, manikins, each other, and simulated patients. In year 3, the paper patient problems are replaced by real patient encounters, as will be described below. Years 4 and 5 are devoted to mostly hospital-based clerkship rotations in different disciplines. During year 6 students participate in scientific research for a period of eighteen weeks and, for another eighteen-week period, they participate in patient care as junior doctors on a ward of their choice, supervised by a member of the clinical staff. The following paragraph describes year 3 of the new Maastricht curriculum more extensively.

The theme of the new year 3, Chronic Diseases, is divided into four subject clusters: abdominal region, locomotor system, circulation and lungs, and psychomedical problems and mental healthcare. Every week students see a patient in the teaching outpatient clinic at Maastricht University Hospital and these encounters are the starting point for learning in the PBL cycle, which comprises a weekly four-hour session of a tutorial group of ten students and their coach.

The PBL cycle in years 1 and 2 consists of three phases: preparation, self-study, and reporting. During the preparation phase students discuss a paper patient problem, activating prior knowledge and identifying gaps in the relevant knowledge they possess in relation to the problem. Out of those knowledge gaps learning issues are generated. In the days following the preparation phase students undertake self-study activities to gain insight into the learning issues, which they report during the next session. The procedure is similar in year 3 of the new curriculum but obviously also different due to the replacement of paper problems by real patients. The first phase of the PBL cycle is now divided into two phases: the 'preparation phase' in which students prepare for the upcoming patient encounter and activate prior knowledge, and the 'patient encounter phase' in which students, in pairs, see a *real* patient instead of a *paper* patient.

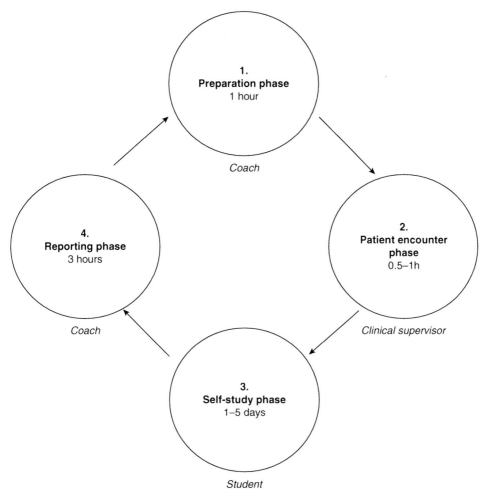

Figure 8.1 PBL cycle with four phases.

From this encounter students derive learning issues for self study. Thus four consecutive phases can be discerned (Figure 8.1): The *preparation phase* takes up the last hour of the tutorial group session; the *patient encounter phase* is scheduled one or two days thereafter; the *self-study phase* covers the time between the patient encounter and the group session in the next week; and the *reporting phase* takes up the first three hours of the session. So, one PBL cycle spans a period of a week, from the last hour of the group session to the last hour of the session in the next week. Apart from the PBL cycle, which is the prevailing educational format in year 3, students attend lectures, skills training, and other educational activities. The content of the four phases will now be discussed in somewhat more detail.

Preparation phase

The students are given a vignette (Box 8.1) describing the problem (or a similar problem) of the patient they will see in the outpatient clinic. The patient problems are elaborated on by the group in order to activate the knowledge they have gained during the preceding two years of the curriculum. During elaboration, attention is also paid to history taking and physical examination.

Box 8.1 Example of a vignette

Example of a vignette used in the abdominal cluster describing a patient problem at the urology outpatient clinic.

A 63-year-old woman presents at the urology outpatient clinic with frequency, nocturia, and urgency. She has had these complaints for two years and by now she knows every public convenience in town.

Additionally, gaps in knowledge identified by the students are converted to learning issues to be studied in preparation for the patient encounter.

By elaborating on the problems of the patient, prior knowledge structures are activated to help students to relate new information to their existing knowledge, which facilitates activation and recall of knowledge. It is the task of the coach to see to it that the elaboration and activation of prior knowledge is of sufficient depth.

Patient encounter phase

One or two days after the preparation phase, student pairs go to the outpatient clinic where they meet a patient and do a history and a physical examination as indicated. The patient's attending physician, who acts as the students' clinical supervisor, observes the students. After about thirty minutes, having completed history and physical, the students consult their clinical supervisor and together they complete the consultation. After the patient has left, the students and the clinical supervisor discuss the patient contact and generate learning issues that will be the driving force for the students' subsequent self-study activities. The role of the clinical supervisor is to observe and give feedback to the students on the consultation, and guide them in defining learning issues.

If a patient (unexpectedly) does not show up at the teaching outpatient clinic, students visit patients on the wards of Maastricht University Hospital or paper patients are used instead.

Self-study phase

During the self-study phase, the students work on the learning issues derived from the patient encounter, using a variety of learning resources, such as books, skills training, and lectures. The student pairs prepare a clinical presentation about 'their patient' for the reporting phase.

Reporting phase

The students report the results of their self-study to the tutorial group in a form resembling that of the clinical presentations commonly held in the hospital, starting with a report of the patient's history and physical examination and ending with a differential diagnosis and a management plan. After the presentations, the students discuss and synthesize what they have learned. The aim of this reporting phase is to promote the integration of theory and practice and to stimulate students to discuss clinical knowledge as well as the underlying biomedical mechanisms. In-depth discussion of the patient problems, in which students elaborate on their new understanding and insights, is of vital importance as it is assumed to facilitate understanding, encoding, and later retrieval of their new knowledge (Schmidt, 1993). The coach guides the students in this phase of learning. He must ensure that elaborate deep discussion takes place in which information is synthesized and a coherent picture is formed in which theory and practice are appropriately linked.

The coach and the clinical supervisor are both clinical staff members of the disciplines involved in the year 3 programme. Prior to performing these teaching roles, both attend a two-hour training in which it is explained to them how to guide the sessions as a coach and as a clinical supervisor.

Logistics

Because it is logistically impossible for the whole year group of 320 students—the current size of student cohorts at FHML—to simultaneously take part in patient consultations in the outpatient clinic, the group is split into four subgroups (eighty students each). The students of the subgroups are allocated to tutorial groups of about ten students each. The subgroups rotate in different order through the four ten-week thematic clusters and the tutorial groups rotate in different order through the outpatient clinics belonging to the thematic cluster.

In the course of a cluster, students visit six different outpatient clinics and see patients at a general practice twice per cluster, i.e., eight times a year. The students are assigned to the same general practice for the duration of the whole year. For the cluster abdomen, for example, the participating outpatient clinics are general surgery, gastroenterology, obstetrics and gynaecology, paediatrics, urology, radiotherapy, and two general practice visits. The last week of each cluster is dedicated to the final reporting phase and assessment. The fact that students see patients in pairs means that five patients must be selected per tutorial group and scheduled to visit the outpatient clinic consecutively. Student pair A meets patient A, thereafter student pair B meets patient B, and so on.

Each cluster has a coordinator, a staff member of one of the participating disciplines, who is supported by a cluster group consisting of staff members from the disciplines. The cluster group is responsible for the organization in their outpatient clinics and selects the clinical supervisors and coaches out of their staff members. The coach stays with the tutorial group during the ten weeks of the cluster. The clinical supervisor is the attending physician of the patient the students see in the teaching outpatient clinic. It is the task of the clinical supervisor to select patients, most of whom are visiting the University Hospital for a regularly scheduled appointment.

Discussion

Programme evaluation data reveal that students are highly satisfied with the real patient encounters as the starting point for learning in PBL (Diemers et al., 2007). Students say their learning benefits from these contacts. The patient encounters are discussed adequately during the reporting phase according to the students and they think integration of theory and practice is actually promoted by this experience (Diemers et al., 2007). Results from focus group studies have revealed that students feel motivated by the real patient contacts and think they help them to understand the impact of illness on patients' lives, enhance their professional socialization process, and lead to improved acquisition and retention of knowledge (Diemers et al., 2008). These findings are all in concordance with the described beneficial effects reported in the literature as cited at the beginning of this chapter.

The students also indicate that they develop both analytical and non-analytical reasoning strategies (Diemers et al., 2008). Encouragingly, the students' perceptions that they use both kinds of clinical reasoning, analytical as well as non-analytical, are supported by observations of tutorial group sessions. These observations additionally showed that the tutorial groups did discuss both basic science knowledge and clinical knowledge (Diemers et al., in preparation). These evaluative and observational findings support the conclusion that using real patients as the driving force for learning early in a PBL medical curriculum can contribute towards a more gradual transition from the preclinical years to the clinical years. Research of the effects of real preclinical patient contacts on this transition phase is in progress.

The results of our studies of the early clinical experience at FHML also pinpointed areas where improvement is needed. First of all, students are less satisfied with the preparation phase (Diemers et al., 2007). An explanation may be that the intended learning processes do not occur; for example, prior knowledge may not be activated. Second, lower satisfaction with the preparation phase may also be due to a patient who fails to show up at the outpatient clinic and is replaced by another patient or a paper patient with a different problem than the one the students prepared for. Using real patients as opposed to paper patients brings the risk of patients not turning up at the appointed time. Being suddenly faced with a patient presenting with a problem different to the one they prepared for demands great flexibility from students and may considerably detract from the effectiveness of the preparation phase. Therefore, patient selection deserves very careful consideration in setting up a programme with a large number of real patient encounters.

The logistics of the implementation of real patient encounters in the ambulatory setting are complex and by no means easy to accomplish. The participating outpatient clinics receive students once a week during the whole academic year, which requires major logistical efforts: patients have to be asked to participate, time schedules have to be adjusted, and clinical supervisors and coaches have to be made available (and thus are not available for patient care at that time). Despite all the changes and efforts, however, the participating disciplines and their staff members are very positive and enthusiastic about the real patient encounters in year 3.

Annotated literature

Dornan, T., Littlewood, S., Margolis, S. A., Scherpbier, A., Spencer, J., and Ypinazar, Y. (2006). How can experience in clinical and community settings contribute to early medical education? A BEME systematic review. *Medical Teacher* **28**, 3–18.

The authors of this paper describe a systematic literature review of empirical research of the effects of early experiences in medical education published between January 1992 and December 2001. The main conclusions are that early experience motivates students, makes them more confident when interacting with patients, and supports the social professionalization process. Early experience furthermore strengthens students' learning and makes clinical practice more relevant to them. It additionally supports students in learning biomedical sciences, behavioural/social sciences, communication skills, and basic clinical skills. Finally early experiences also have beneficial effects for other stakeholders like teachers and patients.

Eva, K. W. (2005). What every teacher needs to know about clinical reasoning. *Medical Education* **39**, 98–106.

In this paper the author reviews the literature on clinical reasoning for clinical teachers. Two ways of clinical reasoning, analytical and non-analytical reasoning, are discussed. In analytical reasoning doctors use causal rules linking symptoms and signs to diagnoses. In non-analytical reasoning clinicians unconsciously compare the current case with previously encountered cases to make judgments regarding the probability that any particular case belongs within a particular diagnostic category. Either method of clinical reasoning is not inferior to the other and it is likely that both contribute to the final decisions made by novice clinicians as well as by experts. Eva describes a model illustrating the interactive role of both types of reasoning when a clinician faces a new patient problem. The use of both leads to greater diagnostic accuracy than the use of either one of them singly. Furthermore he discusses the importance of context specificity which determines the way clinicians work through future cases.

Woods, N.N. (2007). Science is fundamental: the role of biomedical knowledge in clinical reasoning. *Medical Education* **41**, 1173–7.

In this paper Woods describes the different roles biomedical knowledge can have in clinical reasoning. From research Woods suggests that to students biomedical knowledge creates coherence among clinical features leading to improved recall and application of clinical knowledge. Furthermore, it seems that when students are instructed to use basic science knowledge this leads to improved accurate diagnosing, particularly under time constraints and after a time delay resembling performances of expert clinicians. Woods additionally stresses that students are not able to transfer biomedical concepts to clinical problems spontaneously. As a result of these findings she recommends offering students clinical and basic science knowledge in an integrated way at early stages of their medical education to explicitly show the relationship between them.

References

Cooper, H. C., Gibbs, T. J., and Brown, L. (2001). Community-orientated medical education: extending the boundaries. *Medical Teacher* **23**, 295–9.

Diemers, A. D., Dolmans, D. H. J. M., van Santen, M., van Luijk, S. J., Janssen-Noordman, A. M. B., and Scherpbier, A. J. J. A. (2007). Students' perceptions of early patient encounters in a PBL curriculum: A first evaluation of the Maastricht experience. *Medical Teacher* **29**, 135–42.

Diemers, A. D., Dolmans, D. H. J. M., Verwijnen, M. G. M., Heineman, E., and Scherpbier, A. J. J. A. (2008). Students' opinions about the effects of preclinical patient contacts on their learning. *Advances in Health Sciences Education* **13**, 633–47.

Dornan, T., and Bundy, C. (2004). What can experience add to early medical education? Consensus survey. *British Medical Journal* **329(7470)**, 834–7.

Dornan, T., Littlewood, S., Margolis, S. A., Scherpbier, A., Spencer, J., and Ypinazar, Y. (2006). How can experience in clinical and community settings contribute to early medical education? A BEME systematic review. *Medical Teacher* **28**, 3–18.

Eva, K. W. (2005). What every teacher needs to know about clinical reasoning. *Medical Education* **39**, 98–106.

Joseph, G. M., and Patel, V. L. (1990). Domain knowledge and hypothesis generation in diagnostic reasoning. *Medical Decision Making* **10**, 31–46.

Littlewood, S., Ypinazar, V., Margolis, S. A., Scherpbier, A., Spencer, J., and Dornan, T. (2005). Early practical experience and the social responsiveness of clinical education: systematic review. *British Medical Journal* **331(7513)**, 387–91.

Mainhard, T., van den Hurk, M. M., van der Wiel, M. W. J., Crebolder, H. F. J. M., and Scherpbier, A. J. J. A. (2004). Learning in a clinical education program in primary care: The Maastricht adoption program. *Medical Education* **38**, 1236–43.

Norman, G. R., Trott, A. D., Brooks, L. R., and Smith, E. K. (1994). Cognitive differences in clinical reasoning related to postgraduate training. *Teaching and Learning in Medicine* **6**, 114–20.

Norman, G. R., and Schmidt, H. G. (1992). The psychological basis of problem-based learning: a review of the evidence. *Academic Medicine* **67**, 557–65.

O'Brien-Gonzales, A., Blavo, C., Barley, G., Steinkohl, D., and Loeser, H. (2001). What did we learn about early clinical experience? *Academic Medicine* **76**(4, suppl), S49–54.

O'Neill, P. A., Morris, J., and Baxter, C. M. (2000). Evaluation of an integrated curriculum using problem-based learning in a clinical environment: the Manchester experience. *Medical Education* **34**, 222–30.

Parsell, G., and Bligh, J. (2001). Recent perspectives on clinical teaching. *Medical Education* **35**, 409–14.

Patel, V. L., Evans, D. A., and Groen, G. J. (1989). Reconciling basic science and clinical reasoning. *Teaching and Learning in Medicine* **1**, 116–21.

Prince, K. J. A. H., Boshuizen, H. P. A., van der Vleuten, C. P. M., and Scherpbier, A. J. J. A. (2005). Students' opinions about their preparation for clinical practice. *Medical Education* **39**, 704–12.

Prince, K. J. A. H., van de Wiel, M., Scherpbier, A. J. J. A., van der Vleuten, C. P. M., and Boshuizen, H. P. A. (2000). A qualitative analysis of the transition from theory to practice in undergraduate training in a PBL-medical school. *Advances in Health Sciences Education* **5**, 105–16.

Schmidt, H. G. (1993). Foundations of problem-based learning: some explanatory notes. *Medical Education* **27**, 422–32.

Seabrook, M. (2004). Clinical students' initial reports of the educational climate in a single medical school. *Medical Education* **38**, 659–69.

van de Wiel, M. W. J., Schaper, N. C., Scherpbier, A. J. J. A., van der Vleuten, C. P. M., and Boshuizen, H. P. A. (1999). Students' experiences with real-patient tutorials in a problem-based curriculum. *Teaching and Learning in Medicine* **11**, 12–20.

Woods, N. N. (2007). Science is fundamental: the role of biomedical knowledge in clinical reasoning. *Medical Education* **41**, 1173–7.

Chapter 9

Simulated patients

Lonneke Bokken and Jan-Joost Rethans

Undergraduate medical training has traditionally depended heavily on student–patient contacts. However, changes in healthcare delivery, coupled with concerns about the objectivity and standardization of clinical examinations, have led to the introduction of 'simulated patients'. Simulated patients (SPs) are normal people who are trained to portray a patient in an authentic, realistic way. SPs can also be trained to portray a patient in a standardized, consistent way, as is required for (high-stakes) assessments.

At the Faculty of Health, Medicine and Life Sciences (FHML) of Maastricht University, SPs are mostly used for teaching purposes. This means that authenticity of role performance takes precedence over standardization. Teacher–independent SP encounters are used in teaching communication skills and, to a lesser degree, physical examination skills. Additionally, special SP encounters have been developed: adolescent SP encounters, longitudinal SP encounters, and SP encounters combining consultation and procedural skills.

Theoretical considerations

Several developments in healthcare practice and education have given rise to problems with regard to the role of patients in medical education. SPs were developed partly to provide a solution to these problems. Before going into SPs and various aspects of their roles in medical education, some of the developments that have prompted their emergence will be described briefly.

Contacts with real patients have always been an integral part of undergraduate medical education. A fairly recent development has extended the role of real patients to preclinical training, where they have been found to increase student motivation and ease the transition from preclinical to clinical training. Another strong point is that they can teach students 'things that cannot be learned from books', such as empathy, responsibility towards patients, and professional identity (Dornan et al., 2006). Patient contacts also help students build integrated skills for clinical reasoning, communication, history taking, and physical examination (Dornan et al., 2006; Spencer et al., 2000). However desirable extending patient contacts to earlier curricular years may be from an educational point of view, it increases the demand for patient participation in education. Unfortunately, this increased demand coincides with reduced availability of patients for education and training due to changes in healthcare delivery, notably fewer inpatient beds and shorter hospital stays. On top of this, mounting concerns about patient comfort, safety, and confidentiality also restrict the use of real patient contacts, particularly for relatively inexperienced learners (Howe & Anderson, 2003).

Real patients have not only contributed to teaching, they have also featured in assessment. For a long time bedside clinical examination was the accepted method for assessing students' clinical competence. However, wide variations in the level of difficulty presented by patients and variation in the judgements of examiners raised doubts about the reliability of these clinical exams (Collins & Harden, 1998).

The above-described changes in healthcare delivery, ethical issues, and concerns about reliability and validity in assessment provoked a search for alternatives to using real patients. As early as 1964, the neurologist Barrows introduced the 'programmed patient', 'a person without neurological symptoms who was trained to simulate a neurological disorder and to assess third-year medical students' (Barrows & Abrahamson 1964). Over the years, the term programmed patient has come to be replaced by simulated patient and standardized patient, both abbreviated to SP. Although these terms are often used interchangeably, there is a distinction (Collins & Harden, 1998). A simulated patient is defined as 'a normal person who has been carefully coached to present the symptoms and signs of an actual patient' (Barrows, 1985). The emphasis is on authenticity, i.e., faithful simulation of reality (Collins & Harden, 1998). Standardized patients are 'people with or without actual disease who have been trained to portray a medical case in a consistent fashion. They may portray their own problem(s) or ones based on those of other patients' (RCSA, 1993). Consistency is the main concern here. Standardized patients are especially suitable for assessment, high-stakes examinations in particular, which require standardized and consistent role play in order to create equal conditions for all examinees (Barrows, 1993). Another important function of standardized patients is their contribution to healthcare research (Rethans et al., 2007). For teaching purposes, authenticity is more important than consistency, and thus simulated patients are more suitable in this context (Wind et al., 2004).

SPs are considered a feasible, reliable, valid, and cost-effective tool in the evaluation of clinical competence (Vu & Barrows, 1994). Barrows (1993) described many advantages of SPs as opposed to real patients. Their main strengths can be summarized as follows: they can play an active role, they offer a relatively risk-free training environment, and they are adaptable. What do these strengths entail? In addition to the ability of SPs to provide feedback, which is a major benefit, SPs offer safety because students need not feel embarrassed if their interviewing and physical examination skills are imperfect. Mistakes are acceptable, even in difficult and sensitive situations, such as pelvic examination or breaking bad news. Because SPs are adaptable, they are available at any time and in any setting, unlike real patients whose timely presence in hospital or general practice can be difficult to arrange. In addition, SP performance can be tailored to specific educational purposes. For example, an SP encounter can be interrupted to discuss the case or give tips to the student ('timeout') and SPs can be examined repeatedly to allow students to perfect their examination techniques. Also the level of difficulty of the patient encounter can be adapted to match a student's competence level. The use of SPs can minimize undesirable variability in learning by allowing each student to question and examine an SP who simulates the same medical problem in the same way. Finally, SPs can simulate a wide range of physical findings, for example wheezing, abdominal tenderness, muscle weakness, and tremor (Barrows, 1993).

Assumed disadvantages of SPs relate to costs and the amount of time involved in recruitment and training (Lane & Rollnick, 2007). Another issue is negative effects on SPs due to role play, such as exhaustion, irritability, and physical complaints (Bokken et al., 2004, 2006). This will be discussed in more detail in the final section of this chapter. Lack of authenticity compared to real patients is a potential problem brought up frequently. However, experiences with SPs in research appear to contradict this notion. In studies in which incognito SPs visited practising physicians (who were informed that an SP would come to their surgery but not when) detection rates were less than 15% (Rethans et al., 2007). A clear sign that SPs can have quite acceptable authenticity.

Implementation of SPs

The Skillslab of FHML has employed SPs for over thirty years. Their main function has always been in the communication skills programme but they also contribute to assessment. Over the years there have been many developments and work is ongoing to find new modalities and improve current practices. This section describes the ways in which SPs, patient instructors, and real patients contribute to medical education.

A prerequisite for the Skillslab programme is the availability of a sufficient number of SPs to deliver the training programme. Currently, there is a pool of about one hundred SPs. Recruitment of new SPs is mostly by word-of-mouth. Although SPs at FHML predominantly function to support student learning, they also contribute to the assessment of communication skills in the annual Objective Structured Clinical Examinations (OSCE) in the first three and the fifth year of the curriculum. Encounters of one student with an SP are observed and assessed by one examiner, either a doctor or a behavioural scientist. For the OSCE, SPs are specially trained to perform a predetermined, standardized, and more or less fixed role. They do not assess or give feedback on students' performance.

The main part of the contribution of SPs at FHML is to teaching during the three preclinical years of the six-year problem-based curriculum. During these years all students ($N = 340$ per cohort) are offered the opportunity to practise communication and physical examination skills in teacher-independent encounters with SPs in the Skillslab (van Dalen et al., 2001). The SP roles are aligned with the theme of the curriculum unit that runs concurrently with the SP session. Pairs of students take part in three-weekly encounters with a simulated patient, in which one student plays the role of the doctor while the other observes the consultation. With every new contact roles are switched to ensure an equal number of turns as doctor and observer. The student doctor takes a history and/or performs a physical examination and afterwards the SP gives feedback on his or her experiences during the consultation. The SP encounters are recorded by a web-based software program. In the SP programme students work in the same group of some ten students and one teacher for the duration of one academic year. In the week after the SP encounters, students and teachers individually watch the recorded encounters of the students in their group on a secured webpage linked to the Skillslab. In group sessions, the students discuss their own encounter and those of the other students in their group (van Dalen et al., 2001), determining what went well and where more work is needed (see Chapter 10).

Authenticity is considered of the essence when SPs are used for teaching purposes (Wind et al., 2004). It is thought that roles gain credibility if they closely resemble an SP's real situation and character. That is why, at FHML, SPs are trained to perform a patient role by means of 'method acting', an acting style that requires actors to draw on their personal experience in portraying a role. SPs thus portray a patient role tailored to their own personality. In addition to role training, SPs are trained to give feedback using four feedback rules (Box 9.1).

Although students are encouraged to perform a complete consultation, including physical examination, the emphasis is primarily on communication and consultation skills, such as initiating the consultation, gathering information and history taking, giving information (about diagnosis and treatment), and closing the consultation. Basic consultation skills are the focus of attention in the first year, and in the next two years more complex consultation skills are addressed, including breaking bad news or dealing with angry and aggressive patients. To supplement the regular SP programme, special types of SP encounters have been developed: adolescent SP encounters, longitudinal SP encounters, and SP encounters in which consultation skills and procedural skills are combined. These will now be discussed in more detail.

Box 9.1 Feedback rules for SPs

Priority rule—SPs should start their feedback by answering the student's questions about the achievement of his or her individual learning goals. After this, the SP can give feedback on aspects that struck him or her particularly and on other matters.

Domain rule—The SP is only allowed to give feedback with regard to his or her own experiences as a patient during the encounter with the student (i.e., no feedback on medical content).

'I statements' rule—SPs should give feedback from their own personal point of view, using 'I statements', for example, 'I didn't feel comfortable during the conversation because I didn't understand your questions', instead of 'You should be more clear because people don't understand your questions and then they may feel uncomfortable.'

Neutrality rule—SPs should judge the student's performance neither positively nor negatively. Furthermore, SPs should direct their feedback at the individual student and refrain from making comparisons with the performance of other students. For example, 'I felt you really listened to me', instead of 'I felt that you listened to me much better than the other student I talked with.'

Adolescent SP encounters

It is relatively recently that adolescents made their debut as SPs (Blake et al., 2006). At FHML adolescent SPs were introduced in 2002, in the second-year unit 'puberty and adolescence'. An important theme of this unit is communication with adolescents about contraception and sexuality and students can practise this in SP consultations related to this topic. For the SP encounters, girls aged between thirteen and twenty years are trained as simulated patients. There is a pool of adolescent SPs who have participated in earlier years and new SPs are recruited by word-of-mouth. All adolescents play the role of 'Miss Jacobs', who asks her general practitioner (GP) about oral contraception. Although the basic question is similar for all encounters, the reason for the question is different for each SP and the student-doctor can only discover it through careful history, taking and after establishing a good rapport with the patient and gaining her trust. The SPs help to create their own roles, which are largely based on reality. Box 9.2 provides an overview of individualized role scenarios.

Longitudinal SP encounters

At FHML students see SPs mostly in single-case encounters. An important limitation of this format is that students do not learn about continuity of care. Furthermore, it does not reflect real-life healthcare, chronic disease management in general practice in particular, where patient problems are typically managed over a number of consultations. Training in continuity of care requires extensive, longitudinal patient encounters rather than snapshot-like, single-case encounters (Diederiks et al., 2006).

The longitudinal SP encounters developed at FHML are aimed to prepare students for continuity of care. Individual students have four consultations with the same SP spread over an eight-month period with feedback from the SP after each consultation. These encounters are scheduled in the third year in which chronic diseases are the central theme. During the first

Box 9.2 Overview of individualized role scenarios for adolescent SPs

Request for an oral contraceptive for the holidays.

A first-time request for an oral contraceptive but the girl is not sure whether she really wants it; her boyfriend is putting pressure on her.

A first-time request for an oral contraceptive but the girl is not sure whether she really wants it; her boyfriend's parents are putting pressure on her.

'I have painful periods. Would an oral contraceptive help?'

'I would like to start the pill because I think I'm ready for it.'

Girl comes in with a boy (not her boyfriend): 'Last night the condom ruptured.'

'I have painful periods. Would an oral contraceptive help?', but the real reason the girl wants to use an oral contraceptive is to prevent pregnancy. However, she is afraid to tell the GP this outright.

Girl comes in with boyfriend and asks for information about oral contraceptives but the boyfriend is urging her to actually start using an oral contraceptive now.

Girl comes in with boyfriend. They are arguing when they enter the GP's office: he thinks he has an STD and blames it on her. She denies it came from her.

consultation the SP and the new 'GP' are introduced to each other. The encounter focuses on the SP's chronic disease, for example, diabetes mellitus or radiculopathy. During subsequent encounters, the SP presents with new problems on top of the chronic health problem and students have to consider not only the new problem but also the existing chronic illness as well as possible interactions of these problems. New problems can be fever in patients with diabetes mellitus, which can lead to hyperglycaemia, or a sprained ankle, which can lead to deterioration of symptoms in patients with radiculopathy. Extensive documentation and detailed training of the SPs is necessary to match SPs' responses to students in order to guarantee continuity and realism in the consultations.

Integration of communication and procedural skills

Students usually learn communication and procedural skills as separate skills. However, in real practice, when doctors interact with patients during clinical procedures, they should be able to seamlessly integrate the performance of procedure-related technical skills and communication skills. Kneebone and colleagues have reported several studies in which SPs participated in combined communication and procedural skills training (Kneebone et al., 2002). Integration was achieved by combining inanimate models for the teaching of procedural skills, such as venepuncture, wound closure, or urinary catheterization, with SPs to create authentic and realistic simulations. Important advantages of these simulations are that SPs can give feedback on students' performance and students can practise integrating skills in a safe, simulated environment before moving on to consultations with real patients.

Analogous to the work of Kneebone and colleagues, SPs at FHML are used in consultations in which communication and procedural skills are integrated. In 2006, these integrated SP consultations were introduced in the third year of the curriculum.

Real patients and patient instructors

In the Skillslab, patient instructors and real patients contribute to the training of medical students along with SPs. Patient instructors are 'non-physicians who have been taught to simulate an actual patient encounter and who function in the multiple roles of patient, teacher, and evaluator'. For example, patient instructors can provide feedback and teach students skills for the female pelvic examination while the student is actually performing the examination on the patient instructor. Patient instructors can be simulated patients or real patients with stable findings. At FHML, patient instructors play a role in the training of intimate examination skills, such as gynaecological and urogenital examination skills (van Ravesteijn et al., 2007). The usual progression from training with models, via other students, to real patients is considered unsuitable for these intimate examinations. In the presence of a teacher, one patient instructor meets with one student for one hour. After a brief preparatory interview, in which the examination is described and the student's knowledge about the examination is refreshed and tested, the student examines the patient instructor. The patient instructor and the teacher guide the student. Afterwards the patient instructor gives feedback on the technical and communicative qualities of the student's performance.

Real patients are used as the final step in physical examination training. In the Skillslab, students can practise their diagnostic skills on persons with relatively stable dysfunctions, who present with real symptoms. For example, following training sessions in thorax examination, students are offered the experience of 'successfully' diagnosing a real patient with impaired lung function. Besides training in diagnostic skills, real patient encounters offer other valuable experiences to students, such as considering the disease and its impact from the perspective of the patient (Bokken et al., 2009d).

Discussion: experiences and reflections

Students generally value learning with SPs and consider it more effective than traditional teaching methods (Bokken et al., 2008). However, an SP programme requires continuous evaluation, reflection, and improvement. In this section the evaluation of the FHML SP programme is discussed, including the evaluation of SP performance and adverse effects on SPs.

Evaluations of the SP programme at FHML show that students and teachers generally value the programme highly. A study showed that students rated the general performance by adolescent SPs between 7.5 and 8 on a 10-point scale, while teachers and adolescent SPs were also very positive about the programme (Bokken et al., 2009a). Nevertheless, there are ongoing efforts to develop and improve the programme, and several changes have been made based on evaluations by students, SPs, and teachers. Initially, giving feedback was optional for the adolescent SPs; it was emphasized that they should only give feedback when they felt comfortable doing so. They received no feedback training. However, it turned out that the majority did provide feedback. Good feedback too as judged by teachers. As a result, SP feedback was fully integrated in the programme. Concomitantly, feedback training was provided for the adolescent SPs, which resulted in a gradual improvement of feedback over the years. Nevertheless, some of the adolescents quite recently indicated that giving feedback could be difficult for them (Bokken et al., 2009a). That is why feedback remains an important point of attention for the adolescent SP programme. Other changes that have been made are an increase in the number of consecutive consultations per day and easier recruitment of adolescent SPs, while authenticity has been improved by tailoring the SP roles to individual SPs.

As for the longitudinal SP programme, this was appreciated by students, teachers, and SPs (Bokken et al., 2009b; Linssen et al., 2007). The SPs appreciated the increased realism of the longitudinal encounters and the chance to build a good 'doctor'–patient relationship with the students. They felt they were also able to give more detailed feedback. However, despite the favourable evaluations, the programme was considered unfeasible and discontinued after one year, mainly due to lack of cooperation of faculty staff and the huge workload involved.

Ongoing monitoring and evaluation is also required for SP role performance and its impact on the SPs themselves. This will be discussed further in detail.

Evaluation of SP performance

Authentic role play and high-quality feedback are essential for the educational success of an SP programme. To ensure a high quality performance, it is important that SPs receive specific and appropriate feedback on a regular basis. The Maastricht Assessment of Simulated Patients (MaSP) instrument (Figure 9.1) was developed for this purpose (Wind et al., 2004). It has proven to be a valid, reliable, and feasible instrument for annually monitoring the quality of performance of each SP.

Impact of simulation on SPs

SPs generally enjoy their task in the teaching of undergraduate medical students, but there have been occasional reports of symptoms experienced by SPs in relation to role playing. McNaughton et al. (1999) used focus groups to explore the impact on SPs of performing highly affective psychiatric roles. The majority of the SPs mentioned negative effects, predominantly stress symptoms like exhaustion, irritability, sleep disorder, and physical complaints. The likelihood of occurrence of stress symptoms was increased by the type of role and reduced by the type of motivation for being an SP. Woodward and Gliva-McConvey (1995) found that the number of patient roles and amount of experience as an SP affected the probability of symptoms. Role playing by adolescent SPs and its impact on them was examined in a few studies. No negative effects were found (Blake et al., 2006; Bokken et al., submitted). One study on the impact of role playing on SPs identified an effect of acting style on the probability of symptoms (Naftulin & Andrew, 1975). The study showed that SPs who used a 'method acting' style—characterized by strong emphasis on personal experience—were more likely to develop stress symptoms than SPs who adopted a more technical approach, which meant maintaining a greater personal distance from their role. Because a method acting-like approach is used at FHML in training SPs for their roles, it seemed possible that Maastricht SPs might be at risk for negative effects from role playing. In order to examine this, two consecutive studies were performed (Bokken et al., 2004, 2006). The first study examined which immediate stress symptoms occurred, the severity of the symptoms, and which factors affected their occurrence. Although 73% of the SPs reported role-related stress symptoms, reassuringly, the severity of the symptoms was only moderate (2.2 on a 5-point scale). The second study demonstrated that the majority of the SPs did experience some negative effects. However, these effects, which included exhaustion, dissatisfaction with performance, performance-related physical complaints, and inability to snap out of the character afterwards, were all short lived and did not affect SPs' enjoyment of their work. Factors affecting the occurrence of symptoms were the type of role (whether emotionally complex), the number of consecutive performances, the length of the interval between performances, whether the SP had to give feedback, the amount of experience, and students. Box 9.3 provides an overview of measures that can be taken to reduce the impact of portraying a patient role. Debriefing can also be effective in this respect.

Future developments

An important area for future development and research is feedback from SPs. The ability of SPs to give feedback is considered an important advantage, distinguishing SPs from real patients. In a

The MaSP: Maastricht assessment of simulated patients

Name of SP role ....SP role no: ....(1-3) Curriculum year: ....(4-6)

Real name of SP: ....SP no: ....(7-9) Block no:................................(10-11)

The tape was assessed by: (tick as appropriate) (12)
- ☐ Student who interviewed the SP on the tape
- ☐ Student present at interview as observer
- ☐ Other student
- ☐ Physician
- ☐ Behavioural scientist

		Complete disagreement	Moderate disagreement	Moderate agreement	Complete agreement	Not applicable
Authenticity during the consultation						
1 SP appears authentic	1	☐	☐	☐	☐	(13)
2 SP might be a real patient	2	☐	☐	☐	☐	(14)
3 SP is clearly role-playing	3	☐	☐	☐	☐	(15)
4 SP appears to withhold information unnecessarily	4	☐	☐	☐	☐	(16)
5 SP stays in his/her role all the time	5	☐	☐	☐	☐	(17)
6 SP is challenging/testing the student	6	☐	☐	☐	☐	(18)
7 SP simulates physical complaints unrealistically	7	☐	☐	☐	☐	☐ (19)
8 SP appearance fits the role	8	☐	☐	☐	☐	(20)
9 SP answers questions in a natural manner	9	☐	☐	☐	☐	(21)
10 SP starts conversation with the student(s) during time-out	10	Yes ☐	No ☐			(22)
Feedback after the consultation						
11 SP left the room between consultation and feedback	11	Yes ☐	No ☐			(23)
12 SP stimulates student to ask questions.	12	☐	☐	☐	☐	(24)
13 I can judge from the reactions of the SP whether / she listens to the student or not	13	☐	☐	☐	☐	(25)
14 SP communicates how he/she felt during the consultation	14	☐	☐	☐	☐	(26)
15 SP gives feedback about medical issues	15	☐	☐	☐	☐	(27)
16 SP gives examples from the consultation	16	☐	☐	☐	☐	(28)
17 SP speaks about his/her role in the first person (I)	17	☐	☐	☐	☐	(29)
18 SP gives constructive criticism	18	☐	☐	☐	☐	(30)
19 SP compares student with other students	19	☐	☐	☐	☐	(31)
20 SP is friendly to the student	20	☐	☐	☐	☐	(32)
21 What mark (out of 10) would you give the SP for this SPC?	21	....	Mark (1 - 10)			(33-35)

Comments: (concerning SP and/or SPC)

SP: Simulated Patient   SPC: Simulated Patient Contact

Figure 9.1 The Maastricht assessment of simulated patients.

recent systematic review, feedback by SPs has been described as heterogeneous and lacking evidence to underpin feedback methods, domains, and training (Bokken et al., 2009c). It thus seems that the advantages of SP feedback are not being used to the full, which is disappointing considering the crucial role effective feedback plays in clinical learning. Furthermore there is ample evidence on how to provide effective feedback from studies on feedback in general (not specifically by SPs). Effective methods for SP feedback could build on that. As for the domain in which SP feedback can be useful, feedback from the patient's perspective would be consistent with recommendations in the literature.

Box 9.3 Overview of measures to reduce the impact of portraying a patient role

- ◆ Maximum of 7 performances a day, including a 30-minute break after a few performances;
- ◆ Highest number of performances to be scheduled before the break;
- ◆ More short breaks to be scheduled between performances;
- ◆ A standby SP who can stand in when other SPs need a break;
- ◆ Encourage SPs to turn down roles they do not feel comfortable with;
- ◆ Change or adjust a patient role after four years; and
- ◆ More frequent or improved feedback training to make SPs more confident in giving feedback to students.

Future developments might also focus on the complementary use of SPs and real patients. It has been shown that students consider SPs useful in learning communication skills and in preparing them for real patients (Bokken et al., 2008), but less so for other clinical skills, like clinical reasoning or physical examination skills (Bokken et al., 2008; Diemers et al., 2008). This affected students' motivation for preparation and self-study. SPs at FHML are mostly used for communication skills, not for clinical reasoning. However, it cannot be ruled out that an important educational opportunity is being missed here. The use of SPs might be extended to the teaching of complex clinical skills, like clinical reasoning. This may be particularly important in the curriculum's second and third years when most students feel they have mastered basic communication skills (Bokken et al., 2008). The use of SPs might also be extended to a more general educational format, for example, PBL tutorials. In traditional PBL curricula, where paper patient problems are commonly used as triggers for learning, students have reported difficulties in clinical problem solving and integration of knowledge (van de Wiel et al., 1999). Perhaps the opportunities to learn basic science knowledge in the context of clinical cases were not fully exploited. In 2001, real patient encounters were introduced as triggers for learning in the last preclinical year (third year), replacing the paper patients of the first two years (Diemers et al., 2007, 2008). Students were enthusiastic and appreciated how these contacts helped them make connections between theory and practice. For the success of the real patient programme patient selection is crucial (Diemers et al., 2007) and the limited availability of suitable patients can be a problem (see Chapter 8). SPs could be used in addition to real patients as triggers for learning and thus partly resolve shortages of real patients. SP contacts can be introduced early in the curriculum without aggravating the problem of selecting suitable real patients, since SPs are available when needed and adaptable to students' needs. This flexibility also opens up the possibility of presenting cases of gradually increasing complexity to students.

Annotated literature

ASPE: The Association of Standardized Patient Educators (http://www.aspeducators.org).
ASPE is the international organization for professionals in the field of standardized patient methodology. ASPE is dedicated to: (a) professional growth and development of its members; (b) advancement of SP research and related scholarly activities; (c) setting standards of practice; and (d) fostering patient-centred care. ASPE has a yearly SP conference and a number of committees in the different domains of SP methodology.

Barrows, H. S. (1993). An overview of the uses of standardized patients for teaching and evaluating clinical skills. *Academic Medicine* **68**, 443–51.

This is a useful paper on the development of SPs, which evaluates the strengths and weaknesses of SPs as well as future research opportunities. It includes a table of physical findings that can be simulated by SPs.

Bokken, L. (2009). *Innovative use of simulated patients for educational purposes.* Datawyse, Maastricht University Press.

This thesis written by Dr Bokken, who received her PhD degree from Maastricht University in 2009, addresses the practical implications of the perceived advantages and disadvantages of the use of SPs in undergraduate medical education and the advantages and disadvantages of SPs as opposed to real patients, particularly the instructiveness of a real patient encounter or an SP encounter as perceived by students.

Cleland, J. A., Abe, K., and Rethans, J. J. (2009). *The use of simulated patients in medical education.* AMEE Guide.

This AMEE guide gives an overview of the use of simulated and standardized patients with emphasis on practical implications of this methodology. It also has an extensive list of references on SP methodology.

Wallace, P. (2006). *Coaching standardized patients: For use in the assessment of clinical competence.* New York: Springer.

A useful handbook intended as a guide and as a support for those involved in the training of SPs, 'from the art of coaching through preparing SPs for the physical exam, to encourage each coach to develop a system that will deliver the best results and, in the end, help train the most competent doctors'.

References

Barrows, H. S., and Abrahamson, S. (1964). The programmed patients: a technique for appraising student performance in clinical neurology. *Journal of Medical Education* **39**, 802–5.

Barrows, H. S. (1993). An overview of the uses of standardized patients for teaching and evaluating clinical skills. *Academic Medicine* **68**(6), 443–51.

Barrows, H. S. (1985). *How to design a problem-based curriculum for the pre-clinical years.* New York: Springer.

Blake, K., Gusella, J., Greaven, S., and Wakefield, S. (2006). The risks and benefits of being a young female adolescent standardized patient. *Medical Education* **40**(1), 26–35.

Bokken, L., van Dalen, J., and Rethans, J. J. (2004). Performance-related stress symptoms in simulated patients. *Medical Education* **38**(10), 1089–94.

Bokken, L., van Dalen, J., and Rethans, J. J. (2006). The impact of simulation on simulated patients: a focus group study. *Medical Education* **40**(8), 781–6.

Bokken, L., Rethans, J. J., Scherpbier, A., and van der Vleuten, C. (2008). Strengths and weaknesses of simulated and real patients in the teaching of skills to medical students: a review. *Simulation in Health Care* **3**(3), 161–9.

Bokken, L., van Dalen, J., Scherpbier, A., van der Vleuten, C., and Rethans, J. J. (2009a). Lessons learned from an adolescent simulated patient educational program: five years of experience. *Medical Teacher* **31**(7), 605–12.

Bokken, L., Linssen, T., Scherpbier, A., van der Vleuten, C., and Rethans, J. J. (2009b). The longitudinal simulated patient program: Evaluations by teachers and students and feasibility. *Medical Teacher* **31**(7), 613–20.

Bokken, L., Linssen, T., Scherpbier, A., van der Vleuten, C., and Rethans, J. J. (2009c). Feedback by simulated patients in undergraduate medical education: a systematic review of the literature. *Medical Education* **43**(3), 202–10.

Bokken, L., Rethans, J. J., van Heurn, L., Duvivier, R., Scherpbier, A., and van der Vleuten, C. (2009d). Students' views on the use of real patients and simulated patients in undergraduate medical education. *Academic Medicine* **84**(7), 958–63.

Bokken, L., van Dalen, J., and Rethans, J. J. (Submitted). The case of 'Miss Jacobs': Adolescent simulated patients and the quality of their role playing, feedback and personal impact.

Collins, J. P., and Harden, R. M. (1998). AMEE Medical Examination Guide No 13: real patients, simulated patients and simulators in clinical examinations. *Medical Teacher* **20**(6), 508–21.

Van Dalen, J., Bartholomeus, P., Kerkhofs, E., Lulofs, R., van Thiel, J., Rethans, J. J., et al. (2001). Teaching and assessing communication skills in Maastricht: the first twenty years. *Medical Teacher* **23**(3), 245–51.

Diederiks, J. P., Bosma, H., van Eijk, J. T., van Santen, M., Scherpbier, A., and van der Vleuten, C. (2006). Chronic patients in undergraduate education: didactic value as perceived by students. *Medical Education* **40**(8), 787–91.

Diemers, A. D., Dolmans, D. H. J. M., van Santen, M., van Luijk, S. J., Janssen-Noordman, A. M. B., and Scherpbier, A. J. J. A. (2007). Students' perceptions of early patient encounters in a PBL curriculum: A first evaluation of the Maastricht experience. *Medical Teacher* **29**, 135–42.

Diemers, A. D., Dolmans, D. H. J. M., Verwijnen, M. G. M., Heineman, E., Scherpbier, A. J. J. A. (2008). Students' opinions about the effects of preclinical patient contacts on their learning. *Advances in Health Sciences Education Theory and Practice* **13**(5), 633–47.

Dornan, T., Littlewood, S., Margolis, S. A., Scherpbier, A., Spencer, J., and Ypinazar, V. (2006). How can experience in clinical and community settings contribute to early medical education? A BEME systematic review. *Medical Teacher* **28**(1), 3–18.

Howe, A., and Anderson, J. (2003). Involving patients in medical education. *British Medical Journal* **327**(7410), 326–8.

Kneebone, R., Kidd, J., Nestel, D., Asvall, S., Paraskeva, P., and Darzi, A. (2002). An innovative model for teaching and learning clinical procedures. *Medical Education* **36**(7), 628–34.

Lane, C., and Rollnick, S. (2007). The use of simulated patients and role-play in communication skills training: a review of the literature to August 2005. *Patient Education and Counseling* **67**(1–2), 13–20.

Linssen, T., van Dalen, J., and Rethans, J. J. (2007). Simulating the longitudinal doctor-patient relationship: experiences of simulated patients in successive consultations. *Medical Education* **41**(9), 873–8.

McNaughton, N., Tiberius, R., and Hodges, B. (1999). Effects of portraying psychologically and emotionally complex standardized patient roles. *Teaching and Learning in Medicine* **11**(3), 135–41.

Naftulin, D. H., and Andrew, B. J. (1975). The effects of patient simulations on actors. *Journal of Medical Education* **50**, 87–9.

Van Ravesteijn, H., Hageraats, E., and Rethans, J. J. (2007). Training of the gynaecological examination in The Netherlands. *Medical Teacher* **29**(4), e93–9.

RCSA. (1993). Consensus statement of the Researchers in Clinical Skills Assessment (RCSA) on the use of standardized patients to evaluate clinical skills. *Academic Medicine* **68**(6), 475–7.

Rethans, J. J., Gorter, S., Bokken, L., and Morrison, L. (2007). Unannounced standardized patients in real practice: a systematic literature review. *Medical Education* **41**(6), 537–49.

Spencer, J., Blackmore, D., Heard, S., McCrorie, P., McHaffie, D., Scherpbier, A., et al. (2000). Patient-oriented learning: a review of the role of the patients in the education of medical students. *Medical Education* **34**(10), 851–7.

Vu, N. V., and Barrows, H. S. (1994). Use of standardized patients in clinical assessments: Recent developments and measurement findings. *Educational Researcher* **23**(3), 23–30.

Van de Wiel, M. W. J., Schaper, N. C., Scherpbier, A. J. J. A., van der Vleuten, C. P. M., and Boshuizen, H. P. A. (1999). Students' experiences with real-patient tutorials in a problem-based curriculum. *Teaching and Learning in Medicine* **11**(1), 12–20.

Wind, L. A., van Dalen, J., Muijtjens, A. M., and Rethans, J. J. (2004). Assessing simulated patients in an educational setting: the MaSP (Maastricht Assessment of Simulated Patients). *Medical Education* **38**(1), 39–44.

Woodward, C. A., and Gliva-McConvey, G. (1995). The effect of simulating on standardized patients. *Academic Medicine* **70**(5), 418–20.

Chapter 10

Skills training

Robbert Duvivier, Jan van Dalen, Pie Bartholomeus, Maarten Verwijnen, and Albert Scherpbier

Medical training could no longer depend exclusively on patient encounters for the practical aspects of the profession. Patients were not to be reduced to mere teaching aids, with all the obvious risks involved. Furthermore, students should not depend on the accidental hospital population present at a certain time for their clinical encounters. These insights led to the establishment of clinical skills laboratories, educational facilities set up to provide systematic skill training in a safe environment, using effective educational methods and tailored to the level of experience of students.

Introduction: developments in clinical skills training

'Modern medicine, like all scientific teaching is characterised by activity. The student no longer merely watches, listens and memorises; he *does*.'

—Abraham Flexner, *Medical Education in the United States and Canada* (1910)

Since the introduction of formal medical education, training in clinical skills has been provided in several ways. In the early centuries of medical education students were gradually initiated into the secrets of the craft by observing an experienced physician. This apprenticeship approach changed during the first half of the twentieth century after Flexner published his report on the state of medical education (Flexner, 1910). New medical curricula were designed to provide students with a solid theoretical foundation. Contrary to Flexner's observation quoted above, practical medical education served merely as an illustration to the theoretical principles. It was only in the final years of medical training that future doctors encountered the practical components of their profession. Students were introduced to clinical skills during their time on hospital wards: arguably not the most appropriate setting to allow untrained students to practise essential skills (Engel, 1976). During the 1960s the effectiveness of this traditional approach came increasingly under attack from students and staff. It was argued that clinical skills should be an integral part of the curriculum.

The Skillslab

Maastricht University established a Faculty of Medicine in 1974. One of the key principles of the curriculum was to encourage students to formulate their own learning goals. Integration of different elements of knowledge was considered very important. This was reflected in the organization of learning. Problem-based Learning (PBL) became the educational backbone of the theoretical strand of the curriculum. Students were presented with problems rather than discipline-related factual knowledge. The presentation of multidisciplinary problems served as a preparation for reality.

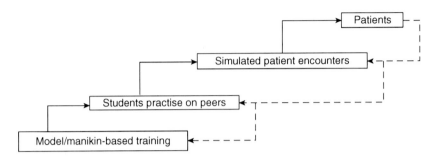

Figure 10.1 Skillslab training loop.

Early exposure to practical elements of healthcare was another important characteristic of the new medical curriculum. One of the implications of this was the need to prepare students for the practical aspects of their profession. Ways for providing skills training were sought. After ample deliberation an independent unit was set up: the first Skillslab to be established in a medical school.

The main reasons for setting up the Skillslab were:

◆ A laboratory setting enables the unravelling of complex practical situations ('whole tasks') into simple teachable skills ('part tasks'): the complexity of learning situations can be controlled.

◆ Students can practise as often as necessary to master a skill and mistakes are acceptable, which is in sharp contrast to training with real patients (Van Dalen & Bartholomeus, 1990).

◆ Clinical skills can be integrated in the curriculum in a longitudinal training programme. Skills training can illustrate theoretical topics. When students sign up for a particular training session, they will be more motivated to study the anatomy of the part of the body they will be examining. This promotes the acquisition of basic and clinical science knowledge and skills (Scherpbier, 1997).

Didactic approach to skills training

The Skillslab offers training in physical examination, laboratory, procedural, and communication skills. Communication skills are addressed in the next chapter. Training in the other types of skills roughly follows a similar didactic approach.

In skills training at least four teaching goals can be distinguished:

1 The technique of a skill should be performed correctly;

2 The skill should be performed in interaction with a patient; communication is part of all procedures;

3 Knowledge and skills are integrated; and

4 Findings must be correctly interpreted.

A variety of training formats can be used. Models and manikins can provide a safe and standardized context to learn the technique of a skill. Training with fellow students, under supervision, allows students to practise with real persons with different characteristics and feelings, who can give feedback about the quality of the interaction. Simulated patients can provide a realistic context where students can integrate their skills and knowledge in realistic doctor–patient encounters. (Real) patients help students interpret their findings. The use of these training formats enables the implementation of various didactic principles:

◆ Gradual increase in complexity of skills, for example

• Learning how to use a stethoscope;

- Using the stethoscope to take another student's blood pressure;
- Deciding whether blood pressure should be taken in a specific case presented by a real or a simulated patient; and
- Interpreting the blood pressure of a patient with hypertension.

- Gradual increase in complexity and realism of training situations; and
- Increasing integration of skills and knowledge, culminating in problem-solving in real doctor–patient encounters.

This approach enables students to gradually acquire a beginning of clinical competence and prepares them for encounters with real patients. Students develop their abilities by mastering every element of a skill before moving on to the next stage. Additionally, transfer of what is learned is maximized when skills are acquired in a wide variety of different situations (Patrick, 1992).

A distinct advantage of the use of models and manikins is the abstraction of reality. Students can concentrate on different technical aspects of a skill before having to deal with interactive aspects. When practising on peers, supervised by a teacher, students will experience what it feels like to undergo a certain examination and learn how to cope. This is an important experience for future professionals, who will have to prepare their patients for examinations. In addition, students discover that a wide range of findings is considered normal. In encounters with simulated patients students learn to integrate knowledge and skills in diagnosing and managing patient problems. At this stage, skill training begins to evolve into the development of initial clinical competence. Clinical competence increases during the most complex type of training offered at the Skillslab, in which persons with relatively stable dysfunctions contribute to skill training.

If at any stage students have doubt about their level of mastery of a particular skill, they can go back to a less complex practising stage for further practise. This training loop can be repeated until the student is confident enough to proceed to the next stage (refer to Figure 10.1).

By practising in many separate steps and in many different situations students acquire dexterity and flexibility of skill performance.

Training sessions

Students sign up for training sessions via the electronic learning environment. They can choose a moment when training is most appropriate with respect to their learning goals. They can also select a training session with the teacher of their choice. Finally, training is not compulsory: the Skillslab offers opportunities for training and it is up to the students to decide whether training can contribute to their competence. Although attendance of training sessions is voluntary, the annual skills test, an objective structured clinical examination (OSCE), is compulsory for all students and has consequences for their study progress. The students who decide not to attend a training session are mostly students who have had prior training. A training session typically lasts ninety minutes and is conducted in groups of eight to ten students. The size of the group depends on the level of complexity of the skill, the risk involved (for example venapuncture on peers), the intimacy of the skill (for example chest examination in mixed groups), and the availability of staff and equipment. Students can prepare by studying recommended reading before training sessions. For individual training sessions a variety of training methods is used, from 'trial and error' to 'find the mistake the teacher has built into the demonstration'. However, a typical training session consists of a four-stage process comprising demonstration of the skill by the teacher, explanation of the skill by the teacher, supervised practice, and corrective critique (Anderson, 1983; Dent & Hesketh, 2004; Van Merriënboer, 1997; Van Merriënboer et al., 2002).

Intimate examinations

Some specific areas of physical examination, like the pelvic examination, are obviously very intimate. Students can practise these skills on patient instructors because it is ethically questionable to perform these examinations on other students. Male and female patient instructors are carefully selected and trained to guide students through the examination, giving feedback along the way. The procedure during a training session follows a set pattern. One student meets with a patient instructor and a supervising teacher. In a brief preparatory introduction the examination is described and the student's knowledge about the area involved is refreshed. Then the student examines the patient instructor with guidance from the teacher and the patient instructor. Afterwards the patient instructor gives feedback on the technical and the interpersonal aspects of the examination.

Integration within curriculum

The longitudinal skills programme starts in the first week of the first year. It is integrated with the other curricular activities. The theme of the unit in which students participate is the overriding organizing principle of the curriculum (see Chapter 4). Horizontal integration ensures the relevance of activities to the unit theme. This way, theory and practice go hand in hand, and skills training serves the additional purpose of helping students to understand theoretical concepts and underlying mechanisms. Vertical integration is addressed in the skills curriculum plan. The skills curriculum has its own structure: some topics must be mastered before the student can move on to another one. This organization is intended to enable students to acquire the necessary skills when they are studying the related theoretical knowledge. In practice, this means continuous interaction between theory and practice. In the unit 'blood loss', for example, tutorial group sessions and lectures deal with theory and the concurrent Skillslab programme addresses the skills of the pelvic examination, rectal examination, urine and faeces analysis, suturing wounds, and infusion therapy.

Apart from the regular, supervised training sessions for which students can sign up, the Skillslab also offers teacher independent training. Whenever students wish to practise a particular skill, to maintain mastery or as extra practice, pairs of students can book a room at the Skillslab with the required training equipment and materials. A special area of the Skillslab is dedicated to these sessions. They enable students to maintain skills throughout the years and work at their own pace.

Evaluation, quality assessment, and staff training

The skills programme is evaluated annually by students and staff. Questionnaires are used to measure student satisfaction with a unit. Students are asked to judge specific aspects of a unit, including skill training sessions. The head of the Skillslab meets regularly with student representatives to discuss the results of these evaluations. Teachers can elicit student feedback on specific issues by special questionnaires. The issues concerned usually originate from the Skillslab teacher training programme. Skills teachers develop their own learning goals in small working groups, check these with their students, and report back on their individual progress (Steinert, 2005). Experts both from within and outside the university are invited to give workshops on various topics. Each staff member has a personal budget that can be used to attend courses or purchase books. Teacher satisfaction and performance are addressed during yearly performance appraisals.

Assessment

Once a year all the students in years 1, 2, and 3 and year 5 are tested on their knowledge and skills. These examinations are standardized according to the OSCE model. Students move through several 'stations' in which they are presented with a specific clinical scenario that requires them to apply their knowledge and demonstrate specific skills. Every student is confronted with the same series of tasks and is graded on a standardized scoring scheme. Planning groups responsible for the unit are also responsible for the contents of the stations in this examination. This implies that planning groups and the Skillslab must collaborate closely on this.

Lessons learned

Maastricht University has accumulated more than thirty years of experience in clinical skills teaching. The lessons learned can be summarized as follows.

Longitudinal organization of clinical skills training has a longer lasting effect

Students should be able to relate skills to their prior knowledge and experience. A useful approach to clinical skills training is an iterative revisiting throughout the medical curriculum. Clinical skills are revisited at different levels of difficulty and new skills are related to previous skills. In addition, teachers frequently refer to underlying principles and clinical relevance when teaching physical examination skills. Young students may have initial difficulties with skills training, but in general it is well appreciated in the early years (Lam et al., 2002). Compared to skills acquired in courses that are organized differently, such as a condensed full-time 'introduction to clinical medicine' unit, skills acquired in a longitudinal programme appear to have a longer lasting effect. Thus, skills training should be longitudinally integrated into a helical curriculum organization (Van Dalen, 2001; Scherpbier, 1997).

Undergraduate skills training helps students to benefit more from clerkships

When they have attended preclinical skills training students are somewhat skilled when the clerkships start. They feel more confident about their skills (Busari et al., 1997) and consequently apply more skills compared to students who have not attended a similar skill programme (Remmen, 1999; Scherpbier, 1997). Moreover, students are able to focus more, and better, on pathological findings.

Instructional materials help to standardize training

At the Skillslab many different teachers moderate the same training sessions. To enhance uniformity of training, sessions are conducted according to a 'standard lesson plan', including didactic guidelines and practical pointers. These are created by the teaching staff. Skillslab staff members collaborate closely with clinicians of the relevant disciplines in order to contribute to a true 'educational continuum'. The contents of the 'standard lesson plans' have led to a series of instruction books on clinical skills for students. Illustrated with photographs showing the correct procedures, these books now serve as the principal learning resource on clinical skills for Maastricht students. When moving images are needed, video clips are accessible via the electronic learning environment.

Staff must be allocated and trained and their time must be protected

Initially teaching staff from different healthcare backgrounds contributed to skills teaching. These staff members were called upon when needed. However, when teaching and healthcare responsibilities are in competition, healthcare inevitably wins. In order to ensure availability of trainers, staff members were appointed specifically to the Skillslab. Nowadays, most skill teachers have their primary affiliation with the Skillslab. The Skillslab teaching staff consists of a small core staff exclusively active in skills training and other staff members who combine their Skillslab tasks with work in other (clinical or research) settings. Time allocated for Skillslab work is carefully guarded. It has proved crucial that all staff assigned to work in the Skillslab receive appropriate training in the methods used, the objectives of the programme, and how these fit into the overall medical curriculum. Skillslab staff members, therefore, also assume other teaching roles in the curriculum, such as unit planner, mentor, or tutor of a PBL group.

The Skillslab must be embedded in the faculty organization

The Skillslab has full departmental status within the Faculty of Health, Medicine and Life Sciences. The department head is responsible for the day-to-day management of the Skillslab. Specific responsibilities are carried out by administrative staff. This setup has the advantage that staff can be appointed on the basis of proven teaching competence. Being a separate department, the Skillslab is at risk of becoming isolated: the link with clinical departments must continuously be nurtured (Scherpbier, 1997). This can be accomplished by collaboration in the development of learning materials and training of skills teachers.

Training with peers is beneficial

Physical examination training on peers has proved to be a very useful experience, particularly prior to exposure to simulated patients. It is not only valuable for the student who performs the examination but also for the student who undergoes the examination. More sensitive examinations (such as chest examination) and more invasive procedures (such as venapuncture) need to be handled with discretion and care by students and staff alike. This in itself is a valuable learning experience. Understandably, students initially show some reluctance to participate in this type of training. However, the overall experiences at the Skillslab are favourable, which is in line with findings described in literature (O'Neil et al., 1998; Power & Center, 2005). Students from different cultural backgrounds may respond differently to examining (and being examined by) peers. The provision of women-only groups is appreciated by students who might otherwise opt out of physical examination training on religious or cultural grounds. If students have concerns about this type of training, they can confidentially discuss any personal issues with an advisor appointed by the Skillslab especially for this purpose.

Real patients have a valuable role in preclinical skills training

Over the years a bank of real patients has been developed and maintained. These patients have proved to be a valuable asset for the teaching of clinical skills, in addition to simulated patients (Chapter 9). Patients with chronic, stable clinical conditions (and their partners!) offer unique learning possibilities (Van Hellemondt, 2001). This is especially true when simulation of physical signs and symptoms is difficult or impossible. Moreover, patients can help students to appreciate the psychological and social impact of their illness. The use of patient encounters in skills training requires careful organization. Real patients, like simulated patients, must be introduced into the curriculum in exactly the same structured and planned way as any other skills training activity. Additionally, patients, like simulated patients, must be trained on how to provide feedback.

Information and communication technology (ICT) can be helpful but its validity must be guarded

Nowadays many sophisticated computerized patient simulators are available, which react to examinations or interventions. The benefits are that students can see and practise procedures at their own pace while the simulator provides feedback. However, caution is needed. Computerized models are often very expensive. Moreover, the validity of the use of these models must be carefully considered. Teachers must avoid teaching 'the delivery of a baby' with a computerized model, test students with that model, and then assume that they are fully prepared to deliver a real baby (McGaghie et al., 2003; Norman, 2003). Most feasible are models that allow students to practise, provide feedback, and simulate situations that could otherwise not be simulated. There are many ICT programmes available that help students to (cognitively) prepare for skills training by challenging them to use their prior knowledge.

Research should be the basis for skills training development

Research and development has always been an integral part of the Skillslab at Maastricht University. Scientific evaluation of existing programmes is carried out to establish and monitor quality and effectiveness. In addition, exploration of new methodologies and assessment techniques guides the development and advancement of clinical skills training as an academic endeavour. The outcomes of research are shared in conference presentations, peer-reviewed publications, and PhD theses. Initially there was not much research into the use of OSCEs for assessment of skills but this gap has been filled by Skillslab-based research (Van Luijk, 1994; Verhoeven et al., 2000; Van der Vleuten, 1996). Next, the added value of a Skillslab for skills training was studied (Van Dalen, 2001; Scherpbier, 1997). The use of simulated patients has been extensively researched (Bokken, 2009). Detailed teacher guidelines for adequate skills training have been developed (Duvivier et al., 2009; Martens et al., 2009) and a research project has investigated the actual evidence base of the skills taught at the Skillslab. These and other studies have assisted in helping skills training develop beyond intuition into a rational programme.

(Inter)national collaboration helps to update the programme

Skillslab staff members are often consulted by medical schools abroad that wish to set up skills training facilities. For example, supported by funding from the Dutch government, the Maastricht Skillslab has facilitated the establishment of Skillslabs in the eight medical faculties in Vietnam (see Chapter 25). Projects like these obviously promote health professions education abroad, but they are also beneficial for the Maastricht programme. Advising other institutions to find solutions to their problems helps the Maastricht Skillslab to become more creative (Kiguli et al., 2006). Moreover, in today's rapidly changing world, with increased mobility, diversity in the population, pandemics, and intercultural interaction, collaboration with institutions in other countries is important to enhance awareness of public health and healthcare issues in other parts of the world. This awareness can help the Skillslab to adapt its programme to better reflect our current, diverse society.

Future developments

Research projects that have been initiated are planned to continue for some time. Ongoing research focuses on the value of physical examination (Simel & Drummond, 2009) and the theoretical underpinnings of skills training. Additionally, the use of e-learning in skills training is being explored. Faculty development will continue to be a focus of Skillslab activities as is continued skills training for vocational training. Some areas, such as interprofessional education and intercultural aspects of healthcare, have not been developed yet, but will be developed in the near future.

Annotated literature

Bradley, P., and Postlethwaite, K. (2003). Setting up a clinical skills learning facility. *Medical Education* **37**, 6–13.

This article provides practical information for establishing a clinical skills centre, ranging from staffing issues to didactical considerations. The authors highlight different aspects of learning in a clinical skills centre, and describe the use of manikins, simulated patients, and real patients with their respective pros/cons.

Dent, J. A. (2001). Current trends and future implications in the developing role of clinical skills centres. *Medical Teacher* **23**, 483–9.

Dent describes the range of teaching methods that can be used in clinical skills centres. Different educational strategies are discussed and there is particular emphasis on the role of assessment in the learning of clinical skills.

References

Anderson, J. R. (1983). *The architecture of cognition*. Cambridge, MA: Harvard University Press.

Bokken, L. (2009). *Innovative use of simulated patients for educational purposes*. Dissertation, Maastricht University Press.

Busari, J. O., Scherpbier, A. J. J. A., and Boshuizen, H. P. A. (1997). Comparative study of medical education as perceived by students at three Dutch universities. *Advances in Health Sciences Education* **1**, 141–51.

van Dalen, J. (2001). *Communication skills: teaching, testing and learning*. Dissertation, Maastricht University Press.

van Dalen, J., and Bartholomeus, P. (1990). Training clinical competence in a Skillslaboratory. In: W. Bender, R. J. Hiemstra, A. J. J. A. Scherpbier, and R. P. Zwierstra (eds) *Teaching and assessing clinical competence*. Groningen: BoekWerk.

Dent, J. A., and Hesketh, E. A. (2004). Developing the teaching instinct. 13: how to teach in the clinical skills centre. *Medical Teacher* **26**, 201–10.

Duvivier, R. J., van Dalen, J., van der Vleuten, C. P. M., and Scherpbier, A. J. J. A. (2009). Teacher perceptions of desired qualities, competencies and strategies for clinical skills teachers. *Medical Teacher* **31**, 634–41.

Engel, G. L. (1976). Are medical schools neglecting clinical skills? *JAMA* **236**, 861–3.

Flexner, A. (1910). Medical education in the United States and Canada: a report to the Carnegie Foundation for the Advancement of Teaching. New York: Carnegie Foundation for the Advancement of Teaching. Available online at http://www.carnegiefoundation.org/files/elibrary/flexner_report.pdf

van Hellemondt, G. D. M. (2001). Echte patiënten in het vaardigheidsonderwijs neurologie: eerste ervaringen. [Real patients in neurological skills training: first experiences.] *Tijdschrift voor Medisch Onderwijs* **20**, 32–6.

Kiguli, S., Kijjambu, S., and Mwanika, A. (2006). Clinical skills training in a resource constrained medical school. *Medical Education* **40**, 459–89.

Lam, T. P., Irwin, M., Chow, L. W. C., and Chan, P. (2002). Early introduction of clinical skills teaching in a medical curriculum –factors affecting students' learning. *Medical Education* **36**, 233–40.

van Luijk, S. J. (1994). *Al doende leert men. [Learning by doing.] Dissertation*, Maastricht University Press.

McGaghie, W. C., Issenberg, S. B., and Petrusa, E. R. (2003). Simulation—savior or saint? A rebuttal. *Advances in Health Sciences Education* **8**, 97–103.

Martens, M. J. C., Duvivier, R., van Dalen, J., Verwijnen, G. M., Scherpbier, A. J. J. A., and van der Vleuten, C. P. M. (2009). Student views on the effective teaching of physical examination skills: a qualitative study. *Medical Education* **43**, 184–91.

van Merriënboer, J. J. G. (1997). *Training complex cognitive skills: a four-component instructional design model for technical training*. Englewood Cliffs, NJ: Educational Technology Publications.

van Merriënboer, J. J. G., Clark, R. E., and de Croock, M. B. M. (2002). Blueprints for complex learning: the 4C/ID-model. *Educational Technology, Research and Development* **50**, 39–64.

Norman, G. (2003). Editorial: simulation—savior or saint? *Advances in Health Sciences Education* **8**, 1–3.

O' Neil, P. A., Larcombe, C., Duffy, K., and Dornan, T. L. (1998). Medical students' willingness and reactions to learning basic skills through examining fellow students. *Medical Teacher* 20, 433–7.

Patrick, J. (1992). *Training: research and practice*. London: Academic Press.

Power, D. V., and Center, B. A. (2005). Examining the medical student body: peer physical exams and genital, rectal or breast exams. *Teaching and Learning in Medicine* 17, 337–43.

Remmen, R. (1999). *An evaluation of clinical skills training at the medical school of the University of Antwerp*. Dissertation, Antwerp University Press.

Scherpbier, A. J. J. A. (1997). *Kwaliteit van vaardigheidsonderwijs gemeten. [Measuring quality of skills training.]* Dissertation, Maastricht University Press.

Simel, D., and Drummond, R. (2009). *The rational clinical examination*. New York: McGraw Hill.

Steinert, Y. (2005). Staff development for clinical teachers. *Clinical Teacher* 2, 104–10.

Verhoeven, B. H., Hamers, J. G. H. C., Scherpbier, A. J. J. A, Hoogenboom, R. J. I., and van der Vleuten, C. P. M. (2000). The effect on reliability of adding a separate written assessment component to an objective structured clinical examination. *Medical Education* 34, 525–9.

van der Vleuten, C. P. M. (1996). The assessment of professional competence: developments, research and practical implications. *Advances in Health Sciences Education* 1, 41–67.

Chapter 11

Communication skills

Robbert Duvivier, Jan van Dalen, and
Jan-Joost Rethans

Communication plays an important role in patient care. Research has shown that communication skills training in a medical curriculum should be longitudinal. Training should preferably be experience-based and take place in small groups with role play and (simulated) patient contacts. It should focus on multiple aspects of communication and increase in complexity over the years. Knowledge of underlying psychological principles is considered helpful, as is integration of medical decision making and clinical reasoning with communication.

Introduction

At Maastricht's Faculty of Health, Medicine and Life Sciences (FHML) the above-mentioned considerations have resulted in a communication skills programme that starts in the first week of the first year of the curriculum. In order to ensure cohesion with the curriculum the subjects addressed in the communication programme reflect the topics and themes of concurrent curricular units. Several stages of increasing complexity can be distinguished in communication training: role playing, training with simulated patients, and training with real patients. At the role-playing stage students receive immediate feedback from the teacher and the peers in their group. The simulated patient contacts are discussed in small groups also with feedback from peers and the teacher. In the communication skills programme, real patients are used to ease the transition from contacts with simulated patients to contacts with real patients in healthcare settings.

Communication skills

Communication is crucial for the delivery of healthcare. The average doctor will conduct some 200,000 patient interviews during his or her professional life, making it the most commonly performed 'procedure' in clinical practice. And a very effective one it is too. A good history can yield about 80% of the data needed for an accurate diagnosis. These figures underscore the significance of communication skills in medicine.

Research over the past twenty years has indicated that effective doctor–patient communication is related to patient satisfaction, compliance, lower costs, and medical outcomes (Kaplan et al., 1989, Reames & Dunstone, 1989). Patient dissatisfaction with medical care and malpractice claims are often related to miscommunication between doctors and patients (Shapiro et al., 1989).

Fortunately, the quality of doctor–patient communication can be enhanced by training. There is sound evidence that training can actually improve doctors' communication skills. Consequently, there has been increasing pressure from medical professional bodies to improve the training and evaluation of doctors' communication skills.

Additionally, it has been demonstrated convincingly that longitudinal training in communication skills is superior to concentrated training (Van Dalen et al., 2002; Flaherty, 1985). There are also indications that without training communication skills do not improve spontaneously and may even deteriorate over the course of the medical curriculum (Bishop et al., 1981; Helfer, 1970; Poole & Sanson-Fisher, 1979). That is why training should ideally be organized longitudinally and in alignment with other curricular activities.

At FHML, communication skills training is integrated with the teaching of underlying psychological theory, training in other clinical skills (i.e., physical examination skills), and the assessment system. The following section describes the development and implementation of the communication skills programme.

Communication skills training

Communication skills training at FHML is primarily experience based. In the first year students learn by role playing and in contacts with simulated patients. The emphasis is not only on *what* to say, but also very much on *how* to say it. Examples of topics of training include exploratory interview and breaking bad news. As with all skill training, communication training increases in complexity over the years.

To promote integration with the other components of the curriculum the communication skills programme runs parallel with the thematic, usually six-week, units. Of the two parts of the communication skills programme, the contacts with simulated patients are mandatory, while students are free to sign up for the other training sessions, which deal with subjects such as 'obtaining information from a patient', 'providing information', and 'intercultural communication'. The elective communication programme also includes a session in which students reflect on their role as a doctor by trying to answer questions like 'What sort of doctor do I wish to be?' (see Box 11.1).

The name of the communication skills programme is CORE, where 'CO' stands for consultation and 'RE' for reflection. The basic CORE philosophy is that it is not only important for students to learn how to communicate as a doctor but also to reflect on their future professional

Box 11.1 Overview of CORE Elective Modules (all related to patient-doctor consultations)

- Registration and reporting on a consultation;
- Intercultural communication;
- Clinical reasoning;
- Non-verbal communication;
- Asking questions respectfully;
- Providing information;
- Dealing with emotions;
- Asking for and receiving feedback;
- Negotiating with patients;
- Obtaining information from patients;
- The patient does not exist;
- Models for the doctor–patient relationship;
- Purposes and boundaries of healthcare; and
- The doctor as a professional.

role as a doctor. The contacts with simulated patients during the CORE programme also make it clear to students that they have to make certain personal choices with regard to that role.

Learning by role playing

For role playing students are given written roles (for patient and doctor separately) describing the setting of the consultation, the patient's signs and symptoms (the reason for the encounter), and some biographical details of the patient. Based on these roles, two students role play a consultation in a group of some ten students and a teacher, who guides the learning process. The group observes and gives feedback. In the course of the programme students play both the doctor and the patient so that they can experience the attendant emotions from both perspectives. The students who observe the consultation learn to analyse the verbal as well as the non-verbal aspects of communicative behaviour.

Learning with simulated patients

Apart from the group sessions, students are offered experiences in individual consultations with simulated patients during the first three years. Students sign up for consultations (in pairs) switching roles as doctor and observer between consultations. In one curricular year each student can take part in a total of ten consultations with simulated patients: five as a doctor and five as an observer. Physical examination is gradually integrated into the simulated patient contacts. For a more detailed description see Chapter 9.

Learning with patients

At the Skillslab the simulated patients are trained to achieve a high level of authenticity in their roles. Nevertheless, the impact of the switch from these relatively safe contacts to contacts with real patients in an authentic healthcare setting is not to be underestimated (Diemers et al., 2007). This transition can be eased by including preparatory consultations with real patients in the communication programme. Patients with chronic, stable clinical conditions offer unique learning opportunities compared to simulated patients, because they present with real abnormal findings on physical examination.

Small-group sessions

Groups of ten students meet every three weeks with a facilitator. The composition of the group remains unchanged during the academic year. In between group sessions the students engage in the above-described encounters with simulated patients. The simulated patients portray a role relevant to the theme of the concurrent unit. For example, during the unit on abdominal complaints the simulated patient presents with acute abdominal pain from appendicitis. One student plays the 'doctor role' during the consultation with the simulated patient, including history, physical examination, and management decisions, while the other student observes. Afterwards the simulated patient gives feedback by describing to the student how he or she experienced the consultation. No teacher is present at the encounters but the encounters are recorded digitally and can be accessed on FHML computers by the members, students and teacher, of the same group. The teacher can do so in his/her own office. All the group members, including the teacher, are expected to have watched the recorded consultations of all group members before the next group session, when the group elaborates and reflects on the consultations. Feedback is given and possible alternative communication strategies are discussed. Ethical issues are addressed as well.

There are three important obligations for students in relation to their encounter with a simulated patient. Firstly, they are required to write personal learning goals before the contact. Secondly, they must write their impression of the contact with the simulated patient directly afterwards and formulate questions to ask the group. Thirdly, after the group session, students must produce a written analysis of their consultation and the feedback from the group. From this analysis new learning objectives are derived for the next contact with a simulated patient. The learning objectives are addressed during communication skills training sessions and simulated patient encounters in subsequent units. The process of simulated patient encounter and feedback session is repeated shortly afterwards to enable the other half of the group to play the doctor role. Only this time the patient's complaint differs slightly; for example, instead of appendicitis the patient's abdominal complaints are caused by Crohn's disease or an ectopic pregnancy. Thus at the end of a unit all students have experienced the doctor and the observer role with a simulated problem related to the unit theme. This cycle is repeated in the following unit. In the course of the communication skills programme in the first three years of the curriculum students can participate in some fourteen consultations as a doctor and directly observe another fourteen consultations. In addition, each student watches at least 120 recorded consultations with simulated patients of the other group members.

It has been shown that the didactic qualities of communication skills teachers are more important than their professional background (Levine, 1995), but CORE tries to recruit as many healthcare professionals as possible as facilitators. Experience with CORE has also taught that a mix of different healthcare disciplines contributes positively to the overall educational goals of the programme. Students value the opportunity to identify with teachers and therefore may prefer doctors. In the course of the curriculum medical knowledge and problem solving are increasingly integrated into the communication skills programme. For these reasons behavioural scientists are only facilitators in the first year of the programme, although a few also facilitate groups in the second year. In the later years, however, the communication skills programme is taught by doctors only.

Some eighty to ninety teachers are involved in delivering the programme to some 1100 students in three year cohorts. Dependent on the year, CORE teachers spend annually about 47 hours (year 3) to 82 hours (year 1) on each CORE group they facilitate. In addition the elective parts of the CORE programme require per group 40 hours of teacher time annually. In total, investment in the teaching of the CORE programme (excluding administrative work) amounts to some 4.5 full-time equivalents (FTE) staff time. CORE is run by a CORE-planning group consisting of five faculty members and a student. In addition there is a CORE secretariat and the simulated patient programme (Chapter 9).

Development of the communication skills programme

During its development the communication skills programme has passed through different phases. Initially, the main activities were directed at the production of teaching materials and after that at designing an adequate assessment tool. The next step was to systematically implement an evaluation procedure aimed at adapting and improving the programme. CORE sought students' opinions about both the programme and the teachers. This information was used to develop a teacher training programme.

Teaching materials

To ensure uniform teaching, a detailed training protocol was written for each session, containing:

◆ The teaching goals;
◆ Preparatory material (recommended reading, handouts);

- A time schedule; and
- A chronological description of the steps to be taken: presentation, introduction of the role play, the role of the patient, the role of the doctor, assignments for students who observe the role play, topics for which the role was written, feedback rules, guidelines on how to stimulate involvement of the observing students, topics to be addressed during feedback, evaluation of the training session, and preparatory advice for the next session.

A schematic example of a protocol for an elective session of the CORE programme can be found in Table 11.1 (adapted from Van Dalen et al., 1989). For the sessions after the simulated-patient encounters, the protocols include specific information for teachers: a description of the complaint portrayed by the simulated patients and the individual variations between the simulated patients, the correct clinical diagnosis, and medical background information.

Assessment procedures

FHML uses different formats to assess students' communication skills. In the first year of the curriculum students keep an electronic CORE portfolio to which they add materials during the academic year. The emphasis is on the documentation of progression and not so much on individual students' achieved levels of expertise in communication skills. At the end of the year the communication portfolio is graded. In the portfolio students describe and analyse their learning process from four perspectives:

1 Analysis of contacts with simulated patients: directly after a contact students write their personal impressions (including their feelings) as well as questions to ask the group in the

Table 11.1 Example of a training protocol (first year)

Training protocol	Listening
Learning goal	Active listening
Sub goals	Showing minimal encouragement;
	Giving regular recapitulations of the information;
	Asking questions within the patient's frame of reference
Preparation	Literature
	• J. van Dalen, Stimulating and blocking reactions, in: Van Dalen (1986)
	• S. Maes, Attending to the patient, in: Maes (1983), Chapter 3
	Videotape: *Listening: a model*

Training design

A	B	C	D	E	F
30 mins.	10 mins.	20 mins.	30 mins.	20 mins.	10 mins.

A—Discussing the recommended readings;

B—Role-playing;

C—Evaluation;

D—Interviews in subgroups;

E—Evaluation of the interviews

F—Evaluation of the training session.

next session. After the group session they write a summary of the feedback they have received, which leads to the formulation of new learning objectives for the next contact with a simulated patient.

2 Reasons to attend elective modules: students describe their reasons for attending a particular component of the elective part of the communication skills programme.

3 Longitudinal comparison: students compare their first and last contact with a simulated patient in one year focusing on aspects in which they have shown improvement.

4 Reflection: students write a short essay on 'What sort of doctor do I wish to be?'

In the second year, the assessment procedure is the same, but additionally students must pass the end-of-year communication test, consisting of an observed contact with a simulated patient followed by the student's analysis of this contact. Students' performance is graded using an instrument specially developed for this test in 1981 and validated in scientific studies for reliability and consistency. The resulting instrument is called MAAS-Global and is used as the principal assessment of communication skills (Van Dalen et al., 1998; Kraan & Crijnen, 1987; van Thiel et al., 1991, 1992).

Furthermore, knowledge about communication skills and underlying psychological principles is assessed in the unit tests and the progress tests (Chapters 21 and 22).

Programme evaluation

Programme evaluation questionnaires have been shown to reliably measure students' satisfaction with a course (Cook et al., 1997; Dolmans et al., 1994; Gijselaers, 1988) (see also chapter 17). The communication skills programme is evaluated annually by students and teachers. Students' individual feedback to teachers is reported back to those teachers. These evaluations are also sent to the heads of the teachers' departments and the CORE coordinator and included in the teacher's teaching portfolio.

Teacher training

Detailed information from the programme evaluations provides course organizers with teaching goals for faculty development. Faculty development addresses the analysis of videotapes of simulated patient encounters, the application of feedback rules, and the stimulation of student involvement. Attendance is mandatory for new teachers.

Discussion: lessons learned

The communication skills programme is firmly embedded in the FHML infrastructure. We will review some of the difficulties in setting up the programme that were encountered over the past thirty years.

From instruction videotapes to video vignettes

Initially, a great deal of time, money, and energy were invested in the making of video instruction tapes to help students prepare for group sessions. It was thought that watching positive or negative role models would make it clear to students what type of behaviour they were expected to show. Those videotapes never really worked. Clothing that was out of fashion very quickly and poor acting soon overshadowed the messages of the tapes. As time passed this problem became desperately urgent and finally it was decided to stop using the tapes altogether. In our experience, a very effective video teaching aid is video vignettes (Blok et al., 1999), nowadays available on

DVD in the university library or accessible via the electronic learning environment. These vignettes are used in group sessions, mostly in the CORE elective sessions. A vignette is a short role-played scene (lasting 10-30 seconds) with an oral introduction in which a teacher explains the setting. For example, 'imagine you are a medical student. It is the first day of your Obstetrics/ Gynaecology clerkship and you sit in with your supervisor at a consultation with a patient. Now the following happens.' Students are asked to write down what they have seen and heard, how it affects them, and suggest a possible adequate professional reaction. Their answers are reported and discussed. These video vignettes immediately capture students' attention and most students see the relevance of this exercise right away.

Entire consultations for first-year students

Originally, different phases of the consultation were learned in different years of the curriculum. 'Clarifying the patient's reasons to visit the doctor', which requires attentive listening by the doctor, is an ideal topic to start with in the first year, because at that stage students have little medical knowledge. As a result they can be unbiased listeners and appreciate and acknowledge the information that patients share spontaneously. As their medical knowledge increases, students find it more difficult to integrate the patient's agenda with their own agenda. Our experience and other studies have shown that students listen less attentively in later curriculum years than in the first year (Bishop et al., 1981; Helfer, 1970; Poole & Sanson-Fisher 1979). In an attempt to counteract this all the contacts with simulated patients were changed into full consultations, for first-year students too. In this way students practised the combination of listening (communication skills) and problem solving (clinical reasoning) from the outset of medical training. A drawback that has emerged is that it has proved quite difficult to create cases that enable first-year students to practise with confidence.

Choice of behaviour as the topic of training

Not all aspects of human interaction can be expressed in observable behaviour. For example, CORE has not succeeded in developing unambiguous criteria for 'eye contact'. It might be argued that CORE pays too little attention to what might be indicated by the word 'attitude'. Although every simulated-patient encounter challenges students to make choices, based on their own norms and values, students and teachers do not always explicate their choices. When they evaluate the programme students regularly say that they want more opportunities to address these issues.

From an optional programme to a mandatory one

Until recently attendance of communication training was not mandatory. However, increased recognition of the importance of communication skills training prompted the decision to make attendance mandatory. It was found that of the many students who were found to not communicate adequately with patients in years 4-6, quite a few had not taken part in the communication skills programme.

Future developments

Without continued training, communication skills tend to deteriorate over the years. Therefore, FHML is currently working to extend the communication programme to years 4–6. Clinical supervisors rarely give feedback on students' communication skills. Since research has shown that in the later years of the curriculum students are more motivated by real patient contacts

(Bokken, 2009), it is being investigated whether it is feasible to use digital recordings of real patient–student contacts for self-assessment and feedback. Another option would be to bring in simulated patients. Also there is a plan to develop elective modules tailored to clinical practice, such as how to deal with an aggressive patient or how to act when faced with medical errors.

Annotated literature

Silverman, J., Kurtz, S., and Draper, J. (2005). *Skills for communicating with patients*, 2nd edn. Oxford/San Francisco: Radcliffe Publishing.

This is one of two companion books on improving communication in medicine which together provide a comprehensive approach to teaching and learning communication skills at all levels of medical education and in both specialist and family medicine. This is considered the standard book on communication skills teaching throughout the world. The complete book is evidence based with many references.

Kurtz, S., Silverman, J., and Draper, J. (2005). *Teaching and learning communication skills in medicine*, 2nd edn. Oxford/San Francisco: Radcliffe Publishing; 2005.

This is the second of the two companion books referred to above. Where the emphasis in the first book is more on the content of communication during a doctor–patient contact, the emphasis here is on how to plan, construct, and develop a programme in communication skills.

References

Bishop, J. M., Fleetwood-Walker, P., Wishart, E., Swire, H., Wright, A. D., and Green, I. D. (1981). Competence of medical students in history taking during the clinical course. *Medical Education* **15**, 368–72.

Blok, G. A., van Dalen, J., Jager, K. J., Ryan, M., Wijnen, R. M., Wight, C., et al. (1999). The European Donor Hospital Education Programme (EDHEP): addressing the training needs of doctors and nurses who break bad news, care for the bereaved, and request donation. *Transpl Int.* **12(3)**, 161–7.

Bokken, L. (2009). *Innovative use of simulated patients for educational purposes*. Thesis, FHML Maastricht, Datawyse.

Cook, D. A., and Brown, L. M. (1997). Skakun EN factors which influence the outcome of student evaluation of teaching. In: A. J. J. A. Scherpbier, C. P. M. van der Vleuten, J. J. Rethans, A. F. W. van der Steeg (eds), *Advances in medical education*. Dordrecht: Kluwer Academic.

Van Dalen, J., Zuidweg, J., and Collet, J. (1989). The curriculum of communication skills at Maastricht medical school. *Medical Education* **23**, 55–61.

Diemers, A. D., Dolmans, D. H., van Santen, M., van Luijk, S. J., Janssen-Noordman, A. M., and Scherpbier, A. J. (2007). Students' perceptions of early patient encounters in a PBL curriculum: a first evaluation of the Maastricht experience. *Medical Teacher* **29(2–3)**, 135–42.

Dolmans, D. H., Wolfhagen, I. H., Schmidt, H. G., and van der Vleuten, C. P. (1994). A rating scale for tutor evaluation in a problem-based curriculum: validity and reliability. *Medical Education* **28(6)**, 550–8.

Flaherty, J. A. (1985). Education and evaluation of interpersonal skills. In: A. G. Rezler and A. Flaherty (eds) *The interpersonal dimension in medical education*. New York: Springer Verlag.

Gijselaers, W. H. (1988). *Kwaliteit van het onderwijs gemeten: studies naar de betrouwbaarheid, validiteit en bruikbaarheid van studentenoordelen.* [*Measuring quality of education: studies of reliability, validity and feasiblity of student judgements.*] Dissertation, Maastricht, University Press.

Helfer, R. E. (1970). An objective comparison of the pediatric interview skills of freshman and senior medical students. *Pediatrics* **45**, 623–7.

Kaplan, S. H., Greenfield, S., and Ware, J. E. (1989). Assessing the effects of physician-patient interactions on the outcomes of chronic disease. *Medical Care* **27**, S110–27.

Kraan, H. F., and Crijnen, A. (1987). *The Maastricht history taking and advice checklist: studies of instrumental utility.* Dissertation, Maastricht, University Press.

Levine, J. H. (1995). Who will teach the skills of history taking and physical examination? *Teaching and Learning in Medicine* **5**, 77–8.

Poole, A. D., and Sanson-Fisher, R. W. (1979). Understanding the patient: a neglected aspect of medical education. *Social Science in Medicine* **13A**(1), 37–43.

Reames, H. R. Jr., and Dunstone, D. C. (1989). Professional satisfaction of physicians. *Archives of Internal Medicine* **149**(9), 1951–6.

Shapiro, R. S., Simpson, D. E., Lawrence, S. L., Talsky, A. M, Sobocinski, K. A., Schiedermayer, D. L. (1989). A survey of sued and nonsued physicians and suing patients. *Archives of Internal Medicine* **149**(10), 2190–6.

Van Dalen, J., Prince, C. J. A. H., Scherpbier, A. J. J. A., and van der Vleuten, C. P. M. (1998). Evaluating communication skills. *Advances in Health Sciences Education* **3**, 187–95.

Van Dalen, J., Bartholomeus, P., Kerkhofs, E., Lulofs, R., van Thiel J, Rethans, J. J., et al. (2001). Teaching and assessing communication skills in Maastricht: the first twenty years. *Medical Teacher* **23**(3), 245–51.

Van Dalen, J., Kerkhofs, E., van Knippenberg-van den Berg, B. W., van den Hout, H. A., Scherpbier, A. J., and van der Vleuten, C. P. (2002). Longitudinal and concentrated communication skills programmes: two Dutch medical schools compared. *Advances in Health Sciences Education: Theory and Practice* **7**(1), 29–40.

Van Thiel, J., Kraan, H. F., and van der Vleuten, C. P. M. (1991). Reliability and feasibility of measuring medical interviewing skills: the revised Maastricht history taking and advice checklist, *Medical Education* **2**, 224–9.

Van Thiel, J., van der Vleuten, C. P. M., and Kraan, H. F. (1992). Assessment of medical interviewing skills: generalisability of scores using successive MAAS-versions. In: R. Harden, I. Hart, and H. Mulholland (eds), *Approaches to the assessment of clinical competence: Proceedings of the Fifth Ottawa Conference* (Dundee: Centre for Medical Education, University of Dundee, Scotland).

Chapter 12

Learning how to learn, teaching how to teach

Emmaline Brouwer and Marijke Kruithof

Theoretical considerations that support a problem-based learning (PBL) approach can be found in cognitive psychology and social constructivist learning theory (see Chapter 24). But theoretical support for a certain educational strategy does not make that strategy and its use self-evident to students. They are likely to need help to find the best way to function or perhaps even survive in an unfamiliar educational system radically different from anything they have come across before. One way to help students understand the underlying principles of PBL is to involve them in the design, implementation, and evaluation of their own education (see Chapter 19). Peer-assisted learning and near-peer teaching are other ways to do so. Such activities can also prepare students for their teaching roles as healthcare professionals. Finally, students can also be involved in faculty development programmes where they can contribute to the development of the educational competencies of their teachers.

Teaching students how to learn

One of the basic assumptions underlying PBL is that it can help students to learn how to learn and become lifelong self-directed learners. Students obviously have prior knowledge and learning skills on entering university, but their preferred ways of studying were developed in secondary education and may not be appropriate for the type of learning required of them in a PBL medical school, where the subject matter is much more extensive and complex and they receive less guidance from teachers. Medical educators have tried to ease this transition for students by describing the required learning skills in accessible language. Such resources can be used as required reading for all students or recommended to interested students (Evans & Brown, 2009, Moust et al., 2007). Maastricht University's Faculty of Health, Medicine and Life Sciences (FHML) has also designed introductory assignments and units for all students to facilitate this process. For students who experience sustained difficulties with the transition from secondary to medical school, student advisors offer individual coaching and remedial teaching workshops.

Yet discussions with 'experienced' students in tutorial groups, education debates, and workshops have indicated time and again that the rationale of the PBL process is largely unknown to students or only partially understood, even though the 'correct' procedures are being followed, with more or less enthusiasm, depending on the dynamics of a student group. The role of the tutor is regularly singled out as one of the reasons students have difficulty grasping the rationale of PBL. This may indeed be the case, as is discussed in more detail in Chapter 6. Another reason given by students is that PBL is explained to them at a point in the curriculum when it is still difficult for them to understand the relevance of the theory. Also, the way in which it is explained may not mesh with their prior knowledge and learning needs.

In order to remedy this unsatisfactory state of affairs a longitudinal programme was developed to give students insight into the principles underlying PBL. This programme has been designed in close cooperation with a group of interested and motivated senior students (Box 12.1). In the future, parts of it will be taught by senior students taking part in the bachelor honours programme in education in health, medicine and life sciences (Box 12.4).

Box 12.1 Principles of PBL in year 1

The current curriculum of the first unit (Unit 1.1) starts with an introductory week. Since 2008, students have been offered several additional learning activities during the first year (one in each of the six units) that deal with different topics related to the theory underpinning PBL.

The formats are chosen for their possibilities to actively involve students in the learning process and help them draw the necessary conclusions.

Unit 1.1 'Point of entry, point of (no) return?'
Two-hour workshops for groups of thirty to forty students, facilitated by a team of a staff member and a senior student. A series of interactive exercises and reflections give rise to discussion of the following topics: *triggers*, *prior knowledge*, *brainstorming*, *schemata*, and *mind maps*.

Unit 1.2 'Scaffolds and safety nets'
An exercise based on three cases related to the topics of the second unit. This activity is carried out during a regular tutorial group session and reminds students of the topics discussed in the first unit and adds the idea of *scaffolding*.

Unit 1.3 'Surfing USA or deep sea diving'
Two-hour workshops as in the first unit in which students can practise drawing mind maps and concept maps and discover their different uses. Exercises also focus on *different learning styles: superficial (rote) learning ←→ deep learning (understanding)*.

Unit 1.4 'Two left hands?'
The structure of a regular skills training session is adapted to guide students to focus on *the similarities of and differences between learning skills and learning theory*.

Unit 1.5 Because of the many official holidays and examinations during this period of the year, no additional activity is planned in this unit.

Unit 1.6 'Practise what you preach'
Two-hour workshops like those in the first unit. The exercises and reflections in these workshops concentrate on the importance of the *context of learning* and the *transfer of learning*.

Learning how to learn

The most obvious way in which students learn with and from each other is in the tutorial groups. The method used in these groups is a type of reciprocal teaching in which students take turns as teacher and learner in a relatively informal way (Ten Cate & Durning, 2007a). By discussing their prior knowledge about the problems presented to them they explore, expand, and accommodate existing knowledge frameworks. When reporting back on the results of their self-study activities, the repetition of the information they have found and the elaboration of their findings during the ensuing discussion with their peers helps them form more explicit and longer lasting connections between prior and newly acquired knowledge (see Chapter 3). Similar processes take place during skills training when students practise in pairs or small groups, giving each other feedback and receiving feedback from the supervising skills teacher. At the Skillslab of FHML this approach was recently formalized in skills training sessions where students repeat a procedure they have learned earlier (e.g., the third year session on the pelvic examination, which refreshes skills from sessions in the second year) by taking turns in instructing one or two other students how to perform a part of the procedure (Box 12.2).

The way students prepare for tutorial sessions and skills training can also serve as an example for the other students in the group, both in a positive and in a negative way. Social cohesion and social control are important elements that can foster positive role modelling. In even less formal ways students can help each other learn by practicing together in the library, pointing out useful resources on the discussion board of the electronic learning environment, or training for skills examinations with each other. The FHML medical student association regularly organizes evening sessions in which clerkship students help junior students to improve their clinical skills. The association also proposed a 'trial OSCE' (Objective Structured Clinical Examination) to enable students to experience the procedure before the real event.

Box 12.2 Third year skills training session 'pelvic examination' in a peer-assisted learning (PAL) format

In the second year students are offered three ninety-minute training sessions in performing a pelvic examination. The first session focuses mainly on speculum examination, the second on bimanual examination, and the third on cases about sexually transmitted diseases (STD), which students are studying in the synchronous tutorial groups, to combine the two examinations and introduce the PAP smear for STD testing.

This final ninety-minute training session on the pelvic examination is part of the third year cluster 'abdomen' and introduces the PAP smear in addition to offering students one last chance to practise the total procedure on a manikin before an individual training session, one or two days later, in which they perform a pelvic examination on a patient-instructor under supervision of a skills teacher. These training sessions prepare the students for their patient contact in the teaching outpatient clinic in gynaecology and obstetrics in the same or the following week (see also Box 12.3).

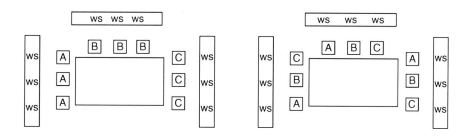

Students are grouped around a central table, with workbenches behind each group on which are arranged two or three workstations (ws) with a gynaecological model, a lamp and all the gynaecological equipment needed for this examination. After a brief introduction of the format of the session the students work in groups of three or four to prepare for teaching other students the different parts of the pelvic examination. Group A prepares to teach external

Box 12.2 Third year skills training session 'pelvic examination' in a peer-assisted learning (PAL) format *(continued)*

inspection and speculum examination, group B bimanual examination, and group C the PAP smear and KOPAC classification. As the latter is a new topic the skills teacher gives special attention to this group, but is also available for answering questions and correcting mistakes and misconceptions in the other groups.

After about twenty minutes the groups split up and new groups are formed composed of one student from each of the previous groups. Student A starts teaching students B and C about the external examination until the speculum is in place. Student C then takes over and explains about the PAP smear and KOPAC classification. Student A then finishes his/her part by teaching how to remove the speculum and carry out the final inspection of the vagina. Student B rounds off the session by teaching students A and C about the bimanual examination. While the students are teaching each other, the skills teacher is available for questions and supervises the groups. The session is rounded off with a summary of the whole procedure with special attention to essential elements and common mistakes. Any remaining questions can also be answered at that point.

Teaching how to learn

A theme issue of *Medical Teacher* in 2007 highlighted the importance of different forms of peer teaching in medical education. Ten Cate and Durning (2007a) distinguish between peer-assisted learning (in which students of the same level and year teach each other), near-peer teaching (in which senior students teach junior students of the same level), and cross-level teaching (in which postgraduate students teach undergraduate students). They also pointed out the importance of role modelling by senior students of the dos and don'ts that are part of the unwritten rules of the 'hidden curriculum'. These are a frequent source of problems experienced by first-year students in the transition to medical school (Ten Cate & Durning, 2007b). The importance of this kind of learning from and with each other became apparent when a group of foreign students entered the FHML undergraduate curriculum in September 2007. This relatively small group followed a new English language programme and as a result they could not ask support from other students and were relatively isolated from the Dutch students. A 'buddy system' was set up, with second-year Dutch students taking a number of foreign students under their wings to remedy this problem.

Other examples of peer-assisted learning or near-peer teaching cited by Ten Cate and Durning (2007b) and other authors in the same issue of *Medical Teacher* focus on clinical skills teaching, anatomy classes, and tutorial groups. In these areas FHML has so far chosen not to work with students but to employ experienced and content expert staff as teachers. Ever increasing student numbers, however, have revived the discussion about what could be learned from other experiences in this area. This is even more pertinent as both theory and practical experiences point towards beneficial effects for both student-learners and student-teachers (Ten Cate & Durning, 2007). One way in which FHML has formalized peer teaching is in the coach group sessions in the third year (Diemers et al., 2007, 2008). Based on real patient consultations in the teaching outpatient clinic, students set learning goals which they pursue during self-study. Students report on the patient case and the outcome of their self-study to the other students in the next session of the coach group (Box 12.3). To most of the third-year students who attended the PBL workshops it was an eye-opener that this education format could actually be considered as 'peer teaching'. They had never realized that they might benefit more from the coach group sessions, if they took time to consider how they could make their presentations more interactive and better tailored to the group's learning needs. The practical placements in the bachelor honours programme during which students participate in the design, implementation, and/or evaluation of FHML education activities are also intended to give students a better understanding of the underlying principles of peer education activities (Box 12.4).

Box 12.3 Early patient encounters as starting point for PBL and peer teaching

One of the main aims of the 'new' curriculum launched at Maastricht medical school in 2001 was to offer students experiences with real patients earlier in the curriculum. In the first two years the PBL tutorials are still mainly based on paper cases, though video-tapes of real and simulated patients are also in use. In the first two units of the first year, students also participate in 'accident simulations' in the Skillslab. These experiences serve as starting points for learning in the tutorial groups and skills training sessions later in those units. In several other skills training sessions in the first two years real patients with chronic diseases and/or stable conditions after CVA are used to enable students to practise interviewing and clinical examination techniques in a group supervised by a skills teacher.

The overall theme of year 3 is 'chronic diseases' and the year is divided into four 'clusters' (instead of units): abdomen, circulation and lungs, locomotor system, and psychomedical problems and mental healthcare. The PBL cycle in the coach group tutorials in this year is based on encounters with real patients in the teaching outpatient clinics.

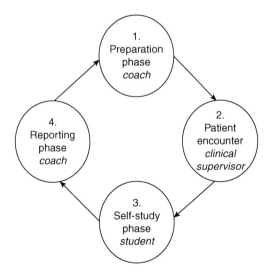

The preparation phase of the usual PBL cycle is split in two. In the preparation phase students discuss a number of vignettes similar to the patients they will see in the outpatient clinic and activate prior knowledge they might need during the patient contact. This is done in a coach group, a special kind of tutorial group facilitated by a coach who is a clinical teacher in one of the clinical domains related to the cluster. Then they go to the teaching outpatient clinic in pairs where they see a patient (history and physical examination) and discuss their

> **Box 12.3 Early patient encounters as starting point for PBL and peer teaching** *(continued)*
>
> findings with the clinical supervisor. After the clinical supervisor has finished the patient consultation and the patient has left, learning goals are generated which the students use as the basis for their self-study. In the following coach group meeting the students report back on the patient they have seen *and* on the results of their self-study. As all pairs in the group see different patients and generate different learning goals this is the moment when they become 'teachers' of their peers. They are the ones with the 'expert knowledge' on that specific case and the students will need that information just as much as the information they have gathered about the patients they interviewed and examined in order to pass the examinations at the end of the cluster.
>
> For a more detailed description of this programme see Diemers et al. (2007, 2008).

Learning how to teach

The Latin word 'doctor' means teacher and the roles of 'communicator', 'health advocate', and 'scholar' in the CanMEDS competency framework (Frank, 2005) also emphasize the importance of teaching, as do the references to physicians as patient educators and teachers of future generations of health professionals in other competency frameworks (GMC, 2003; Metz et al., 2001). Yet until recently this topic had received very little attention in undergraduate education. Dandavino et al. (2007) reviewed the (medical) education literature and found reports on three main issues:

1 That students with a better understanding of teaching and learning principles can become better learners themselves;
2 That students can be better patient educators as future professionals; and
3 That students will have teaching roles as future residents and clinical teachers.

It is these latter two points, which fit under the heading of *learning how to teach*, that are the main focus of the bachelor honours programme 'education in health, medicine and life sciences' (Box 12.4). Even though most medical schools in the Netherlands offer some kind of faculty development programme, it was not until a few years ago that interfaculty agreement was reached on a basic teaching qualification that will be recognized nationally (see Chapter 18). At present, only Utrecht University Medical Centre offers a parallel training programme to students, enabling them to earn a similar qualification. Other faculties offer specific training courses for teaching roles undertaken by students (student-tutor, student-assistant in lab practicals or anatomy training, assistant skills teacher). From the academic year 2009–10, FHML offers a bachelor honours programme for all interested students in the second and third years of the regular bachelor programme. During the first year of the honours programme students are provided a general overview of teaching and learning theories, strategies, and methodologies. In the second year students are encouraged to pursue more in depth a topic of their choice by combining a literature review, practical placement, and honours thesis supervised by an experienced medical teacher.

Box 12.4 Honours Programme Education in Health, Medicine and Life Sciences (FHML-HPEd)

The FHML-HPEd offers motivated and talented students the opportunity to broaden and deepen their knowledge in the field of education. It is a two-year programme running parallel with the regular second- and third-year programmes of all of the four FHML bachelor programmes and started in September 2009 with a first group of students.

In the first year of the honours programme students will be given a broad overview of the following themes and topics:

Implementation		Evaluation		Design	
Teaching and learning	Roles of the teacher	Student assessment	Programme evaluation	Developing learning materials	Course/ curriculum design
Context of learning		Educational research methodology		Instructional design process	

The main format for the first year is 'expert meetings': Three-hour evening sessions with local or external staff with specialized knowledge in these areas. The format will be either interactive lectures or workshops.

Students prepare for these plenary sessions through self-study (literature review) and discussions in small groups (Ox-Bridge 'tutorials': three to four students with one tutor). Students undertake three short placements which will introduce them to the roles of the teacher in the three main areas: design, implementation, and evaluation of educational programmes. Where possible these placements will run parallel with the themes of the expert meetings.

In the second year of HPEd students work more independently to acquire a more profound understanding of a chosen topic. They are supervised by a coach or mentor. To achieve efficiency within the limited time available, students are encouraged to choose the same—or at least a similar—topic for their (long) placement, literature review, and/or honours thesis. The course in writing scientific English will be timed to give students the opportunity to receive feedback on their thesis while following the course.

In both years students are stimulated to participate in any of the activities organized by the School of Health Professions Education (SHE) and the Department of Educational Research and Development of FHML, which are open to outside participation and relevant to the honours programme (e.g., visitors' workshops, summer course, MHPE thesis presentations, thematic lunches). Exchange programmes with other faculties in the Netherlands and elsewhere that are also active in this field will also be part of the programme.

This is a two-year programme which runs parallel to the regular second and third year of all four FHML programmes (Medicine, Health Sciences, Molecular Life Sciences, and European Public Health).

Teaching how to teach

In a recent teacher training workshop it was suggested that the well-known Miller's pyramid (knows → knows how → shows → does) should be extended, on top, by two additional levels: 'teaches' and 'teaches teachers' (Miller et al. 1990). This would also complete the continuum referred to in the title of this chapter: from *learning how to learn* to *teaching how to teach*. Although it seems an unlikely role for students to teach teachers, they can actually contribute to this. For, in the same way in which simulated patients can be used to train students how to communicate with patients, simulated students can contribute to the training of teachers (Pasquale & Cukor, 2007). At FHML simulated students make an important contribution to the visitors' workshops, the Master of Health Professions Education (MHPE) programme, and in-house teacher training courses for clinical teachers.

Within the quality assurance system of FHML students are regularly surveyed about different aspects of the education programme (see Chapter 17). On top of this, each year group appoints a student evaluation committee (SEC), which gives narrative feedback based on comments received from other students. Some years ago a system was developed in which specially trained student-coaches give feedback to lecturers on their performance (Stalmeijer & de Grave, 2008) (Box 12.5).

Box 12.5 Observation of and feedback on teaching by students

Chapter 19 gives extensive descriptions of the way in which students at FHML are involved in evaluating educational activities. Besides regular formalized feedback through evaluation questionnaires, students also give narrative feedback through the Student Evaluation Committees (SEC) in each year group. The Skillslab evaluation committee gives more specific feedback on the skills training programme.

Since 2007 the students on these committees have attended a special training course to learn how to give more concrete and detailed feedback to individual teachers about lectures and/or practicals. The course provides them with background information about PBL and discusses criteria for analyzing teacher performance based on video-taped examples. The students also receive extra training in giving feedback and how to deal with awkward situations that may arise when they are giving feedback to staff.

They then use the acquired knowledge and skills to evaluate the educational activities they attend in the course of the regular curriculum. Before evaluating a lecture, they introduce themselves to the lecturer and ask whether there are any specific points on which the teacher wishes to receive feedback. After the lecture the students give oral feedback and a couple of days later they also send written feedback to the lecturer.

A first evaluation of this process (Stalmeijer & de Grave, 2008) has shown that both students and staff judged that it was a positive and important innovation that could help to improve the teaching skills of the staff. The teachers also acknowledged that the students were able to give concrete and specific feedback. Not all teachers found it easy to accept feedback from students, though, and it is considered advisable to schedule more time for students and staff to talk about the process before and after the lecture. Another suggestion for improvement was to add observation by peers and/or education experts to make it possible to validate and triangulate the student feedback.

In conclusion

Student involvement in the design and evaluation of the education process has been a key element of the PBL curriculum at Maastricht University from the days of its foundation in the mid-seventies of the past century until the present day (see Chapter 15). But even these active and motivated students are not always well informed with regard to the theoretical underpinnings of the PBL process. In educational debates and PBL workshops these students have expressed their need for better communication with all students on this topic. FHML has so far always managed to recruit a sufficient number of motivated and capable tutors and teachers to facilitate small-group tutorials, teach lab practicals, and run skills training. But ever-increasing numbers of students are putting a noticeable strain on the system. Furthermore, theoretical proof of the benefits of (near-)peer teaching provides another reason for increasing the involvement of students in the education process. These students would also benefit from teacher training courses like those developed for the faculty development programme (see Chapter 18).

Over the past years a number of initiatives have strengthened the existing PBL process and introduced new ways of teaching and learning. This chapter offers but a sample of these developments and as education seems to be slowly coming out of the shadows of research and service, hopefully many more such initiatives will be developed in the near future.

Annotated literature

Moust, J. H. C., Bouhuijs, P. A. J., and Schmidt, H.G. (2007). *Introduction to problem-based learning: A guide for students*. Groningen: Wolters Noordhoff.
Most recent edition of the English language version of the book used to introduce problem-based learning to first year students at Maastricht University. A real 'primer' on helping students 'learn how to learn'.

Dandavino, M., Snell, L., and Wiseman, J. (2007). Why medical students should learn how to teach. *Medical Teacher* **29**, 558–65.
Extensive literature review about this topic (Medline 1966-2006; CINAHL 1982-2006; ERIC 1966–2006). Three main answers emerge:

1 Medical students are future residents and faculty members and will have teaching roles;

2 Medical students can become more effective communicators as a result of such training as teaching is an essential aspect of physician–patient interaction; and

3 Medical students with a better understanding of teaching and learning principles may become better learners.

Ten Cate, O., and Durning, S. (2007). Dimensions and psychology of peer teaching in medical education. *Medical Teacher* **29**, 546–52.
An article in a special issue on peer teaching in medical education, focussing on the categorization of different forms of peer teaching and discussing the theoretical framework for peer teaching from two different viewpoints: comparing the cognitive and social-psychological perspective and comparing the benefits for student-learners versus student-teachers.

Ten Cate, O., and Durning, S. (2007). Peer teaching in medical education: Twelve reasons to move from theory to practice. *Medical Teacher* **29**, 591–9.
An article in a special issue on peer teaching in medical education, reviewing reports on peer teaching in the medical education literature in 2006, giving an overview of twelve distinct reasons to apply peer teaching identified in the reviewed literature.

References

Dandavino, M., Snell, L., and Wiseman, J. (2007). Why medical students should learn how to teach. *Medical Teacher* **29**, 558–65.
Diemers, A. D., Dolmans, D. H. J. M., van Santen, M., van Luijk, S.J., Janssen-Noordman, A. M. B., and Scherpbier, A. J. J. A. (2007). Students' perceptions of early patient encounters in a PBL curriculum: a first evaluation of the Maastricht experience. *Medical Teacher* **29**, 135–42.

Diemers, A. D., Dolmans, D. H. J. M., Verwijnen, M. G. M., Heineman, E., and Scherpbier, A. J. J. A. (2008). Students' opinions about the effects of preclinical patient contacts on their learning. *Advances in Health Sciences Education, Theory and Practice* **13**, 633–47.

Evans, D., and Brown, J. (2009). *How to succeed at medical school: an essential guide to learning*. Oxford: Wiley-Blackwell.

Frank, J. R. (ed.) (2005). *The CanMEDS 2005 Physician Competency Framework*. Available at http://rcpsc. medical.org/canmeds/CanMEDS2005/CanMEDS2005_e.pdf

General Medical Council (2003). *Tomorrow's doctors*. London: General Medical Council.

Metz, J. C. M., Verbeek-Weel, A. M. M., and Huisjes, H. J. (eds) (2001). *Raamplan 2001*. Nijmegen, Mediagroep. Available at http://www.vsnu.nl/Universiteiten/Publicaties.htm (retrieved 5 November 2009).

Miller, G. E. (1990). The assessment of clinical skills / competence / performance. *Academic Medicine* **65**, S63–7.

Moust, J. H. C., Bouhuijs, P. A. J., and Schmidt, H. G. (2007). *Introduction to problem-based learning: A guide for students*. Groningen: Wolters Noordhoff.

Pasquale, J. S., and Cukor, J. (2007). Collaboration of junior students and residents in a teacher course for senior medical students. *Medical Teacher* **29**, 572–6.

Stalmeijer, R., and de Grave, W. (2008). De student als observator en feedbackgever voor docenten. *Tijdschrift voor Medisch Onderwijs* **27**, 247–56. (Observation of and feedback on teaching by students: process evaluation. *Dutch Journal of Medical Education*.)

Ten Cate, O. (2007). A teaching rotation and a student teaching qualification for senior medical students. *Medical Teacher* **29**, 566–71.

Ten Cate, O., and Durning, S. (2007). Dimensions and psychology of peer teaching in medical education. *Medical Teacher* **29**, 546–52.

Chapter 13

E-learning in problem-based learning

Jeroen Donkers, Daniëlle Verstegen, Bas de Leng, and Nynke de Jong

Whether e-learning should be used in problem-based learning (PBL) is no longer an issue. Information and communication technology (ICT) has entered all aspects of our world, including education. The real questions are why, when, and how e-learning should be used. There are many reasons for opting for e-learning. It can enable learning activities that would otherwise not be feasible, such as practising risky procedures and the collaboration of students and staff at different locations. E-learning can make learning activities more efficient or more effective, for example by providing multimedia resources to students in tutorial groups or during self-study, by enabling students to reflect on the recorded performance of themselves and other students, or by automatically providing individual feedback (on relatively simple learning tasks) to large groups of students. E-learning can also be used to overcome practical problems. For example, using e-learning, a staff member can deliver a lecture while on sabbatical leave and students in a distance learning programme can participate in on-campus activities.

Introduction

The term 'e-learning' is used in many different ways in spoken and in written language. In this chapter, a broad interpretation is adopted, suited to the context of PBL. In this interpretation, e-learning refers to the use of software to:

A. Support the learning of specific knowledge and skills;

B. Support communication and group work; and

C. Support assessment and reflection.

The specific reason for employing e-learning determines whether its implementation can be deemed successful: if the goal is to enable distance learning, the criterion for success is whether the learning of the students in the distance course is comparable to that of the students in the on-campus programme. If the goal is to overcome defects or gaps in an existing curriculum, the criterion is improvement of students' learning. Experience has shown that saving money or staff time is generally not a very good reason for adopting e-learning. The development of programs, the maintenance of hardware and software, the training of teaching staff, and the additional effort required to manage e-learning activities usually cost as much as one can hope to save. A more efficient use of time, however, can be a valid reason: with e-learning, teaching staff can engage in teaching activities at a convenient time rather than at the time scheduled for a face-to-face session. When students come better prepared to a session as a result of e-learning, the precious (expensive) time of tutors and teachers can be spent on difficult questions, discussions, reflections, and other activities that promote in-depth learning.

In this chapter, examples of each of the three categories of the use of e-learning are given in order to illustrate the experiences with e-learning at the Maastricht Faculty of Health, Medicine and Life Sciences (FHML). Each section ends with a short reflection. At the end of the chapter advantages and potential disadvantages of e-learning in a PBL environment are discussed and a peek into the future of e-learning in PBL is offered. This chapter does not pretend to give an exhaustive overview of e-learning, nor does it describe its most advanced forms. In many cases, FHML has adopted e-learning to support and enhance existing learning activities, not to radically restructure the curriculum.

Supporting the learning of specific knowledge or skills

This section focuses on four ways in which e-learning can support students in learning specific knowledge or skills: learning objects, virtual patients, virtual reality, and gaming. The concept of learning objects is illustrated by a description of virtual slides. Various aspects of virtual patients are presented, including their use in the development of clinical reasoning skills. And, finally, virtual reality and gaming are described briefly.

Learning objects for specific domains

Digital resources for learning are often called learning objects. Specific learning objects can support or (partly) replace a book or a training session. An example within FHML is virtual slides for lab practicals in microscopy (Figure 13.1). Virtual slides are digitally scanned microscopic images of tissue samples that can be browsed online like the maps of Google Earth. They are easier to use than real tissue samples, because fewer facilities are needed. Another advantage is that virtual slides remain accessible to students after lab sessions. Furthermore, all students can study exactly the same tissue sample. This makes for a far more efficient use of time during sessions. Virtual slides are also used during group activities (see below under 'Supporting communication and group work').

Other examples of learning objects are simulations of complex physiological processes using mathematical models that mimic the behaviour of (part of) a living system. For instance, the program 'Weight' was developed at Maastricht University to model global body composition

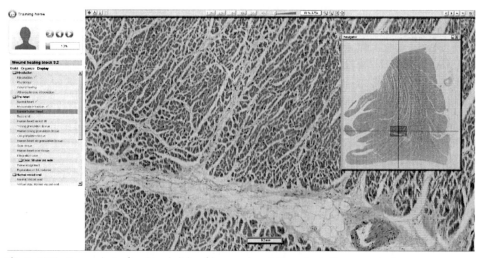

Figure 13.1 Screenshot of a virtual slide of human heart tissue including a navigator pane.

in terms of fat and lean body mass as a function of food intake and energy use by activity (Westerterp et al., 1995). Such a model allows students to experiment with and reason about complex processes.

An increasing number of learning objects, ranging from multimedia materials to entire lessons or modules, is available for free. Examples of open or subscription-based repositories in the medical domain are medischonderwijs.nl (in Dutch),[1] MedEdPortal,[2] MedEdWorld,[3] IviMeds,[4] Open Education,[5] and general sources like Wikipedia. These repositories can be used by teachers but also by students for self-directed study, in line with the PBL principle that students should be stimulated to find a varied set of resources for themselves.

Virtual patients

Traditionally, the presentation of paper patient cases in PBL has been enhanced by the use of audiovisual materials, such as pictures or videos of patients, X-rays, and audio files of a patient's breathing. Virtual patients are interactive electronic medical cases that offer additional support for learning.[6] Depending on the type of virtual patient system, feedback on the students' decisions can consist of pre-entered texts, comparison of students' decisions with those of an expert at the end of a diagnostic cycle, or simulation of the effects of students' diagnostic and management decisions. Virtual patients can provide an authentic practice setting to support contextual learning, as is done in the simulated consultations on nutrition developed by Maiburg et al. (2003) for general practitioners. A range of software packages for constructing and using virtual patients has been developed. They all support the development of case-based simulations, but differ in many ways. Some are elaborate and take a lot of time, allowing students to study complex situations. Others are fairly simple and short, so that students can study many different cases, which can foster a better understanding of a standard population with similar complaints. At Maastricht University the latter scenario is being explored in the domain of diabetes to help students grasp the—difficult—probabilistic relations between certain complaints and background factors.

Some virtual patient systems present cases with a timeline, allowing students to study how their actions affect the course of a patient's problem. Others are less time dependent, such as virtual patients aimed at the acquisition of clinical reasoning skills (cf. de Leng et al., 2009a). Many virtual patients are primarily developed for self-study or assessment, but other scenarios are thinkable. The following uses of virtual patients are explored at Maastricht University: a replacement of paper-based cases in PBL sessions, online or offline group discussions to stimulate clinical reasoning, preparation for skills training or communication training, and reflection during clerkships. In principle, all PBL cases can be presented as virtual patients, as is done elsewhere. Maastricht University has not gone so far yet, because of the potential consequences for the educational concept and the discussion in tutorial groups. de Leng et al. (2007) examined ways to apply video cases as authentic stimuli in PBL.

---

[1] http://www.medischonderwijs.nl
[2] http://www.aamc.org/mededportal
[3] http://www.mededworld.org
[4] http://www.ivimeds.org
[5] http://opened.creativecommons.org
[6] For an overview of recent research on virtual patients, see Cook & Tirola (2009), Roterman-Koniecza (2009), and http://www.virtualpatients.eu.

Virtual reality and gaming

Serious gaming can be said to occur whenever a learning event is enhanced by the introduction of a game factor. At FHML, serious games involve role playing and standardized and simulated patients. They can, but do not have to, be combined with virtual reality. Virtual reality techniques can also be used to extend simulations and virtual patients by simulating not only the relevant processes but also—as much as possible—aspects of the environment. A virtual reality environment like the popular 'Second Life' can simulate the physical appearance of the patient, the room, the team members, and of course, the student. Virtual reality technologies have already led to low-cost applications in molecular biology[7] and anatomy,[8] which have found their way (almost) to the FHML curriculum.

A word on e-learning to support the learning of specific knowledge or skills

There are many potential benefits from the use of e-learning to support learning. E-learning can, for example:

- Offer enriched and more authentic study materials;
- Offer the possibility of selecting from a large collection of learning objects;
- Offer individualized feedback and learning paths; and
- Provide a controlled and safe environment for practising tasks or preparing for face-to-face activities

etc.

It should be noted, however, that e-learning is not always the best idea. Experience at FHML has shown, for instance, that the majority of (on-campus) students will attend lectures even if these are recorded and made available online. One might question, therefore, whether it is worth the expense to record all lectures and make them available online, especially when, unlike the face-to-face lecture, the recorded lecture offers no provisions for asking questions or discussion. Obviously, the situation is different where distance-learning students or lecturers from other universities are concerned.

With more advanced forms of e-learning, such as virtual reality and advanced games, cost is an important consideration. Development is very expensive in terms of both money and domain experts' time. Other solutions are often cheaper. There are also indications that increased realism does not necessarily lead to enhanced learning (cf. Bayne, 2008). Students can be distracted and heavily disturbed by near-perfect reality, whereas clearly imperfect reality can lead to a higher perception of authenticity and greater learning gain.

Careless use of e-learning can be detrimental to the PBL concept, for instance when existing e-learning solutions originally developed for individual learning are used. When teaching staff enthusiastically add existing e-learning materials (lessons or training packages) to a course, students may be tempted to limit their self-study to those materials. If that happens, all students study the same materials and there will be less discussion, which can hamper the occurrence of deep learning processes in the tutorial group. Another illustration is the use of virtual slides, as described earlier. Before virtual slides were available, pairs of students shared one microscope which guaranteed some form of collaborative learning. After the introduction of virtual slides,

---

[7] As an example there are freely available 3D molecule viewers such as Cn3D: http://www.ncbi.nlm.nih.gov/Structure/CN3D/cn3d.shtml.

[8] E.g., http://www.visiblebody.com.

students worked individually at their own computers. To solve this problem, a shared whiteboard facility with chat facilities is currently being developed to enable students to jointly view and annotate virtual slides. Finally, some tutors have reported reduced interaction in tutorial groups when a computer and beamer are used for note-taking. They felt there was less discussion when all students were watching the screen (where the notes are shown) instead of looking at each other. The same holds for laptop use by students. The precise effects and possible solutions remain to be researched.

Supporting communication and group work

This section starts with a general discussion about the role of virtual learning environments. Next, some specific aspects of the role of e-learning in supporting group activities and online communication are described and, finally, a brief glimpse into the future of Web 2.0 for education is offered.

The role of a virtual learning environment in problem-based learning

In present-day PBL, a virtual learning environment (VLE) plays an important role. Maastricht University uses a localized version of Blackboard (see also Chapter 20). For students and teaching staff, the VLE is the central point of curricular information. It contains specific course information, such as schedules, assignments, learning materials, resources, and an e-reader with important literature (provided by the university library). It also contains more general information, such as references to handbooks, specifications of procedures for general medical skills (e.g. VIG online[9]), and links to information on the Internet.

Consistency in the structure and layout of courses is stimulated by the provision of templates. Experience has shown, however, that many staff members have difficulty filling and adapting templates, which makes it difficult for students to find information (de Leng et al., 2006). In the medical curriculum this problem has been solved by designating a staff member to tightly support the construction and use of course pages in the VLE, thereby enforcing a consistent structure and layout. Another useful measure is to explain to students at the start of each course where information can be found and how it is to be used during the course.

Supporting group activities

VLEs can support group work and communication in many ways. Currently, students (and teachers) use designated group spaces to record the results or minutes of group sessions, exchange information, and review each others' work. Discussion fora are used more or less extensively by students, sometimes on their own and sometimes moderated by teachers.

Discussion fora facilitate asynchronous collaboration and can be used for complex problem-solving tasks that require reflection. Advantages include the possibility of discussing specific topics, organizing the discussion in threads, and freezing the content of the discussion by archiving. Polaris (Ronteltap & Eurlings, 2002) is a discussion forum building block in Blackboard that was developed at Maastricht University to explicitly overcome some remaining barriers to collaborative knowledge construction. First, Polaris provides specific functionality for orientation and navigation to prevent information overload during intensive group work, for example the labelling of contributions, a clear structure, and the use of colours and icons to provide a quick overview of the various discussions and their status. Second, Polaris gives learners individual control of the distributed process, allowing them to manipulate the information in the community's workplace

---

[9] See www.vig-online.nl (in Dutch) or www.skillsinmedicine.nl.

and distribute and share the results of these manipulations. This enables interaction among students focused on distributed knowledge building rather than the mere exchange of information.

E-learning tools for supporting communication and group activities are not only useful for distance learning but also for preparing for or supporting face-to-face learning. An example being piloted at FHML is the use of discussion fora by students during clinical clerkships to reflect and prepare for group sessions. Another example is the use of online interactive feedback during face-to-fase practical sessions on diagnostic reasoning. A tool that collects log-data from a virtual patient system has been developed (de Leng et al., 2009b). It allows the teacher to quickly provide an overview of the choices made by students during a virtual patient session. This can focus the plenary discussion, e.g., on the diagnoses made or the tests omitted by the majority of the students.

Sometimes, the biggest advantage of e-learning tools is of a logistic nature. An example of this is the consultations of students and simulated patients that are discussed during practical sessions in communication skills training (Chapter 11). Formerly, the simulated patient encounters were videotaped and teachers and students had to go to the library to watch the tapes. Today, students and teachers can watch the encounters at their own workplace, because the encounters are automatically recorded, stored on a streaming media server, and made accessible online.

Supporting distance learning

There is an increasing demand for distance learning, for example from international students who attend (part of) a master course from their own country and professionals who combine (part-time) work and learning. In principle, the participation of students from different backgrounds and levels of experience can enrich PBL. It can lead to more elaborate discussions and richer information. PBL distance courses vary in the way they use media or e-learning tools for synchronous and asynchronous communication. Some courses combine distance learning with a limited number of face-to-face meetings in order to enable students and teaching staff to get to know each other and to provide skills training. This format is called blended-learning (B-learning).

Closest to 'traditional' PBL is web conferencing for synchronous communication in tutorial groups, as used in the master track in Health Services Innovation (HSI) (de Jong, 2009). This approach requires technical support and some skills from both students and tutors. Moreover, all students must be available at the same time (see Box 13.1).

An intermediate form of distance learning was applied in the course on Health Care in Europe (2005–6), delivered by Maastricht University to Swiss students in Aarau. The students in a tutorial group were divided into subgroups of three students, which used synchronous communication (chat, Skype, telephone) for the first five steps of the pre-analysis phase. Each subgroup placed their learning goals on Polaris for joint asynchronous discussion in the full group. At the end of the designated period (1.5 days in this case) the tutor filtered out the important learning goals and started a new discussion thread for each goal. The students then studied individually, placed information about their learning goals on the Polaris forum, and discussed their findings until all learning goals had been answered satisfactorily.

Collaborative learning, the next generation

Since the advent of Web 2.0, there has been a dramatic increase in the use of social software in daily life (such as Facebook), blogs (web logs), microblogs (e.g., Twitter), and wikis, especially by the so-called millennium kids or Generation Y. Web 2.0 tools open up new possibilities for online collaboration and may prove valuable for collaborative learning as well. Worldwide,

Box 13.1 Web conferencing in the HSI master

The masters in Health Services Innovation (HSI), a specialization of the masters in Public Health, is offered both full and part-time. The part-time version is offered as a blended learning course: students meet at least twice (at the beginning and at the end of a course). The tutorial groups are provided with web conferencing connections (see Figure 13.2). The VLE of Maastricht University is used to distribute literature, to exchange documents, and for discussion in the fora in Polaris. Recorded lectures are made available in the VLE as streaming video. Web conferencing is also used to enable distance students to attend lectures and presentations of their fellow students. In the 2008–9 academic year, eight Dutch students and seven German students participated in the HSI masters track. Most of the students combined the course with work. Students found it advantageous that they could see and hear each other during tutorial sessions with web conferencing. They appreciated that they did not have to do a great deal of travelling for the course and that they could occasionally invite others to participate in discussions. Web conferencing as such was not difficult for them, but there were technical problems, e.g., with headsets and webcams at home, and the connection was sometimes poor. Students also reported some disadvantages regarding communication patterns: there was not enough time and there was less discussion because they had to wait until someone else had stopped talking. It is more difficult to react spontaneously when you must wait your turn. The reactions to the online lectures were similar: easy to use, no travelling, and lectures could be replayed, but less optimal interaction. The lecturer could only see part of the students (those who attended) and asking questions was somewhat awkward (de Jong, 2009).

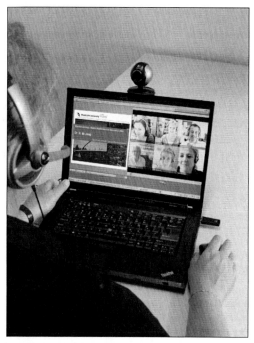

Figure 13.2 A web conferencing tutorial group.

there is a multitude of initiatives to introduce Web 2.0 tools into education.[10] Maastricht University is currently starting to implement the systematic use of some Web-2.0 facilities that are becoming available in Blackboard and most other VLEs: wikis, blogs, and virtual classrooms that combine web conferencing, chat, and document sharing.

A word on e-learning to support communication and group work

The availability of a VLE is quite standard nowadays even though some teaching staff remain somewhat reluctant to use it. However, even those who are prepared to work with VLEs often limit their use to minimal, standard options, for example to distribute information and hand in assignments. More advanced VLE facilities or other e-learning tools are used on a small scale only. This is a pity, because e-learning has a potentially important contribution to make to one of the main pillars of PBL: collaborative learning. E-learning can directly by supporting group work by providing shared workspaces and easy communication, or indirectly support better preparation for sessions and more efficient use of face-to-face time. One important aspect to keep in mind, however, is the workload of students and teaching staff, especially when they simultaneously attend different courses where different software packages, facilities, and use-scenarios are employed. The costs of new tools like blogs and wikis are low, but they require time, effort, and fast adaptation. One year too late, and the technology is out of fashion. It is not easy to foresee which will stay and become part of the mainstream.

E-learning is used extensively for distance learning in many ways. Since a wide range of factors influence the optimal scenario and use of media, it is advisable to carefully consider course goals and the target group of students, and to test any e-PBL design before it is implemented on a large scale. Literally translating a face-to-face concept to an e-learning format is unlikely to be the best solution in most cases, because any kind of mediation inevitably changes the interaction and communication among students and teachers. Moreover, the advantages and extra facilities can only be fully realized when pedagogical concepts are reconsidered carefully.

Supporting assessment

Assessment is an essential component of (problem-based) learning. A range of different ICT tools is used for student assessment within FHML. In this section, these ICT tools are considered as e-learning if they involve direct interaction with students. So, a separate item bank or test-construction tool is not considered e-learning, but an online test is. At FHML, e-learning tools are used for progress testing, case-based testing, workplace-based testing, and the reflective portfolio. (See Chapter 22 for a detailed description of how e-learning is applied to progress testing.)

Current developments point in a clear future direction: more and more information for formative and summative assessment will be collected electronically. In the future, this information may be integrated into a system that can provide student-tailored feedback and facilitate student-driven learning.

Computerized case-based testing (CCT)

The development of CCT at Maastricht University started in the 1990s (Schuwirth et al., 1996). The goal is to test the ability of students to apply knowledge quickly, especially concerning essential decision moments in medical practice. The system consists of a central authoring system/item bank and a student user-interface.

The CCT system offers short patient case descriptions, enhanced by authentic images or other materials. After reading a case, students answer a question, after which additional information on the case may be displayed. When new information has been shown, the student cannot return to

---

[10] See for instance http://www.wikieducator.org and http://web2educationuk.wetpaint.com.

the previous question. One case can contain several pieces of information and several questions. This approach allows for providing correct answers in between questions, which is not possible in a paper-based test. This is the first advantage of the system. Another advantage is that the results can be processed rapidly. CCT allows for the following types of questions: Multiple choice, correct-incorrect-don't know, long-list menu, and open questions. The latter must be checked manually. Other question types have been dismissed because case authors did not use them.

CCT is currently applied for summative assessment during the clerkships in years 4 and 5 of the medical curriculum. The cases are written by content specialists in a standard word processor. Each case is reviewed during a meeting of an educational expert, a medical expert, and two clinical specialists. After review, the case is entered into the item bank by an educationalist. An Angoff method is used to set a standard for each new case. When a case has been used for some time, the standard is revised based on an analysis of the collected scores. Individual case standards are used to set the combined standard for a test. The system records the time used by students to answer each question. This can be used to assess the quality and validity of questions (together with the collected scores). The system enables automatic test construction based on a blueprint.

Since the construction of cases is expensive, CCT is not used for formative assessment: the current set of cases is too small and students tend to become less motivated if they are confronted with the same case over and over. There is an additional use of the CCT system: in year 3 it is also used for summative assessment. Although the same structure is used, the items are not cases but focus on medical facts.

Portfolio

During the first and fifth year of the medical curriculum, students are asked to record their learning and development in a reflective portfolio. Until recently, the portfolios were paper-based. Since 2007, the Blackboard Content System has been used for the electronic portfolio in the first year. The main reason for switching to the electronic system was to diminish the paper flow and speed up procedures. So the electronic portfolio was restricted to a shoe-box of 'digitized paper'. As expected, however, multiple printouts are made of the portfolios, increasing the use of paper. More research is needed to investigate ways to use ICT more efficiently: helping students to plan, structure, and complete their portfolio, keeping track of versions and changes, and helping teachers to read, analyse, and assess the portfolios (Driessen et al., 2007).

Workplace-based testing

Workplace-based learning is closely related to PBL. After the first two years of the medical curriculum, PBL is increasingly supported by clinical (workplace) learning. Workplace-based learning is the core of postgraduate education. Problems related to workplace-based learning are the lack of structure and the measurement of progress. ICT can improve workplace-based learning by supporting workplace-based assessment and development portfolios.

Based on a system developed at Manchester University, the Manchester–Maastricht Test Service System (MMTSS)[11] is an online system to support workplace-based assessment during residency training (Govaerts et al., 2009). The core of the system is formed by electronic competency-based assessment forms and the feedback generation module. Feedback mainly consists of the development per competency as measured by the assessment forms. It is presented against the aggregated development of the peer group. MMTSS also supports multisource feedback. The MMTSS system has recently been extended to support the registration and reporting of activities. Reflection forms and other forms are added to the system to support a general development portfolio.

---

[11] The MMTSS system is called 'ePASS' as from April 2010. See www.epass-maastricht.nl.

Reflection on supporting assessment

Currently, not all assessments and reflection are supported by ICT and support by e-learning tools is rare. Although some parts of the assessment programme would be fairly easy to automate, automation of other parts is quite difficult mainly due to logistic and educational consequences.

The current danger in the use of e-learning for assessment and reflection is that many different systems are introduced independently. Information is stored at so many different places and in so many different formats that it is impossible for students, teachers, and advisors to keep track of a student's overall progress. The development of assessment programmes (see Chapter 21) should therefore include the development of supporting e-learning tools. If data collection is better aligned and linked, it becomes possible to provide not only a better overview to students and teachers but also tools for improving learning. For example, it would be possible to apply statistical and machine learning techniques to combined data to identify student patterns, weaknesses in the curriculum, and current trends. This knowledge can then be used to provide tailored feedback to students, staff, and school management.

Conclusions

E-learning is here to stay. This chapter has shown how more and more facets of the PBL curriculum of FHML are supported by e-learning. As students, staff, and management become increasingly aware of the opportunities of e-learning, the use of e-learning tools in the curriculum is bound to increase. At the same time, new emerging technologies, such as Web 2.0, gaming, and virtual reality simulations, are vying for attention and waiting to replace earlier generations of tools.

When applied wisely, e-learning can support PBL principles (contextual, collaborative, constructive, and self-directed learning) effectively and efficiently. It can potentially support collaboration and communication, enrich study materials, individualize feedback and learning paths, and offer more authentic situations and a controlled and safe environment to perform tasks or prepare for face-to-face activities. In general, it is not a good idea to transfer learning activities unchanged to a different medium. Plans for the implementation of e-learning call for a review of the entire instructional design and the learning activities designed for students. The question is not whether e-learning is good or bad; the real challenge lies in questions like:

- Can we use e-learning to make the tasks of students and/or staff easier?
- Can we use e-learning to enable learning activities that are not possible without technology?
- Can we use e-learning to improve learning by enhancing the pillars of PBL: constructive, contextual, collaborative, and self-directed learning?

There are, inevitably, also dangers and disadvantages to the use of e-learning. Apart from general concerns, such as costs and technical facilities, some specific concerns in relation to e-learning in PBL should be mentioned here. Especially in a non-discipline-based curriculum, the integration of course components is of the essence. Consequently, e-learning should be embedded in useful and structured learning activities, which must be linked to other parts of the curriculum. This means that teaching staff not only need (technical) skills to apply e-learning but also—and even more importantly—knowledge about the useful and purposeful implementation of the varied possibilities of e-learning in the curriculum as a whole.

A further complication is that, in the PBL curriculum of FHML, content is scattered over different courses, which are developed and taught by many different groups of staff members. It may therefore be hard to reach consensus on the purchase or development of—often quite expensive—e-learning applications. Of course, this problem does not apply to small learning objects for studying specific content or practising specific tasks; increasingly, these learning objects are available for free. Finding a suitable module or piece of software, however, is not always easy, because they are available in dispersed spaces and may not be clearly tagged. Once found, they are often not completely suitable and adjustment is needed. One specific issue in repurposing existing e-learning modules is that modules may be too directive, especially when they were not developed for PBL. Another issue is that students may become confused when many different e-learning modules or programs are used.

In order to prevent e-learning chaos and e-learning disasters, it is important that policy-makers incorporate e-learning into the entire educational system. E-learning should be on the list of topics to be addressed by those involved in designing a curriculum, an assessment programme, or a faculty development programme. The following questions need to be answered: Why do we need e-learning (does it really support our educational framework)? When do we need e-learning (probably not always)? How do we apply e-learning (what is the most effective way, preferably evidence-based)?

Annoted literature

Savin-Baden, M., and Wilkie, K. (eds) (2006). *Problem-based learning online*. Maidenhead: McGraw Hill.
 This book contains a collection of experiences with e-learning in the context of problem-based learning (in different domains).

Barab, S. A., Kling, B., and Gray, J. H. (eds) (2004). *Desiging virtual communities in the service of learning*. Cambridge: Cambridge University Press.

Beetham, E., and Sharpe, R. (eds) (2007). *Rethinking pedagogy for a digitial age—desining and delivering e-learning*. London: Routledge.

Clark, R. C., and Mayer, R.E. (2003). *E-learning and the science of instruction—proven guidelines for consumers and designers of multimedia learning*. San Francisco: Pfeiffer.

These three general books approach e-learning from an evidence-based position, which might be particular valid for the context of PBL.

An important journal in the area of e-learning that might be of interest for the readers interested in applying e-Learning in PBL is *Computers and Education* (Elsevier, ISSN 0360-1315), which is a general journal focusing on the application of ICT in a broad area of education. It contains both descriptive and experimental papers. Many journals focus on a specific aspect of e-learning. Good examples are: *American Journal of Distance Education* (Routledge, ISSN 1538-9286); *International Journal of Artificial Intelligence in Education* (IOS Press, ISSN 1560-4306); *International Journal of Computer-Supported Collaborative Learning* (Springer, ISSN 1556-1607).

References

Bayne, S (2008). Uncanny spaces for higher education: teaching and learning in virtual worlds. *Alt-J, Research in Learning Technology* **16**, 197–205.

Cook, D. A., and Tirola, M. M. (2009). Virtual patients: a critical literature review and proposed next steps. *Medical Education* **43**, 303–11.

Driessen, E. W., Muijtjens, A. M., van Tartwijk, J., and van der Vleuten, C. P. M. (2007). Web- or paper-based portfolios: is there a difference? *Medical Education* **41**, 1067–73.

Govaerts, M., Donkers, J., Brackel, H., Verhoeven, B., van der Vleuten, C., and Dornan, T. (2009). Making sense of competency-based assessment in the workplace through the use of an e-portfolio. *AMEE 2009*, short communication.

de Jong, N. (2009). Blended learning—HSI: Study year 2008–2009. Paper presented at the preconference of SURFonderwijsdagen 2008.

de Leng, B. A., Dolmans, D. H. J. M., Muijtjens, A. M. M., and van der Vleuten, C. P. M. (2006). Student perceptions of a virtual learning environment for a PBL undergraduate medical curriculum. *Medical Education* **40**, 568–75.

de Leng, B. A., Dolmans, D., van de Wiel, M., Muijtjens, A. M. M., and van der Vleuten, C. P. M. (2007). How video cases should be used as authentic stimuli in problem-based medical education. *Medical Education* **41**, 181–8.

de Leng, B. A., Donkers, J., Brasch, C., Huwendiek, S., and Kononowicz, A. A. (2009a). Evaluation instruments to support educators in making deliberate choices when they use virtual patients to teach clinical reasoning (International Conference of Virtual Patients, Kraków, Poland, 2009), *Bio-Algorithms and Med-Systems* **5–9**, 45.

de Leng, B. A., van Gent, R., Donkers, J., Hess, F., Heid, J., and van der Vleuten, C. P. M. (2009b). Can virtual patients be used to promote reflective practice as part of pediatric trainees' diagnostic reasoning strategies? In: *Research in Medical Education—Chances and Challenges 2009*. Düsseldorf: German Medical Science GMS Publishing House. Doc09rmeF1. DOI: 10.3205/09rme30, URN: urn:nbn:de:0183-09rme304

Maiburg, B., Koehorst, A. M., van Leeuwen, Y. D., Mathus-Vliegen, L. M. H., and van Ree, J. W. (2003). Development of a computer-based instruction on nutrition, simulating consultations by general practioners. In: B. Maiburg (ed.), *Computer-based nutration education for general practice: development of a training program and effect assessment by standardized patients*. Maastricht: Maastricht University Press. Pp. 37–49.

Ronteltap, C. F. M., and Eurlings, A. (2002). Activity and interaction of students in an electronic learning environment for problem-based learning. *Distance Education* **1**, 11–22.

Roterman-Koniecza, I. (ed.) (2009). Proceedings of the International Conference of Virtual Patients, Kraków, Poland, 2009 (Special issue), *Bio-Algorithms and Med-Systems* **5–9**.

Schuwirth, L. W. T., van der Vleuten, C. P. M., de Kock, C. A., Peperkamp, A. G. W., and Donkers, H. H. L. M. (1996). Computerized case-based testing: a modern method to assess clinical decision making. *Medical Teacher* **18**, 294–9.

Westerterp, K. R., Donkers, J., Fredrix, E. W. H. M., and Boekhoudt, P. (1995). Energy intake, physical activity and body weight; a simulation model, *British Journal of Nutrition* **73**, 337–47.

Chapter 14

Alternative instructional problem-based learning formats

Jos Moust and Herma Roebertsen

Problem-based learning (PBL) has been the dominant educational approach at Maastricht University for almost four decades. A central component of PBL is the tutorial group in which students analyse and synthesize information using the so-called 'seven-step' procedure. Although successful, this procedure has been showing signs of erosion in recent years. Students seem to get bored using the same procedure time after time, and start to skip important steps, thus generating considerable difficulties in integrating and applying new information. In response, problem designers have offered students questions, keywords, and lists of resources along with the problem text. Unfortunately, this elicited traditional learning behaviour from students and thus jeopardized the development of their self-directed learning behaviour. In order to combat the phenomenon of erosion and to ensure continued stimulation of independent learning, alternative learning designs have been developed both in and outside the classic PBL format.

Why change a winning team?

Problem-based learning appears to be a successful educational innovation. Four decades after PBL was introduced at McMaster University (Canada) and Maastricht University (the Netherlands) numerous institutions of higher as well as secondary education around the world have implemented PBL in their curriculum. National, annual evaluations of the quality of teaching in the fourteen Dutch universities have consistently placed the Maastricht faculties working with PBL in the top three (Steenkamp et al., 2004, 2006, 2008).

Despite these quite successful outcomes, however, various signs of erosion have been observed in recent years (Dolmans et al., 2001; Moust et al., 2005a; Vermunt, 2000, 2003). In Maastricht's medical school Dolmans et al. (2001) identified ritualism in various learning processes in and outside the tutorial groups. For instance, students were reluctant to present their thoughts and ideas to the group as fully as possible and some students were free-riders. Confronted with problems in group work, tutors reacted inadequately. Dolmans and her colleagues describe tutor behaviour that seems more teacher- than student-directed. Using the teacher-directed model that prevailed during their own professional training, tutors transmitted information by lecturing in the tutorial groups. Moust et al. (2005a) found that students in the School of Health Sciences too did not work as effectively and efficiently as possible in and outside the tutorial groups. Students quite often skipped parts of the seven-step procedure, which are intended to help them to analyse and synthesize the subject matter knowledge offered by the problems. Superficial problem analysis became a barrier both to the critical processing of new knowledge and to arriving at a deep level of understanding during self-study. Students also experienced difficulties in integrating subject matter offered in multidisciplinary courses. When some of the seven steps were skipped, for instance the elaboration of prior knowledge in the analysis phase, the synthesis phase of new information tended to be reduced to a presentation of the main results with no attempts at critical appraisal of opinions and viewpoints, let alone integration and application of the findings. Students appeared to focus rapidly on one solution or 'the right answer', a strategy that can easily result in prejudices or misconceptions (Houlden et al., 2001).

In an attempt to counteract this undesirable surface learning approach, staff members gradually developed problems with directives like questions, or keywords, or recommended literature resources. This directive reaction, however, provoked a contrary effect. Students confined themselves to answering the questions and selectively studied the recommended literature. Students' growth as independent learners was at risk and they were becoming more and more teacher dependent. With respect to these signs of deterioration in their approaches to learning, Vermunt (2000) observed that 'classic' PBL fails to change with the growing self-directed learning attitudes of students. In his opinion, what should be aimed for is a decrease in the amount of guidance, such as that offered by teachers in their roles as group tutor, designer of problems, assessor of students' achievements, and an increase in students' independent learning behaviour (Figure 14.1). According to Vermunt, this is not achieved when the traditional pattern of two sessions per week, two problems per session, groups of some ten students, a fixed role for the tutor, and a fixed procedure to analyse problems, remains unchanged over the years of the curriculum. To first-year students classic PBL may pose a considerable challenge, compared to the traditional approach in most secondary schools. However, to second- and third-year students repeating the same routine tends to get stale. Students are not challenged to develop more sophisticated self- and team management competencies. Vermunt noticed a certain amount of growth in independent learning in the first year of the PBL curricula in the faculties of Medicine and Health Sciences but a deceleration of self-directedness in the following years (Figure 14.2).

New working formats within as well as outside the classic PBL environment have been explored. In the next section, some variations on the seven-step procedure will be discussed. Subsequently, other formats that while differing from the seven-step approach are nevertheless in line with the basic learning principles of PBL as a constructive, contextual, and collaborative learning environment will be presented.

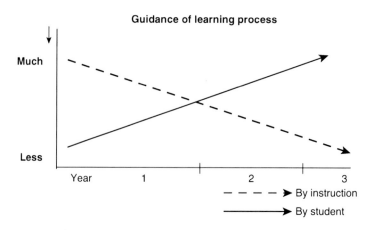

Figure 14.1 Decrease of external guidance, increase of self-directedness.

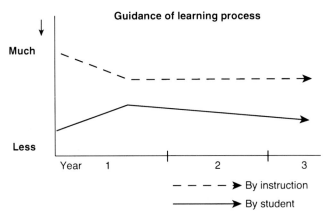

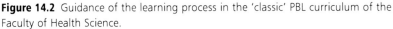

Figure 14.2 Guidance of the learning process in the 'classic' PBL curriculum of the Faculty of Health Science.

Various learning formats within a conventional PBL environment

As said previously, students and staff seem to stick quite rigorously to the seven-step procedure as described in the literature. Unfortunately, recommendations for using this procedure are sometimes interpreted as fixed instructions that must be followed to the letter. As was stated earlier, this can have adverse effects, but these effects can be prevented, for instance by introducing some variety. Once students have gained some experience in working with problems, it can be refreshing for them to try different formats. In this section, some of these formats, such as variations in problem analysis, in the distribution of work among group members during self-study, and in synthesizing new information, will be discussed (Moust et al., 2007).

Variations in problem analysis

Brainstorming with 'post-its'

This is an alternative to the brainstorming technique in which group members express any idea that springs to mind. The procedure is as follows:

1 Each group member writes some initial ideas on post-it notes, one idea per post-it.

2 All post-its are stuck on a board and group members can write additional comments.

3 The group clusters together related ideas.

4 The group sits down and discusses in-depth the clustered ideas.

5 Learning objectives are formulated.

Problem analysis in subgroups

In many fields of study there are clear distinctions between professional points of view and/or professional roles, such as those between professionals involved in health promotion and health policy in health sciences and the perspectives of cure and care in medicine. A tutorial group can be split into subgroups, each subgroup representing a particular point of view or a certain professional role. The procedure is as follows:

1 Divide the group into two or three subgroups according to the number of perspectives.

2 Each subgroup analyses the problem from their perspective.

3 Each subgroup prepares a short presentation of their analysis.

4 Each subgroup presents their presentation to the whole group.

5 The whole group discusses the outcomes of the analysis.

6 The whole group formulates learning objectives.

Nominal group technique

This approach is characterized by minimal interaction among the group members during the initial problem analysis.

1 Each group member writes down their individual problem analysis without consulting other group members.

2 Each group member presents their analysis, which is then summarized on the blackboard and clustered if possible. There is no discussion.

3 All suggestions are clarified by their originators.

4 Each group member revises his/her initial analysis based on what has been presented by the other group members.

5 The most popular explanations or solutions are discussed by the group.

The virtual tutorial

Problem analysis in an electronic learning environment is a variation on the approach just described. An important difference is that students prepare their first analysis at home, post it on the group space in an e-learning environment (e.g., as a wiki), where they can also post comments and questions about contributions from other group members. During the next group meeting, the group develops possible explanations and solutions, and formulates learning goals.

Problem analysis using decision-making software

When analysing complex policy and technological problems, professionals often use software that enables multiphased discussion and decision making. Such working environments can also be utilized in a PBL course. All group members in the 'decision room' are connected online to each other and to a moderator. The moderator invites initial ideas and comments. At regular intervals the moderator asks the students to rank the ideas, based on how much they support or are interested in them. The software then provides a group ranking. In this way, without direct person-to-person discussion, complex problems can be analysed and broken down into components for further exploration.

Variation in dividing the work among group members

In the traditional seven-step procedure all students pursue the same learning objectives formulated at the end of the analysis phase. Here too, variation is possible.

Rely on your peers

A problem may be too complex to study comprehensively within the time available. Dividing the work between group members provides a way to clarify or solve a problem in less time. In this way PBL changes into a micro-project, with students specializing in different components of the problem. This means that students have to rely on the (summary) explanations of other students to understand all the components of the problem.

Look for your own resources

Similar to the use of subgroups during the initial problem analysis, subgroups can study a problem from a particular point of view or perspective and present their findings in the next tutorial.

Variations in the synthesis phase

Some suggestions for different ways of integrating and applying new information are:

'What I didn't understand'

Rather than presenting the outcomes of their self-study, each group member presents an issue that is not clear to them and the other group members then try to clarify the issue, based on what they have discovered.

Critical peer review

Professionals are often required to present their findings to a critical audience of peers. As preparation for this situation, one student presents a problem. The presentation is followed by critical questions from the other group members, who have studied the same problem.

Learning formats in a non-classic PBL environment

In this section some alternative working formats which are nevertheless in line with the ideas of the classic PBL environment are presented. All alternatives have the same educational characteristics in that they foster constructive, contextual, and collaborative learning. These learning formats are also intended to help students to become more proficient and versatile self-directed learners. There is no need to offer the various working formats to students in a fixed order.

PBL with study teams

The first learning format developed within the PBL context is 'PBL with study teams'. Students are offered quite complex problems which require them to study various perspectives, solutions, or disciplines. In line with these complex problems an abundance of learning resources is at the students' disposal. As in the conventional PBL track, groups work together during the analysis phase. They define the problems, brainstorm, and elaborate ideas that can clarify or solve the problem and formulate learning objectives to be addressed during individual self-study. The study team approach differs from the traditional format in that students do not work individually or in informal groups during self-study, but in teams composed of three students from the same tutorial group. The members of the study teams together decide which learning resources they will use. It is important to notice that the learning objectives are not distributed between or within study teams. As in conventional PBL groups, students have the opportunity to synthesize and apply newly acquired information on more or less the same basis. In the period, usually a week, between the analysis and synthesis phase, the study teams have several opportunities to discuss the outcomes of their self-study. They can discuss issues they do not understand and formulate points for discussion during the next plenary group meeting. Additionally, each study team is required to prepare an overview of the contents of their team discussions for presentation in the next plenary group meeting. The presentation can be a concept map or a series of transparencies giving an overview of the material studied. Additionally, each study team must formulate critical questions about the literature they have discussed. In the next plenary group meeting each team gives their presentation to the group. Points which appear unclear are discussed. In a general round-up, the critical questions of every study team are answered and the solutions of the teams are integrated to solve the problem from various perspectives. Table 14.1 offers an overview of the similarities and differences between classic PBL groups and PBL groups with study teams. Figure 14.3 visualizes a PBL learning environment with study teams.

Table 14.1 Similarities and differences between classic PBL and PBL with study teams

Similarities
A member of the tutorial group acts as chairperson during the analysis phase and the synthesis phase.
The principal method of discussion in the tutorial group meeting is the seven-step procedure.
The tutorial group is guided by a tutor.
All the learning objectives are studied by all group members.

Differences	
Classic PBL	PBL with study teams
Two group sessions (2 hours) per week.	One group session (2.5 hours) per week.
The problem consists of a few concepts and connections between the concepts.	The problem consists of many concepts and connections between the concepts.
The problems are concise and well structured.	The problems are complex, ill-structured, and require more than one solution or explanation.
Students are free to collaborate with other students of their study team during the period of self-study.	Students are obliged to meet with the students during the period of self-study.
Students are free as to how they prepare for the synthesis phase.	The members of a study team have to prepare an overview to present at the next group meeting.
Preparation for the synthesis phase is highly student-dependent.	Preparation for the synthesis phase is structured by the discussions in the study team and the presentation the students must prepare.
The synthesis phase is not structured.	The synthesis phase is structured by the presentations of the various study teams and the discussion between the members of the study teams.
Individual assessment by a set of open questions at the end of the unit.	Individual assessment by a set of open questions at the end of the unit and group assessment of the presentations in the group meetings.
Attention for the process of collaboration in the tutorial group is tutor- and student-dependent.	Attention for the process of collaboration in the study team and the tutorial group is explicated in the unit portfolio.

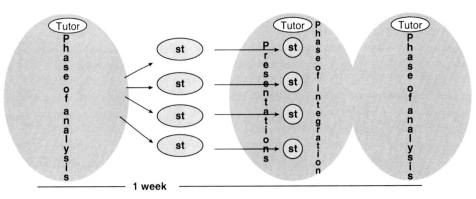

Figure 14.3 A schematic overview of a 'PBL with study teams' learning environment. 'st' = study team.

Tutor on demand

'Tutor on demand' is a more elaborate form of PBL with study teams (Figure 14.4). It can be used when students are able to work inside and outside a tutorial group at quite a high level of self-directedness. Although the tutor is normally absent when students are analysing a problem and synthesizing new information, the tutor is at the students' disposal all the time. When students feel they are getting stuck, they can ask the tutor to help them either in collaborating or in dealing with content matter. Students must report to the tutor regularly by submitting the minutes of their meetings. The advantage of this approach is that one tutor can guide two or three tutorial groups at the same time.

PBL with expert teams

Another format that can be used in a PBL environment is PBL with expert teams. Students are offered a quite complex problem that can be studied from the perspectives of different disciplines, theories, stakeholders, or societal groups with an interest in the solution. At the end of the analysis phase, when students have formulated learning objectives, the students split into homogeneous expert teams (A, B, C, D), each consisting of three or four students and representing one of the perspectives. Within these expert teams students collaborate to clarify and solve the problem from the perspective of their group. They are asked to present the resulting views and solutions as a concept map, a set of handouts, a presentation, or a paper. Next the students are re-assigned to heterogeneous expert teams of three or four members (W, X, Y, Z) in which they offer clarification and solutions from the perspective of their particular expert group. Within these teams the students must synthesize the various perspectives in a critical way. The synthesis process can be stimulated by offering the heterogeneous teams an analogous problem, forcing them to integrate and apply the different perspectives. At the end of the learning period all the students and one or more tutors with relevant expertise meet in a joint session in which they review, discuss, and critically appraise the information and solutions discussed by the teams (Figure 14.5).

Project work

Project work can be described in general terms as an educational format in which external clients (e.g., a for-profit or not-for-profit organization) submit real problems encountered in their work for the students to solve in small groups. The students are expected to analyze the problem and commit themselves to finding one or more suitable solutions which can be useful to the client.

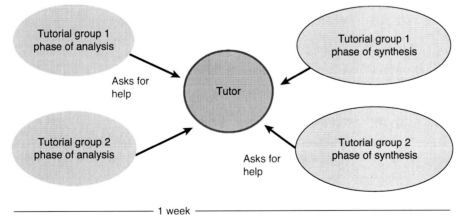

Figure 14.4 Tutor on demand.

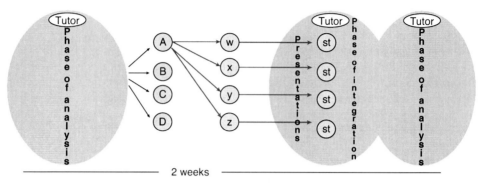

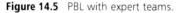

Figure 14.5 PBL with expert teams.

In weekly meetings with their teacher the students discuss intermediate outcomes and the collaborative process in their group. During these meetings the teacher gives feedback on problem content as well as the work process. At the end of the project the students present a finished product, like a device or a report. The product is evaluated by the teachers and the client. Grades can be given for the quality of the product as well as for the process of group collaboration.

Project work is a relatively old instructional format using collaborative and contextual learning. Project work was implemented in higher education in the 1960s and was shown to be quite successful in some studies. In the last decades of the twentieth century, however, it seems to have 'died'. Project work at that time did not live up to the expectations with regard to the fostering of understanding of problems. Today, project-based learning has made a comeback. In some studies, especially in technical domains like engineering, architecture, and industrial design, project-based learning is used from the start of the curriculum (Kolmos, 1996). In other studies (de Graaff & Kolmos, 2003), this method was not implemented in the curriculum until students had become quite experienced in learning in a collaborative setting. One of the difficulties associated with starting too early with project-based learning seems to be that students focus too much on the process of building a relationship with an external client, while still needing to learn a great deal about the subject matter related to the problem. Another frequent problem is that of 'free-riders', students who profit from the work of others and try to earn high grades with low effort.

Project-based learning should not be offered until students have experienced other formats of constructive, collaborative, and contextual learning, like the approaches described above. This enables students to gradually build their competence as self-directed learners. They can also experience in a relatively safe and trustful learning environment how to work in groups, which group dynamics support and hinder effective and efficient collaboration, and how to manage interpersonal cooperation. Table 14.2 offers an overview of the crucial elements of the various formats, discussed in this chapter. Figure 14.6 shows how these formats can be built into a curriculum that supports students' independent learning over the various years of their study.

Evaluation and reflection

Students have been seen to become rather bored with the repetitious routine of working through problems using the 'seven-step' procedure in classic PBL. As this procedure tends to become ritualized, students start to skip one or two steps or try to chunk parts of the procedure. As a result, the process of meaningful learning suffers. It seems that students fail to integrate, criticize, and apply new information at an appropriately deep level. Teacher-centred reactions, such as the provision of questions, keywords, and literature resources together with the problem text or

Table 14.2 An outline of various working formats to be used in a PBL environment

Type	Number of students	Number of meetings	Output	Assessment
Classic PBL	Ten students in one group	Twice a week	Concept maps, schemes, summaries which offer either clarifications of underlying theories, principles, and mechanisms, or theoretical solutions. Students discuss with their groups what they have found during self-study.	Independent of the group meetings. Individual assessment. Grading by the teacher.
PBL with study teams	12–16 students in one group	Once a week	Presentations (handouts, concept maps) which offer either clarifications of underlying theories, principles and mechanisms, or theoretical solutions. Students discuss with the group what they have found during self-study and the discussions in their study team.	Independent of the group meetings; students also must reflect and report on their collaboration. Assessment at individual and group level. Grading by the teacher.
Tutor on demand	10 students in one group, several groups per tutor	Once a week	Presentations (handouts, concept maps) which offer either clarifications of underlying theories, principles, and mechanisms or theoretical solutions. Students of one tutorial group discuss with the members of one or two other tutorial groups what they have found during self-study and discussions in their tutorial group.	Independent of the group meetings. Individual assessment. Grading by the teacher.
PBL with expert teams	12–16 students in one group	Bi-weekly	Presentations (handouts, concept maps, papers) which offer either clarifications of underlying theories, principles, and mechanisms or theoretical solutions from specific perspectives. Students of one heterogeneous team discuss the results of their self-study and discussion with members of other heterogeneous teams.	Independent of the group meetings; students also must reflect and report on their process of collaboration. Assessment at individual and group level. Grading by the teacher.
Project work	16–32 students, subgroups of 8 students maximum	Two to eight weeks with regular meetings	A well-defined product, either a report or a device. Students should offer reflections on content matter and on the process of collaboration.	Independent of the group meetings; students also must reflect and report on their process of collaboration. Assessment at individual and group level. Teacher, client, and students involved in grading.

lecturing to the group, are detrimental to deep as well as self-directed learning. Moreover, these reactions seem to elicit traditional learning responses from students, who confine themselves to answering the questions and focus selectively on the recommended literature. Given the opportunity, students are quick to go along with a 'teacher-centred' approach, which then becomes a barrier to constructive, contextual, and collaborative learning. Additionally, self-directed learning behaviour decreases and may even disappear altogether. Students' development as independent learners is thus halted. According to Vermunt (2000), the 'classic' problem-based learning format is new when students are fresh from secondary school, but ceases to be challenging when it does not change together with students growing self-directedness. A decrease of guidance by teachers does not appear to enhance students' independent learning behaviour. In the long run the traditional PBL approach does not challenge students sufficiently to develop more sophisticated self- and team management competencies.

There are several ways to maintain or even improve students' level of self-directedness. One way to prevent erosion in students' learning behaviour is to offer more open and ill-structured problems (see Chapter 5). When given more complex problem formats, students are forced to consider more diverse hypotheses which clarify underlying mechanisms as well as various solutions for the problems. Students should become aware that information may be missing from the problem text or that they may identify information that can put them on the wrong track. The complexity of problems can also be raised by offering students various types of problems in one problem text. In a realistic problem, described over several pages, students can be invited to clarify the various phenomena by referring to underlying mechanisms and processes. They might be asked to discuss moral aspects related to a problem or to think about various solutions.

A second way to bring more variation to a PBL context is to offer students different ways of analysing and synthesizing a problem within the framework of the seven-step procedure, for instance by using post-it notes, splitting the tutorial group into subgroups, the nominal group technique, the virtual tutorial, and problem analysis using decision-making software.

Designers of PBL programmes, however, might also think of ways of inviting students to work in alternative PBL settings. In this chapter several formats such as PBL with study teams, PBL with expert teams, and project work have been described. Research on the effectiveness of these alternative formats for the classic Maastricht PBL design is scarce, however. In a study of study teams in a PBL setting, Moust et al. (2005b) reported findings about students' appreciation, study time, and achievement. The students generally appreciated this format (although a high standard deviation suggested considerable variety of opinion among the students), they spent considerably more time on self-study, and their results on the end-of-unit test were slightly better than those of students using the classic PBL format. Data on students' growth in self-directed learning were not provided. The same outcomes were found when students worked on projects in a PBL setting. Nearly all students got very involved with the problem they had to solve. Working with real life issues stimulated students' motivation as well as time-on-self-study. In one experiment a student expressed it as 'Project work is really useful. I have never learned so much and I have never spent so much time studying' (Voortgangsrapportage, 2004).

Although there is little evidence from research of these formats so far, these alternatives seem to be making a valuable and promising contribution to widen the PBL approach. If educators want students to become lifelong learners, staff of PBL curricula will have to build in stimuli to support sustained growth of students' levels of independent learning competencies.

What next?

The variations on the classic PBL design in Maastricht focus on two topics: offering students learning content that supports authentic learning and helping them to become lifelong learners. The diversity of working formats described here is aimed at gradually dismantling the scaffolding

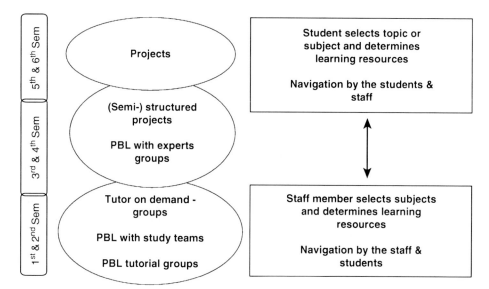

Figure 14.6 A schematic overview of various PBL formats in a PBL environment.

offered by teachers and building up students' skills to steer their own learning and collaboration processes in and outside a tutorial group. The various formats offer opportunities to enable students to take control of their learning environment. As teachers want to develop learning environments that expand students' learning dispositions, they should stretch students' capacity to learn. Claxton and Carr (2004) distinguish an epistemic culture which offers this possibility: a so-called potentiating environment, which forces the students to exercise their learning muscles in an appealing and challenging way. These potentiating milieus should have the following features to increase the likelihood that students will want to take it seriously (Claxton, 2007, p. 126):

◆ Rich: there is much to be explored;

◆ Challenging: the topic contains real difficulty;

◆ Extended: there is time and opportunity to go into it in depth;

◆ Relevant: the topic connects with students' own interests and concerns;

◆ Responsibility: students have some genuine control over what, why, how, and when they organize their learning;

◆ Real: solving the problem or making progress genuinely matters to someone;

◆ Unknown: the teacher does not already know the 'answer'; and

◆ Collaborative: most students enjoy the opportunity to work together on such tasks.

Claxton and Carr (2004) conclude: 'In a potentiating environment there are plenty of hard, interesting things to do, and it is accepted as normal that everyone regularly gets confused, frustrated, and stuck' (p. 90).

Annotated literature

Claxton, G. (2007). Expanding young people's capacity to learn. *British Journal of Educational Studies* **55**, 115–34.

Being an effective learner is not just a means but a valuable end for education in its own right. Students must become effective, powerful real-life learners to adjust and handle the large challenges to be faced in the twenty-first century. In reality, nowadays, most schools are not able to expand the capacity to learn beyond the school gates. Being a 'successful learner' often means offering students hints and tips on how to organize, retain, and retrieve information in order that they do well in exams. In this thought-provoking article Claxton offers a clear conceptual framework about what the capacity to learn involves and a pedagogy that is directly targeted at expanding the capacity to learn.

De Corte, E., Verschaffel, L., Entwistle, N., and Van Merriënboer, J. (2003). *Powerful learning environments: unravelling basic components and dimensions.* Oxford: Pergamon Press.

This book offers new theoretical frameworks, design principles, and research methodologies focusing on the construction, implementation, and evaluation of learning environments which support deep level learning of students. Three intersecting sub-domains within the broader field of research on learning and instruction, instructional psychology, technology, and design are interwoven in the thirteen chapters written by leading European scholars in the field.

Dolmans, D. H. J. M., and Schmidt, H. G. (2006). What do we know about cognitive and motivational effects of small group tutorials in problem-based learning? *Advances in Health Sciences Education* **11**, 321–36.

This article reports findings of studies on students collaborating in small groups within a PBL setting. A distinction is made between studies focusing on cognitive effects of group learning and studies focusing on motivational effects of group learning. Studies concentrating on the cognitive effects of small-group PBL seem to demonstrate that activation of prior knowledge, recall of information, causal reasoning or theory building, cognitive conflicts leading to conceptual change, and collaborative learning construction take place in the tutorial group. Studies focusing on the motivational effects of PBL demonstrate that group discussion positively influences students' intrinsic interest in the subject matter under discussion. The studies also demonstrate that a haphazard discussion in the tutorial group or a discussion that just scratches the surface, probably due to diminished motivation of students, inhibits student learning. Several studies are providing suggestions on how to optimize group work in PBL.

Moust, J., Roebertsen, H., Savelberg, H., and de Rijk, A. (2005). Revitalising PBL groups: evaluating PBL with study teams. *Education for Health* **18**, 62–73.

This article describes a study on PBL with study teams in two courses over a period of two years within the former Faculty of Health Sciences. In this study the achievement as well as the appreciation of students participating in a PBL environment with study teams is compared with that of students working in a conventional PBL environment. The study shows an increase in self-study time of the students working in study teams and considerable differences among students in their appreciation of the new environment.

References

Claxton, G. L. (2007). Expanding young people's capacity to learn. *British Journal of Educational Studies* **55(2)**, 115–34.

Claxton, G. L., and Carr, M. A. (2004). A framework for teaching thinking: the dynamics of disposition. *Earl Years* **24**, 87–97.

Dolmans, D. H. J. M., Wolfhagen, H. A. P., van der Vleuten, C. P. M., and Wijnen, W. H. F. W. (2001). Solving problems with group work in problem-based learning: hold on to the philosophy. *Medical Education* **35**, 884–9.

De Graaff, E., and Kolmos, A. (2003). Characteristics of problem-based learning. *International Journal of Engineering Education* **19(5)**, 146–53.

Houlden, R. L., Collier, C. P., Frid, P. J., John, S. L., and Pross, H. (2001). Problems identified by tutors in a hybrid problem-based learning curriculum. *Academic Medicine* **76**, 81.

Kolmos, A. (1996). Reflections on Project Work and Problem-based learning. *European Journal of Engineering* 2, 141–8.

Moust, J., Van Berkel, H., and Schmidt, H. (2005a). Signs of erosion: reflection on three decades of problem-based learning. *Higher Education* 50, 665–83.

Moust, J. H. C., Roebertsen, H., Savelberg, H., and de Rijk, A. (2005b). Revitalizing PBL groups; evaluating PBL with study teams. *Education for Health* 18, 62–74.

Moust, J. H. C., Bouhuijs, P. A. J., and Schmidt, H. G. (2007). *Introduction to problem-based learning: a guide for students.* Groningen: Wolters-Noordhoff.

Schmidt, H. G. (1993). Foundations of problem-based learning: some explanatory notes. *Medical Education* 27, 422–32.

Steenkamp, F., de Moor, A., and van Beek, M. (2004). *De keuzegids hoger onderwijs 04/05 (The higher education guide 04/05).* Leiden, the Netherlands: Hoger Onderwijs Persbureau.

Steenkamp, F., de Looper, H., and Bliekendaal, M. (2006). *De keuzegids hoger onderwijs 06/07 (The higher education guide 06/07).* Leiden, the Netherlands: Hoger Onderwijs Persbureau.

Steenkamp, F., Dobber, L., and Jansen, M. (2009). *De keuzegids hoger onderwijs 08/09 (The higher education guide 08/09).* Leiden, the Netherlands: Hoger Onderwijs Persbureau.

Vermunt, J. (2000). About the quality of learning. In: W. Gijselaers and J. Vermunt (eds), *Studies for new scholars.* Maastricht University. Inaugural lectures.

Vermunt, J. D. (2003). The power of learning environments and the quality of student learning. In: E. de Corte, L. Verschaffel, N. Entwistle, and J. van Merriënboer (eds), *Powerful learning environments; unravelling basic components and dimensions.* Kidlington: Elsevier Sciences (Pergamon Press).

Voortgangsrapportage 2004 (Progress report 2004) Evaluation of unit 2.6.a 'Health Technology Assessment'. Dijkstra, J., Van Berkel, H., Evers, S., Jaspers, P., and Ament, A. (Internal publication of the Faculty of Health Sciences—Maastricht University).

Chapter 15

How to organize the transition from a traditional curriculum to a PBL curriculum

Martin Paul

Some say that nothing is more difficult than to change a traditional curriculum into a problem-based one. Maastricht University has been lucky in that it was able to start with problem-based learning (PBL) curricula right from its foundation. However, most universities that wish to adopt a PBL curriculum will have to take a more difficult path. Some universities have walked this path successfully and it is worthwhile to learn from their experiences. This chapter is based on involvement over the past 25 years in different models of PBL curricula, at Harvard Medical School, the University of Heidelberg, the Charité Medical Center in Berlin, and Maastricht University. It presents practical advice on the transition from a traditional to a PBL curriculum.

Introduction

Wilhelm von Humboldt, the famous Prussian politician who reformed education in his state in the nineteenth century, is usually quoted as the originator of the concept of the unity of academic research and education, which is still considered to be the mission of most universities. In many medical faculties, however, this unified concept has paradoxically resulted in a strong focus on research and comparative neglect of innovative educational concepts. This has been detrimental to innovation within medical education, which in its classical form does not differ much, conceptually, from the teaching structures in elementary and secondary schools and is teacher-oriented rather than student-focused. Disciplines and subjects are usually taught in a non-integrative way with a clear separation of preclinical subjects, such as physiology, biochemistry, and anatomy, and clinical disciplines, which are taught at a later stage of medical education but also in a rather theoretical way without focus on the skills and competencies required of physicians. This system creates an artificial separation of basic science on the one hand and clinical experience, knowledge, and skills on the other. It is artificial since the end product of our educational efforts, the physician, must be able to deal with problems in an integrative manner, interweaving knowledge, experience, and medical skills in a complex manner during his or her work as a professional. Therefore, learning how to deal with this complexity should be a primary focus of medical education. It should also be taken into account that students, aged 18–25 years, our typical clientele in medical schools, are at the peak of their intellectual and creative capabilities and should not be underestimated in their potential to integrate complex ideas and concepts. At the same time we, as educators, must support them in taking charge of their own education, a concept of lifelong learning and continuing (self-)education that is essential for every practising physician to keep pace with medical innovation and evidence-based medicine.

Why change?

Students are not only our customers: they are the essence of every academic institution and important stakeholders in defining education programmes. Many evaluations have demonstrated that students are unhappy with traditional medical curricula, complaining about the overwhelming dominance of theoretical knowledge and severe shortcomings in clinical education (Cumming & Ross, 2007). As a consequence students may slide into disillusionment with the education system, resulting in chronic absenteeism from lectures and resorting to short-term memory training before exams. In fact, the traditional system focusing predominantly on the scientific basis of medicine does a poor job of preparing students for the reality of working as a physician. This argument should not be misinterpreted: the acquisition of basic science knowledge must be a vital part of every medical education programme, and basic science teaching is usually of high quality in traditional curricula. The point is that basic science education should not be isolated and fragmented but integrated with the other components of the medical curriculum. Despite awareness of these shortcomings within medical faculties, there have been few stimuli to induce change, since educational quality has typically not been a parameter for faculty funding. With the introduction of national and international ranking systems of the educational quality of universities and faculties, which are partly based on students' views, and the attention these rankings received, the problems of traditional curricula became obvious and visible. For example, one of the most recognized and methodologically sound rankings, performed by the Centrum für Hochschulentwicklung (CHE) revealed that traditional curricula performed worse than problem-based curricula (http://www.che.de). This led to the realization in many ministries and government bodies responsible for university funding that quality of education should become an important determinator of public funding of universities. In some countries, including Germany, this rethinking has prompted a call for an 'excellence initiative' to reshape and modernize concepts in higher education. As a result, many medical faculties are in the process of redefining (i.e., modernizing) their teaching and education concepts.

How to induce change?

Successful implementation of a problem-based curriculum depends on parallel coordination of bottom-up and top down processes, which requires the involvement of the faculty leadership as well as the students (Smith & Dollase, 1999). The first step in the transition from a traditional to a PBL curriculum is an *open discussion based on facts*. This can be prepared by a working group evaluating the strengths and weaknesses of the current curriculum. Such a group should consist of students, (junior) faculty members, and representatives of the dean's office and the faculty administration. A questionnaire examining student (customer) and teacher (provider) satisfaction can be very useful for quantifying shortcomings and identifying points that need attention. This can be helpful in focusing the ensuing discussions on facts rather than emotions. To change a curriculum requires work, dedication, and enthusiasm—a process that can be painful and unwanted to those who want to continue in their 'old ways', which are stress free and more comfortable for those who consider education a secondary issue in a research-based environment.

Secondly, the organization and implementation of educational strategies and structures must be based on *financial transparency*. The classical concept of integrated, i.e., non-transparent, funding of research and education within one budget, usually results in the predominance in the budget of research spending . Supporters of such an approach tend to misunderstand von Humboldt's concept of the unity of research and education, if they extend it to budgetary matters. The first administrative step in reorganizing a curriculum is to create *independent budgets* for research and education, which of course must both be based on quality assurance and include components of performance-based funding. Departments within the faculty can then be funded from both resources (research and education) according to their actual perform-ance and quality in these respective fields. The responsibility for the distribution of funds and evaluation of performance should be localized within the dean's office or under its direct supervision.

Thirdly, the introduction of a problem-based curriculum should—from the beginning—be based on a *quantitative analysis of learning quality and outcome*. Those critical of a new organiza-tion of learning will always question whether change is really an improvement and—again—the discussion should be directed by evidence, not emotion. In some faculties, the strategy of running a problem-based curriculum (*Reformstudiengang*) in parallel to a traditional curriculum (*Regelstudiengang*) was chosen to allow comparison between the two systems in terms of learning outcomes and student performance and satisfaction. Obviously, such an approach presents a huge organizational challenge. In Berlin, for example, the extra costs of running this experiment were covered by extramural funding. It is one of the examples that yielded scientific evidence that PBL curricula are not inferior to traditional ones and that students are very well capable of approach-ing knowledge accumulation and medical skills in an integrated fashion, while—at the same time—being highly motivated and satisfied with their study programme. Nevertheless, this approach posed not only an organizational challenge; it presented the additional difficulty of having to integrate the two programmes after the study period was over.

Berlin's Charité reformed medical curriculum as an example

The idea to modernize medical education in Berlin came initially from students and developed during a protest strike in 1988 where students across Germany openly criticized the rigid and mainly theory-based curricula of the country's universities as well as the study conditions, char-acterized by low teacher–student ratios. At the Freie Universität Berlin, medical students were actively developing new ideas of a modern, interdisciplinary, and integrated curriculum. The dean of the medical faculty at the time was sympathetic to these ideas and initiated an interdisci-plinary working group to develop a reform-oriented, problem-based, integrated, and skills-oriented medical curriculum. After a merger of faculties and university hospitals in Berlin these plans were carried out at the Charité, a medical school now belonging to both the Freie Universität and the Humboldt University Berlin and thus responsible for all of medical education in Berlin.

Since the legal framework of medical education in Germany did not allow for deviation from the then-defined structure of the medical curricula, the state of Berlin applied for an experimental clause within the law, regulating medical education to enable the introduction of model curricula that could integrate new and innovative learning concepts and prepare students for the medical licensure exams. In 1999, the new law was passed and Berlin's reformed curriculum started as a model project to compare the outcomes of problem-based medical education with those of stu-dents in the regular curriculum. Consequently, the Charité was running both programmes in parallel, with the majority of students still studying the regular curriculum and sixty students per year entering the reformed curriculum. To support the scientific character of the outcome study, the reformed curriculum was funded by the government as well as by private foundations with the goal of investigating the feasibility, costs, and outcomes of its introduction. Both the federal and state governments in Germany expected important information to result from the experiment.

The Berlin curriculum was based on the PBL curricula developed by McMaster University and Maastricht University and overcame the classical separation of a theory-driven preclinical pro-gramme in the first two years and a more clinically oriented programme that followed lacking significant elements such as skills training and competency-based education. The Berlin reformed medical curriculum, by contrast, took an integrated approach characterized by the so-called

N-model (a model describing the harmonic interplay between basic theoretical knowledge and clinical training and physician skills). This meant that medical students in the reform track at the Charité were exempt from the preclinical exam (Physikum) that marks the transition from the preclinical to the clinical years in Germany's medical education system.

The reformed medical curriculum was monitored and supported by an international advisory board consisting of renowned medical education experts with extensive experience in reformed curricula and problem-based learning. The advisory board evaluated the reformed medical curriculum after one and five years, assessing its quality and giving helpful suggestions for developing what started as an experiment into a solid programme that has won national and international praise (Engel et al., 2005). It has led to the recognition of the Charité as a medical school with a clear reform agenda, not only in medical education but also in other fields, such as career development and innovation of research. The latter effect is important to note since it demonstrates clearly that a commitment to reform education can also be an eye-opener with regard to innovation in other defining areas of a successful medical faculty. The reform markedly increased the attractiveness of the Charité to prospective students. After the implementation of the reformed medical curriculum, the number of students making the Charité their first choice of university increased greatly (by the way, the same effect was seen for the regular curriculum).

On the level of national policy-making in education, the interest in PBL and the positive reports from Berlin led to important changes within the legal system regulating medical education. Within a few years, the regular curricula also were geared towards more practice-oriented education, although without overcoming the classical gap between preclinical and clinical education and without the comprehensive implementation of PBL. The increased flexibility of the new legislation allowed faculties to make more adaptations and some faculties, such as those at the universities of Heidelberg, Munich, and Hannover, followed the Berlin example and implemented reform-based curricula. However, to date, none of these universities have implemented the pure PBL teaching seen at the Charité.

The experiment in Berlin has continued to provide important information on the sense and value of PBL curricula in medical education and has yielded important answers and trends. The observations in Berlin (Burger, 2006) correspond largely to the findings from a systematic analysis of problem-based versus traditional medical curricula published by Koh et al. (2008). All in all the following conclusions can be drawn:

- Students educated within the reform curriculum perform at least as well as those in the traditional curriculum.
- After completion of their studies, the students' competencies, skills, and readiness for professional practice are clearly superior.
- Apart from specific investments in setting up a PBL curriculum, such as a skillslab, the personnel costs for running a PBL curriculum are not necessarily higher than those of a traditional curriculum.
- The PBL programme has increased the overall attractiveness of the institution that implements it, both to prospective students and to politics and society.

The leadership of the medical faculty of the Charité was encouraged by these results to plan the development of a new model curriculum, based on the reformed curriculum, for all students before 2010. As of this writing, however, this plan is still awaiting implementation.

Key features in implementing a PBL curriculum

Implementation of change almost always arouses opposition from those who prefer to leave things as they are. This is also true for the implementation of problem-based curricula.

Despite clear demands from the most important stakeholders, i.e., the students, reluctance to change the traditional curriculum is almost always present among teaching staff, especially those concerned they may lose control over 'their' discipline within the medical curriculum. Such segmental, discipline-oriented thinking is clearly in conflict with the integrated approach of PBL. In order to overcome these and other obstacles the implementation of a PBL curriculum demands an open, transparent, and constructive process, based on rational arguments and not on emotion, and is aimed at persuading stakeholders rather than imposing change. In effect it demands the integration and coordination of 'top-down' and 'bottom-up' processes. The following points should be taken into consideration:

- *Legal issues*: In most countries medical education is regulated by national or state laws and/or regulations that determine structure, content, required exams, and many other aspects of medical education. Therefore, the legal framework of curricular changes should be examined at the earliest possible stage. It is mandatory for curriculum developers to make sure that any planned changes are feasible within the defined legal framework. If this is not the case one should examine the possibility of an 'experimental' clause. Early contacts with government bodies to explore these options are essential. Politicians need to be convinced of the potential benefits of educational innovation.

- *Best practice*: PBL has been introduced internationally in medical education and experiences with such curricula are readily available. The implementation should be based on best practice and evidence from other model projects and established PBL curricula. The early phase of problem-based curricula is over and there are not only many scientific publications which can be consulted, but also institutions that have implemented PBL systems and are usually quite willing to share their experiences and data. Colleagues from such institutions could, for example, be persuaded to form an advisory board for the implementation process. This external advisory board will be able to give advice based on personal experience with the implementation, management, and assessment of problem-based programmes.

- *Governance*: The driving force for the development of a PBL curriculum should have a broad base, which should include students, teachers, and faculty leadership, including the dean. Without such a broad base the chances of successful implementation are bound to be slim. The implementation of a PBL curriculum requires content- and strategy-oriented management structures. To organize this it is helpful to create a central management team, which should consist of staff and students and report directly to the dean's board or any other established structure, for instance an education centre established by the faculty. Whatever the local tradition, it is critical that such a team should work closely with and have direct support from and access to the dean and the executive board of the faculty. The management team carries out the central tasks for the running of the PBL programme, such as planning, delivery, and development of the educational programme, assessment structures, exams, assessment, evaluation, education research, and management of the skillslab. Apart from this team, which is involved in the immediate process of running the programme, it is helpful to have steering groups appointed by the faculty council or the faculty board in a more supervisory role. Depending on the local structures, the supervisory role can take different forms, but, as a minimum, such a group should provide internal control in such important questions as curriculum development, implementation, and assessment.

- *Transparency and communication*: Open innovation is a prerequisite for academic progress. PBL, although by now quite well established internationally, can still be met with resistance by those who do not feel ready for change. It is therefore of the utmost importance to create and maintain an open atmosphere within the faculty about the planned curriculum changes and to initiate an open and fair discussion on the advantages of PBL. Two points can be very helpful in this discussion process: (1) use only academic and scientific arguments from the many studies evaluating the success of other PBL curricula; and (2) ensure broad student involvement in this process. In the end they are not only our customers but also our partners in education.

◆ *Financial matters*: Many of those critical of changing to a PBL curriculum will argue that PBL requires more resources and is simply more expensive than traditional non-PBL programmes. In order to counter such criticisms the implementation should be supported by a solid business plan. Educational structures are directly related to teaching staff capacity, which in some countries such as Germany is regulated by law. Published experiences from other programmes, such as the one in Berlin, show that, apart from one-time investments such as setting up a skillslab and managerial staff for the programme, the actual running costs of PBL and non-PBL curricula are comparable, particularly in terms of personnel costs (Burger, 2006). A mistake frequently made is a non-complete switch to PBL, i.e., the parallel running of teaching systems or programmes. Because this is inevitably more expensive and requires more resources than one programme, it is preferable to make a complete changeover to a PBL curriculum and not succumb to partial solutions, even though these may be easier to achieve 'politically'. Another issue is the allocation of funds for research on one hand and education on the other. In many places the financial stream of these two main tasks are not separated and not transparent. Typically, this causes misdistribution of funds to the research domain. The development of a solid business plan will also help to establish the costs of education and thus provide the required transparency. Ideally, separation of funding should be achieved, since in the end this is the only guarantee that funds will be used appropriately.

◆ *Assessment and quality control*: Since optimal medical education for students is our product, we (also as academics) need to adopt a process-oriented view and pay careful attention to detail. A crucial component of this process is assessment of the contents, quality, and learning outcomes of the curriculum. It is critical in this respect that assessment is congruent with the aims of education within a PBL context and is tailored to its integrative approach.

◆ *Educational competence*: We are all familiar with the structural organization of research within universities and faculties. This is typically assigned to institutes, departments, or research schools with earmarked budgets. Interestingly, comparable structures for education are generally lacking within faculties and education has very often an 'also done' reputation among staff. It is crucial that educational structures are created according to the same principle as the research structures. It is highly advisable, for both internal and external recognition, to create an education institute or centre of excellence within the faculty, which should be managed and budgeted according to the same basic principles as the research-oriented departments. Furthermore, it is important that education research should also be integrated within such a structure. This will not only increase recognition but also provide the basis for scientific evaluation and assessment of the programme.

◆ *Recruitment strategies*: Hiring new staff is an essential investment in the future of academic institutions. In many cases this is based mainly on candidates' research reputations and performance. It is strongly recommended that *additionally* account should be taken of the educational vision of potential recrutees. Of course it is not necessary for every individual professor to be integrally involved in education, but having an open mind about education, modern ideas about teaching concepts, and an open ear to students' interests should be a basic quality in each appointee. Faculties should make it a principle that these qualities are tested when recruiting new staff.

- *Career development*: The notion of unity of research and education is often misunderstood as implying an equal role for every staff member in both research and education on a fifty-fifty basis. In practice, the notion of unity generally results in a marked preference for research. This is natural since most of the achievements that enhance the prospects of a successful university career are related to research performance. It is of the essence that both education and research attainments are considered, but this should be done on an individual basis. Indeed research AND education are the integral tasks of universities but this concept applies to the organization as a whole, not to each faculty member individually. We clearly need principal investigators within our research programmes but we equally need principal educators to ensure the quality of educational performance. This view implies that career frameworks that make it attractive for faculty members to choose an educational career path need to be worked out. Nothing is deadlier for educational progress than the notion that teaching is for those whose research performance is below par. In contrast, both career paths should be based on competence within the respective fields. It goes without saying that this is not a matter of all or nothing, because there are many brilliant researchers who are also outstanding educators and vice versa. Participation in research and education should therefore be seen as a gradient of engagement by faculty staff.

- Apart from this, efforts should be undertaken to train staff in modern education principles and strategies. The decision to engage (or not engage) in the development of educational expertise should not be left to the initiative of individual staff members. There are many national and international programmes, such as masters of medical education programmes, and the faculty should support or even co-finance participation in such programmes. Building a dedicated and engaged academic staff cannot be achieved without firm faculty support.

- *No half-hearted solutions*: One of the biggest mistakes that can be made in the implementation process of a PBL curriculum is to create a mixture of a traditional and a PBL curriculum. Although this may seem an attractive compromise after controversial discussions within a faculty, this 'PBL light' option (integrating components of both PBL and non-PBL-based methods) is more expensive, confusing, divisive, and cumbersome to implement than an all-out transition to a PBL approach. When in doubt or unable to implement a complete changeover, one would be wiser to stick with the conventional curriculum as a whole.

Conclusions

The extensive list in the previous section may seem rather daunting. Is it really worth all the effort and trouble to switch to a PBL curriculum? Is it worth it to choose 'the road less travelled'? In answering these questions, we should not forget that we are dealing with a group of young, motivated, and enthusiastic individuals, who after the *baccalaureat* or high school exam are at the top of their mental and intellectual capabilities. The best advice for educators in medicine is to remember their own time as a medical student. Without a doubt many have shared the experience of a traditional medical curriculum having an anti-stimulatory effect during this otherwise exciting phase of personal development. After the feeling of freedom and positive energy on completing secondary education, it is clearly undesirable for students to be forced into a rigid, old-fashioned, and drill-oriented teaching system which threatens to steadily dilute the competencies achieved during primary and secondary education. Many will have resorted to 'autodidactic' strategies to prevent deterioration of the integrative, 'holistic' competencies that a physician needs. Lifelong learning is also a concept to be embraced by the educators: learning from one's own experiences is an excellent basis for the mission to build education programmes that enable modern institutions to train the best possible physicians for our society. Everybody who has seen the positive impact a PBL curriculum has not only on students, but on staff and the faculty as a whole, will never want to turn back.

References

Burger, W. (2006). The Berlin reformed medical curriculum at the Charité. Experiences with the first cohort. *Bundesgesundheitsbl-Gesundheitsforsch-Gesundheitsschutz* **49**, 337–43.

Cumming, A., and Ross, M. (2007). The Tuning project for medicine learning outcomes for undergraduate medical education in Europe. *Medical Teacher* **29**, 636–41.

Engel, C., Obershain, S., Sefton, A., and van der Vleuten, C.P.M. (2005). *Towards a twenty-first century medical curriculum: report by the International Advisory Board, 2005.* Available at: http://www.charite.de/lehre/downloads/gutachten_rsm_05.pdf

Koh, G. C.-H., Khoo, H. E., Wong, M. L., and Koh, D. (2008).The effects of problem based learning during medical school on physician competency: a systematic review. *Canadian Medical Association Journal* **178**, 34–41.

Smith, S. R., and Dollase, R. (1999). Planning, implementing and evaluating a competency-based curriculum. AMEE Education Guide No. 14 Part 2, *Medical Teacher* **21**, 15–22.

Chapter 16

Curriculum governance

Ineke Wolfhagen and Albert Scherpbier

Problem-based learning (PBL) is a student-centred approach to education that differs fundamentally from the traditional, teacher-centred approaches in which programmes are organized by discipline and teachers are primarily transmitters of knowledge. PBL, by contrast, is organized thematically and multidisciplinary and students actively direct their own learning stimulated by an inspiring learning environment. For teachers this means having to take on a role for which their own experience offers at best only a few models. They must be facilitators and stimulators of students' learning processes, in addition to the familiar role of disseminator of knowledge (Chapter 3). In PBL, the roles of medical teachers have diversified. This situation calls for high-quality professionalization and support for teachers.

In accordance with the PBL principle of multidisciplinarity, teachers from different disciplines jointly develop, implement, and deliver courses and educational programmes. Inevitably, this means reduced autonomy of individual departments and, consequently, more central governance.

Matrix organization

Multidisciplinarity is a key characteristic of PBL (Chapter 4), requiring staff from various disciplines to work together in different configurations depending on the theme of a specific educational unit. In fact, the construction and delivery of a unit can be regarded as a project carried out by a group that changes in composition, over time and depending on the activities at various project stages. If an educational programme and its parts are produced by flexible multidisciplinary groups, it is not feasible to adhere to an organization model in which individual departments have full autonomy. A medical school with a multidisciplinary PBL programme, like that of the Faculty of Health, Medicine and Life Sciences (FHML) of Maastricht University, is better off with a matrix organization, a dual structure in which individual actors are accountable to different persons and different organizational levels for different activities. With regard to an educational unit in the medical curriculum, this means that the participating departments are primarily responsible for supplying discipline-related expertise, while the project group, or the planning group as it is named in the medical curriculum of FHML, is responsible for the development and delivery of the unit. The manpower for the project organization is supplied by the collaborating departments.

Central management

In a matrix organization, several collaborative arrangements are thinkable, all organized as projects. If a matrix organization is to be effective the departments involved must cooperate and be willing to assign their best staff members to educational tasks for a certain period of time. Obviously, an organization of this kind requires central management to commission and oversee

Illustration

Educational units are constructed and delivered by unit planning groups. Take the unit on ageing in the undergraduate medical curriculum of FHML. The members of the unit planning group are appointed for four years, after which they rotate. The unit coordinator, who chairs the group, is a staff member of the Department of Internal Medicine. The three group members are from the departments of Family Medicine, Rehabilitation Medicine, and Anatomy. All bring their own special expertise based on their professional background but together they decide on educational formats, learning materials, assessment, etc. The chair of the planning group is in charge of the planning the unit and group members are accountable to him/her. So the final responsibility for the unit rests with the group chair and not with the heads of the contributing departments.

all the educational projects that together constitute the programme and to monitor the education performance of the departments accountable to the central organization.

This responsibility can be given to an Educational Board. If such a board is to function effectively, it must have an adequate mandate and be authorized to make decisions in relation to the educational programme and implement them in the organization.

Illustration

FHML has chosen to install an Education Institute with a central Education Board headed by a scientific director in the rank of full professor. The director has substantial autonomy in overseeing all aspects of the educational programme. Various responsibilities are delegated to other levels. Each of the FHML programmes—undergraduate medical education, health sciences, and life sciences—is headed by a programme director. One level down, the bachelor and master coordinators are in charge of their respective programme components, while the year coordinators are accountable to the bachelor or master coordinator depending on the year in question, and the unit coordinators report to the relevant year coordinator. The picture that emerges is one of a multilayered organization in which each layer has its own well-defined tasks and responsibilities.

A central Education Board cannot fulfil its tasks without support from an effective administrative, policy, logistical, financial and quality assurance infrastructure. The critical role of a strong professional support staff in the smooth running of an organization is inestimable. This applies very strongly in the case of a PBL curriculum, with its complexity due to the huge diversity of projects, schedules, teaching roles, rotation of teaching staff, and variation in the numbers of staff hours allocated to education by the different departments.

Illustration

The FHML Education Board is supported in carrying out its tasks by a professional department comprised of the following units: Educational Affairs (administration and organization of exams, ICT, and logistics); Business unit (management support and finance); and Strategy and Policy unit (supports the education board in strategic and tactical matters mostly beyond the local level).

Diversity of teacher roles

Since a PBL curriculum is characterized by a plethora of educational roles, the Education Board must stay up to date with the different roles and their associated tasks and competency and time requirements. This is essential not only for ensuring that tasks are allocated to the most suitable teachers but also for keeping track of the time the departments invest in education, which the Education Board compensates for by allocating staff time and financial means.

Illustration

There is a description of each teaching role in the FHML programmes so that staff members know what is expected of them. The same template is used for each role. By way of illustration the task description of a unit coordinator is presented:

Task description

- Is responsible for planning, implementation, delivery, assessment, and evaluation of the unit;
- Chairs the planning group, allocates tasks, and appraises the performances of the planning group members;
- Supplies information requested by the education organization; and
- Tutors student groups.

Functional requirements

- Staff member with extensive experience in education;
- Has attended all mandatory training courses;
- Has knowledge of the content of the curriculum; and
- Has good interpersonal and organizational skills.

Recruitment

- Open procedure in which all departments can participate. Candidates can express interest by filling out the application form.

Appointment

- The education director appoints unit coordinators on the advice of the bachelor coordinator.

Number of hours

- 200 hours, not including the tutor role.

Duration

- 3 years, reappointment for one additional term is possible.

Evaluation

- The bachelor coordinator appraises the performance of the block coordinators in the bachelor programme.

Category

Educational development and/or organization of major programme components.

Teachers in a PBL programme fulfil many roles, not all of which are specifically related to their personal professional expertise. Education roles vary widely from tutor to coordinator of a bachelor or master programme. A solid faculty development programme offering basic courses

(PBL) as well as courses tailored to specific roles is prerequisite to ensuring that staff members are well prepared for their education tasks (Chapter 18).

Task forces

Within PBL, teaching staff from different disciplines need additional educational support to develop and sustain a high-quality programme. Educationalists contribute to the development of new programmes, modification of existing programmes, quality improvement, faculty development, application of new technologies in education, and the development of the assessment programme.

Illustration

Within the Education Institute there are task forces on e-learning, quality improvement, assessment, faculty development, and student guidance, each with specific responsibilities and domains of expertise. The task forces support all aspects of the education programme and monitor new developments in their area. Additionally, task forces ensure that new developments find their way to the educational programme and they guide teachers in the implementation of innovations.

The task group on assessment, for example, supports unit planning groups in designing an assessment plan for their unit by putting forward new ideas about assessment, but also by making suggestions for standard setting, question formats, and wording of test items.

Quality assurance

In order to sustain high-quality curricula a solid quality assurance system is needed to supply data to underpin criticism of and praise for, as well as to monitor the quality of, the programme and its teachers. In this way quality assurance systems can both *improve* and *control* the quality of education and teachers (Dolmans et al., 2003). The notion that quality assurance is vital to the organization should permeate at all levels. Individual staff members should engage in continuous educational improvement, based on a shared set of norms and values and commitment to education. On the other hand the institution should facilitate the measurement component of quality assurance and give it its unequivocal backing (EUA, 2006). Evaluation data on programmes and teachers are indispensable for achieving the objectives of quality assurance. Teachers can use evaluation data to improve their courses and teaching based on the strengths and weaknesses revealed by the evaluation. After the implementation of change, its effects must be monitored to ensure that improvements are actually achieved (Chapter 17).

The Education Board is responsible for the quality of all aspects of FHML's education efforts. In order to meet this responsibility the Education Board must scrutinize evaluation data and discuss them with the departments. Feedback on and discussion of evaluation data with the departments is important because it emphasizes the weight placed on the evaluations. Whenever it is deemed necessary, department heads must take action in response to evaluation data, for instance by confronting staff members whose performance was below par but also by commending staff for excellence in education. Evaluation can also reveal that a department is not meeting its required contribution to the curriculum. This calls for an investigation of potential causes. Perhaps it is a sign of insufficient attention paid to the domain in question in the curriculum and/or a matter of department members not fulfilling their share of education roles.

Illustration

At FHML, all components of the education programme and many teaching roles are evaluated regularly, mainly based on student judgments. The data are sent to the unit coordinators, who make a plan of action, based on the evaluation outcomes, to improve their unit. The coordinators discuss their plans with the bachelor coordinator. In the following year, it is evaluated whether the desired effects have occurred.

Department heads receive an annual review of their department's contribution to education in terms of staff hours allocated as well as the quality of the performance of staff members. The scientific director meets annually with department heads to review the qualitative and quantitative evaluation data of their departments. Both positive and negative aspects are subject of discussion. Any agreements reached on steps to be taken to ensure improvement are documented.

Human Resources Management (HRM)

High-quality education can only be achieved in an organization that invests in human resources management. An important premise should be that education tasks are taken at least as seriously as research or service tasks. In order to promote that educational achievements have an equal impact, they should be considered in career decisions. Clearly, an explicit career policy is needed. In other words it should be possible for staff members to be promoted to a professorial rank on the basis of their educational achievements. Faculty who wish to improve their educational skills or who aspire to a career in education must be given the opportunity to develop their skills and expertise by attending faculty development activities.

Illustration

At FHML, faculty can be promoted to any professorial rank based on excellence in education. The aim of this policy is to strengthen the scientific base of education to foster continuous innovation of the educational profile. Faculty eligible for promotion must have made a marked contribution to education and show potential for further personal development in the education domain. To date these cases are fairly rare but more focused policies are being developed and a career track in education is being set up.

Future developments

The education market is in a state of flux: it is becoming increasingly difficult to recruit the right students, in sufficient numbers, to the right education programmes. Additionally, the demand for different education programmes is likely to change in the future. The Education Institute will be facing huge challenges as a consequence.

On the one hand efforts must continue to improve the FHML curricula in order to maintain and enhance their quality and prepare them to meet changes in the environment. On the other hand the financial prospects for higher education are not entirely favourable. Human resources management and continuous education (lifelong learning) are crucial for the future to ensure a large pool of well-trained teachers who can help to bring about the necessary changes. A logical consequence is that it must become much more self-evident than it is today that teachers' efforts in education and training translate into promising education career prospects.

In conclusion

This chapter focused on what is considered the most appropriate organizational and management structure in a PBL curriculum. Examples from the FHML medical curriculum have illustrated how governance is implemented there. In the ten years since it was formed, the FHML Education Institute has developed into an independent organization with well-defined powers and responsibilities. Some of the faculty feel that today there are too many organizational layers and too much central management. This may reflect a loss of teachers' sense of ownership. It is imperative that this be prevented, because the commitment of teachers is crucial to the quality of education.

High-quality education is paramount for FHML. Well-trained professional teachers have an essential contribution to make in this respect and therefore faculty development is high on the agenda. Staff should be offered realistic opportunities to pursue a career in education. Excellence in education must be taken into consideration in decisions on promotion and appointments. There is therefore broad support for a strong development of human resources management in this area.

It is a positive result of the developments of the past ten years that the Education Institute has gained an important position within FHML, a position that places the institute on an equal footing with the research schools.

References

Dolmans, D. H. J. M., Wolfhagen, H. A. P., and Scherpbier, A. J. J. A. (2003). From quality assurance to total quality management: how can quality assurance result in continuous improvement in health professions education? *Education for Health* **16**, 210–17.

EUA (2006). *Quality culture in European universities: a bottom-up approach*. Belgium: European University Association (EUA).

Chapter 17

Quality assurance

Renée Stalmeijer, Diana Dolmans, Henk van Berkel, and Ineke Wolfhagen

Quality assurance in higher education has gained significant importance, and both internal and external quality assurance are high on the agenda of higher education institutions (HEI). Rising student numbers and the concomitant increase in costs, increased emphasis on efficiency and effectiveness, and more autonomy for higher education in general have incited a need for quality assurance (Becket & Brookes, 2006). Although the need is clear, many HEIs find themselves struggling to develop and implement a system for internal quality assurance and create a quality culture within their institutions (Harvey & Stensaker, 2008).

Why quality assurance? Accountability and improvement

Quality assurance can be defined as the planned and systematic activities put in place to ensure that quality requirements for a product or service are fulfilled (Bowden & Marton, 2000). Translated to an educational setting this definition implies that quality assurance can focus on the quality of teaching staff, faculty development, and quality of assessment, but also on managerial processes; input, throughput, and output of students; and human resource management. In general, two main goals of quality assurance can be discerned: providing information to account for the quality of an educational programme and generating data that can help to improve the quality of education (Vroeijenstijn, 1995). Accounting for quality is directed at detecting and signalling weaknesses within the process or system by monitoring the quality of education. Quality improvement, on the other hand, is concerned with diagnosing weaknesses and generating suggestions for improvement. In higher education an overall shift from accounting for quality to improving quality has been reported. Elton (1992; cited in Houston, 2008; McKay & Kember, 1999) described this change as a shift in focus from 'quality A's'—assurance, accountability, audit, and assessment—to 'quality E's'—enhancement, empowerment, enthusiasm, and excellence. However, the balance between accountability and improvement differs between individual institutions and countries, depending on external quality directives and the internal quality assurance culture within institutions.

Programme evaluation

One of the processes for supporting quality assurance is programme evaluation. Programme evaluation is defined as 'a process consisting of defining, collecting, and presenting useful information with the aim to judge alternative decisions' (Stufflebeam et al., 1971). Ideally, it is a cyclic process comprising: (1) defining and measuring quality; (2) judging quality against predefined standards to determine strengths and weaknesses; and (3) making improvements based upon the information collected. After improvements have been made, the effectiveness of these improvements needs to be measured, and the cycle of measuring, judging, and improving starts all over again.

Quality assurance and programme evaluation at FHML have a long history. In 1983, a system of programme evaluation was designed in order to collect more information about the educational process (Dolmans et al., 2003; Gijselaers, 1990). Up till then quality assurance had mainly relied on assessment results, i.e., student outcomes. However, at that point it was argued that quality assurance should provide faculty and decision makers with more information to monitor and improve the curriculum (Dolmans et al., 2003; Gijselaers, 1990). Currently, quality assurance at FHML is focused on both accounting for and improving the quality of education, and is quite firmly embedded in organizational and curriculum development processes.

Measuring quality: systematically defining what you need to measure

The cyclic process of quality assurance starts with defining the objective of evaluation: collecting data for accountability or improvement purposes. This decision influences which type of instrument is to be used. For example, when the goal is to *account* for the quality of education, instruments are usually designed to generate a general impression or quick scan of the current status of educational quality (for example, a questionnaire filled out by students at the end of a unit or semester). However, *improvement* requires rich data, usually collected through more diagnostic-type questionnaires (open-ended questions), interviews, focus groups, observations, and document analysis. During the development of evaluation instruments, care should be taken to involve stakeholders and make use of theory about educational quality. Stakeholder involvement will not only enhance the content validity of the instrument in question, it will also enlist support for its use (Bowden & Marton, 2000; Guba & Lincoln, 1989). All in all it is important to approach the measurement phase in a systematic manner to ensure that all key educational aspects are part of the evaluation process (Dolmans et al., 2003).

At FHML, evaluation is guided by both accountability and improvement goals. For accountability purposes several standardized student evaluation questionnaires have been developed, which serve as 'thermometers' to gauge and/or monitor the quality of education. These questionnaires are limited in length (twenty items maximum), consist mostly of Likert-type questions, and signal strengths and weaknesses. Whenever weaknesses are detected, in-depth data collection may be initiated to seek information to guide improvement.

At FHML, several instruments are used for monitoring and/or improvement purposes. An example of a monitoring instrument is a questionnaire that measures the quality of a PBL unit. Research has indicated several key issues that determine the success or quality of a PBL unit (Figure 17.1): the linkage between the contents of the unit and students' prior knowledge, the quality of the problem tasks, the time spent on self-study, the functioning of the tutorial group, and the functioning of the tutor (Gijselaers & Schmidt, 1990). This theoretical framework has guided the development of a written questionnaire that monitors the quality of PBL units in the first and second year of the FHML curriculum (Appendix 1). It is administered when students sit end-of-unit tests. Another evaluation instrument used with every PBL unit is a questionnaire for evaluating the tutor. Because the tutor is one of the most important elements in a PBL curriculum, a lot of attention is focused on monitoring and improving the quality of tutors. At the end of each unit a questionnaire is administered to generate feedback for individual tutors. This questionnaire is based on a theoretical framework of effective tutor behaviour based on extensive research (Dolmans & Ginns, 2005). In the internal quality assurance system of FHML, clerkships also receive ample attention. Research aimed at defining a theoretical framework for good clinical teaching within clerkships was the starting point for the development of a questionnaire which is filled out by students at the end of each rotation (Wolfhagen et al., 1997). The results of this questionnaire

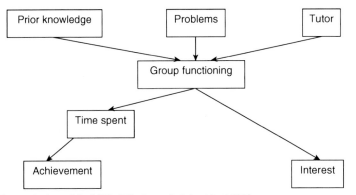

Figure 17.1 Theoretical model of PBL (Gijselaers & Schmidt, 1990).

relate to the rotation just completed but in order to enable comparisons between different rotations, all students fill out the same questionnaire. Recent efforts to provide specific feedback to individual clinical teachers on their teaching skills have resulted in the Maastricht Clinical Teaching Questionnaire (MCTQ) (Stalmeijer et al., 2008). This questionnaire consists of statements about effective clinical teaching behaviour during clerkships, and is based on the cognitive apprenticeship model (Collins et al., 1989).

Judging quality: defining criteria, setting standards, and interpreting the data

After quality measurement, the evaluation process proceeds by judging the quality of education based on the data collected. The measurement phase answers the question 'What is quality?', resulting in several indicators of what should be measured and how. In the judgement phase, criteria and standards are set to aid the interpretation of the collected data in order to inform decisions about desired and necessary actions. A distinction is usually made between absolute and relative criteria (Table 17.1). Absolute criteria define a norm against which a measurement can be gauged. Relative criteria relate to a point of reference that depends on whether judgement is passed in relation to accountability or improvement. For example, at FHML, the evaluation of an unit is compared with the evaluation of the same unit in previous years but also with the evaluations of other units in the same year.

In terms of data reporting, several aspects are important: which data are reported, who should receive which information, and finally in what format should the data be reported? At FHML, a general evaluation report is produced at the end of each unit. Dolmans et al. (2003) stress the need for structural data collection to stimulate the continuous process of quality assurance. In other words evaluations are carried out at regular intervals and with proper frequency. The report published at the end of a unit provides a summary of the evaluation results (based on the PBL evaluation questionnaire and an overview of the tutor ratings) and an overview of suggestions for improvement (Tables 17.2 and 17.3).

This report is sent to all those involved in the delivery of the unit (unit coordinator, planning group, tutors) and to the faculty administration. The unit report is intended as information for accountability and improvement, and unit coordinators are responsible for formulating plans for improvement based on the evaluation results. The clerkship reports are distributed in a similar fashion to all those involved in clerkship coordination and to the management of teaching hospitals.

Table 17.1 Evaluation criteria used at FHML

Absolute standard
1–5 Likert scale
< 3.0: unsatisfactory (−)
< 3.5: needs improvement
≥ 4.0: good (+)
Relative standard
Compared with the same unit in previous years
Compared with other units in the same year

Feedback for individual teachers (i.e., tutors and clinical teachers) is sent to the teachers individually with personal and specific feedback. Department heads receive general information on how their staff has performed as teachers together with an overview of their general functioning.

Improving quality: the importance of defining responsibilities

The final step in the evaluation process is to initiate improvements based on the results from the measurement and the judgement phases. In order to ensure that quality assurance is a true cyclic process that results in continuous improvement, quality assurance should be integrated within regular organizational working patterns (Dolmans et al., 2003). This means that the evaluation activities should form a coherent whole and that, most importantly, clear responsibilities are defined in relation to improvement activities.

Table 17.2 Example of unit report with absolute criteria

		N	Min	Max	Mean	SD
1	Unit contents fitted in with the knowledge I already had.	343	2	5	3.5	0.8
2	There was good coherence among the different parts of the unit.	343	1	5	3.3	1.1
3	Objectives of the unit were clear to me.	343	1	5	3.3	1.3
4	The tasks stimulated useful group discussion.	343	1	5	3.4	1.2
5	The teasks encouraged self-study.	343	1	5	3.3	1.3
6	Skillslab training sessions were in alignment with the unit contents.	343	2	5	3.9	0.9
7	Skillslab trainig sessions were useful.	343	2	5	4.1+	1.1
8	Recommended resrouces were usefyl in studying the learning goals.	343	2	5	4.1+	1.0
9	The unit assignments were in alignment with the unit contents.	342	2	5	3.9	1.0
10	The end-of-unit test reflected the unit contents.	325	1	5	3.4	1.4
14.1	Overall quality of the organization of this unit.	342	1	5	3.7	1.1
14.2	Educational quality of the unit.	343	1	5	4.0+	0.8
14.3	Tutorial group productivity.	343	2	5	3.9	0.6
14.4	Usefulness of ELEUM.	343	1	5	4.0+	0.8

N, number of students; Mean, on 1–5 Likert scale; Min, lowest rating; Max, highest rating; SD, standard deviation.

Table 17.3 Example of unit report with relative criteria (compared with the same unit in previous years)

	2006/7	2007/8	2008/9
Quality of organization	3.7	3.5	3.7
Educational quality	3.9	3.9	4.0 +
The productivity of the tutorial group	3.8	3.8	3.9
Number of hours of self-study per week (median)	18.0	18.0	18.0
Total number of hours per week (median)	28.0	28.0	28.0

At FHML, responsibilities for the education programme are distributed across different management roles. There is a task force programme evaluation, whose task it is to develop evaluation instruments, collect and report data, and provide suggestions for improvement of the unit. The responsibility for the improvement of a unit, based on the evaluation results, rests first and foremost with the coordinator of that unit. This also means that the unit coordinator is the first person to talk to tutors who are underperforming. Unit coordinators are requested to write an action plan setting out how they wish to improve their unit for the next year. Secondly, there is a Bachelor and a Master coordinator who make sure that unit and clerkship coordinators actually follow up on their action plans. And thirdly, the education dean oversees the whole process. In order to further build a quality culture within FHML (Harvey & Stensaker, 2008) the education dean meets annually with the heads of academic and clinical departments at FHML and other teaching hospitals to discuss the evaluation results. During these meetings plans for improvement are finalized and department heads are requested to make sure the plans are carried out by discussing them with the staff members concerned.

Lessons learned

Using a theoretical framework for instrument development

The development of evaluation instruments is often taken lightly and regarded as 'just putting some questions together'. Bowden and Marton (2000) indicated that the use of a theoretical framework as the basis for evaluation helps to establish the direction in which efforts to improve teaching should be headed. A theoretical framework therefore can stimulate continuous improvement of educational quality.

Combining instruments and respondent groups

Many HEIs rely heavily on student ratings as the main input for their quality assurance system. Although student ratings have proven to be reliable and valid (Wachtel, 1998), research has indicated that exclusive reliance on student questionnaires is no guarantee for real improvement of education quality (Penny & Coe, 2004). Since quality is a relative concept (Harvey & Green, 1993), different stakeholders need to be involved to obtain a holistic view of the quality of education. Consequently, a combination of different instruments and respondents is needed to guide evaluation for accountability and improvement purposes. For example, Berk (2005) has described as many as twelve strategies for evaluating teacher effectiveness, including peer ratings, self-evaluation, and student interviews. Recent initiatives at FHML are focus groups with skills trainers to evaluate a new skills programme and specially trained students who observe lectures and provide oral and written feedback to lecturers. Both initiatives are highly appreciated by staff as these methods are considered to provide more specific feedback and concrete suggestions for improvement.

Involvement of students

Another lesson learned at FHML is the importance of communicating (some of the) evaluation results to students. Because of the heavy reliance on student ratings in most HEIs, students will have filled out many questionnaires by the end of their university career and 'evaluation fatigue' is not unheard of (Svinicki & Marilla, 2001). One of the ways to counter this is to engage students more in the evaluation process by involving them in the development of new instruments and communicating (some of) the evaluation results to them (Nulty, 2008). In that way the importance of evaluation can be conveyed to students, which may stimulate response rates, because students feel involved and see that things actually change as a result of their evaluations.

Future developments

Several authors have described the advantages of electronic evaluation as compared to paper evaluation (Nulty, 2008; Sorenson & Johnson, 2003). Electronic evaluation is said to result in less administration, more complete data collection, longer and more thoughtful student responses, reduced processing time and costs, more accurate data collection and reporting, and more detailed, user-friendly reports (Johnson, 2003). However, the major and serious disadvantage of electronic evaluation is the drop in response rates (Sorenson & Reiner, 2003). This drawback and the fact that FHML relies heavily on student ratings for accounting for and improving the quality of the curriculum explain why FHML remains hesitant to collect evaluation data electronically. Nevertheless, in order to be able to benefit from the advantages of electronic evaluation, future projects will investigate ways of achieving response rates that will ensure the validity and reliability of the instruments. One of the ways to do so is increased involvement of students in the evaluation process (Nulty, 2008). Not only by involving them in the development of instruments or by reporting evaluation results to them, but also by engaging them as trained observers in the curriculum as described earlier. Ensuring the completion of the evaluation cycle of measuring, judging, and improving in such a way that continuous improvement is achieved also depends on strong collaboration with and commitment from faculty. Additionally, collaboration with other expert groups in faculty development and assessment can further stimulate the implementation of improvements based on quality assurance data. By completing the evaluation cycle and building a quality culture (Harvey & Stensaker, 2008) FHML hopes to continue to make progress towards excellence in quality assurance.

Annotated literature

Harvey, L., and Green, D. (1993). Defining quality. *Assessment and Evaluation in Higher Education* **18**, 9–34. This is one of the most cited articles in the literature on quality assurance within higher education institutions. Quality is a relative concept and can mean different things to different stakeholders and in different contexts. Harvey and Green discern five types of quality: (1) quality as exceptional or excellence; (2) quality as perfection or consistency; (3) quality as fitness for purpose; (4) quality as value for money; and (5) quality as transformation. They argue that in order to determine criteria for measuring and improving quality, an understanding of the different conceptions of quality is needed.

Morrison, J. (2003). ABC of learning and teaching in medicine: evaluation. *British Medical Journal* **326**, 385–7.
The ABC of Learning and Teaching in Medicine series is a very practical and compact guide that gives an overview of the different purposes of evaluation, tools, procedures, respondents, and other relevant elements. This publication can get readers off to a good start in designing their own system of programme evaluation.

Sallis, E. (2001). *Total quality management in education*. London: Kogan Page.

This book by Edward Sallis describes total quality management as a philosophy that can help educational institutions not only to implement quality assurance within their institutions but also to manage change. A framework for quality management is provided and described.

References

Becket, N., and Brookes, M. (2006). Evaluating quality management in university departments. *Evaluating Quality Management* 14(2), 123–42.

Berk, R. A. (2005). Survey of 12 strategies to measure teaching effectiveness. *International Journal of Teaching and Learning in Higher Education* 17(1), 48–62.

Bowden, J., and Marton, F. (2000). Quality and qualities. In: J. Bowden and F. Marton (eds), *The university of learning*. London: Kogan Page.

Collins, A., Brown, J. S., and Newman, S. E. (1989). Cognitive apprenticeship: teaching the crafts of reading, writing, and mathematics. In: L. B. Resnick (ed.), *Knowing, learning, and instruction: Essays in honor of Robert Glaser*. Hillsdale, NJ: Lawrence Erlbaum. Pp. 453–94.

Dolmans, D. H. J. M., and Ginns, P. (2005). A short questionnaire to evaluate the effectiveness of tutors in PBL: validity and reliability. *Medical Teacher* 27(6), 534–8.

Dolmans, D. H. J. M., Wolfhagen, H. A. P., and Scherpbier, A. J. J. A. (2003). From quality assurance to total quality management: how can quality assurance result in continuous improvement in health professions education? *Education for Health* 16(2), 210–17.

Gijselaers, W. H. (1990). Curriculum evaluation. In: C. van der Vleuten & W. Wijnen (eds), *Problem-based learning: perspectives from the Maastricht experience*. Thesis, Amsterdam.

Gijselaers, W. H., and Schmidt, H. G. (1990). Development and evaluation of a causal model of problem-based learning. In: Z. M. Nooman, H. G. Schmidt, and E. S. Ezzat (eds), *Innovation in medical education: an evaluation of its present status* New York: Springer. Pp. 95–113.

Guba, E. G., and Lincoln, Y. S. (1989). *Fourth generation evaluation*. Newbury Park, London: Sage.

Harvey, L., and Green, D. (1993). Defining quality. *Assessment and Evaluation in Higher Education* 18(1), 9–34.

Harvey, L., and Stensaker, B. (2008). Quality culture: understandings, boundaries and linkages. *European Journal of Education* 43(4), 427–42.

Houston, D. (2008). Rethinking quality and improvement in higher education. *Quality Assurance in Education* 16(1), 61–79.

Johnson, T. D. (2003). Online student ratings: Will students respond? *New Directions for Teaching and Learning* 96, 49–59.

McKay, J., and Kember, D. (1999). Quality assurance systems and educational development: part 1—the limitations of quality control. *Quality Assurance in Education* 7(1), 25–9.

Nulty, D. D. (2008). The adequacy of response rates to online and paper surveys: What can be done? *Assessment and Evaluation in Higher Education* 33(3), 301–14.

Penny, A. R., and Coe, R. (2004). Effectiveness of consultation on student ratings feedback: A meta-analysis. *Review of Educational Research* 74(2), 215–53.

Sorenson, D. L., and Johnson, T. D. (eds) (2003). Online student ratings of instruction. *New Directions for Teaching and Learning* 96.

Sorenson, D. L., and Reiner. (2003). Charting the uncharted seas of online student ratings of instruction. *New Directions for Teaching and Learning* 96, 1–24.

Stalmeijer, R. E., Dolmans, D. H. J. M., Wolfhagen, I. H. A. P., Muijtjens, A. M. M., and Scherpbier, A. J. J. A. (2008). The development of an instrument for evaluating clinical teachers: involving stakeholders to determine content validity. *Medical Teacher* 30(8), e272–7.

Stufflebeam, D. L., Foley, W. J., Gephart, W. J., Guba, E. G., Hammond, R. L., Merriman, H. D., et al. (1971). *Educational evaluation and decision making*. Itasca, IL: F. E. Peacock.

Svinicki, M. D., & Marilla, D. (2001). Encouraging your students to give feedback. *New Directions for Teaching and Learning* **87**, 17–24.

Vroeijenstijn, A. I. (1995). *Improvement and accountability: navigating between Scylla and Charybdis.* London: Jessica Kinglsey.

Wachtel, H. K. (1998). Student evaluation of college teaching effectiveness: a brief review. *Assessment and Evaluation in Higher Education* **23(2)**, 191–212.

Wolfhagen, H. A. P., Gijselaers, W. H., Dolmans, D. H. J. M., Essed, G. G. M., & Schmidt, H. G. (1997). Improving clinical education through evaluation. *Medical Teacher* **19(2)**, 99–103.

Appendix 1

Evaluation questionnaire PBL unit
Unit Evaluation Year 1 and 2, FHML, Medicine

Unit:	1.1	1.2	1.3	1.4	1.5	1.6	2.1	2.2	2.3	2.4	2.5
	☐	☐	☐	☐	☐	☐	☐	☐	☐	☐	☐

Tutorial group number:

1	2	3	4	5	6	7	8	9	10
☐	☐	☐	☐	☐	☐	☐	☐	☐	☐
11	12	13	14	15	16	17	18	19	20
☐	☐	☐	☐	☐	☐	☐	☐	☐	☐
21	22	23	24	25	26	27	28	29	30
☐	☐	☐	☐	☐	☐	☐	☐	☐	☐
31	32	33	34	35	36				
☐	☐	☐	☐	☐	☐				

		Totally disagree				Totally agree
		1	2	3	4	5
1	The unit contents fitted in with the knowledge I already had.	☐	☐	☐	☐	☐
2	There was coherence among the different parts of the unit.	☐	☐	☐	☐	☐
3	The objectives of the unit were clear to me.	☐	☐	☐	☐	☐
4	The tasks stimulated useful group discussion.	☐	☐	☐	☐	☐
5	The tasks encouraged self-study.	☐	☐	☐	☐	☐
6	The Skillslab training sessions were in alignment with the unit contents.	☐	☐	☐	☐	☐
7	The Skillslab training sessions were useful.	☐	☐	☐	☐	☐
8	The recommended resources were useful to study the learning goals.	☐	☐	☐	☐	☐
9	The unit assignments (that were part of the end-of-unit examination) were in alignment with the unit contents.	☐	☐	☐	☐	☐
10	The end-of-unit test reflected the unit contents.	☐	☐	☐	☐	☐

	1	2	3	4	5
	too easy	easy	just right	difficult	too difficult

11 The contents of the unit were
☐ ☐ ☐ ☐ ☐

12 What was the **average number of hours per week** you spent on **self-study** during this unit? (**Excl.** scheduled hours)

☐ ☐ ☐ ☐ ☐ ☐ ☐
< 5   6–10   11–15   16–20   21–25   26–30   > 31

13 What was the **average number of hours per week** you spent **in total** during this unit? (**Incl.** scheduled hours)

☐ ☐ ☐ ☐ ☐ ☐ ☐
< 15   16–20   21–25   26–30   31–35   36–40   > 41

14 Give a mark between 1 and 10 (6=satisfactory; 10= excellent) for:

	1	2	3	4	5	6	7	8	9	10

a) the overall quality of the organization of this unit
☐ ☐ ☐ ☐ ☐ ☐ ☐ ☐ ☐ ☐

b) the educational quality of this unit
☐ ☐ ☐ ☐ ☐ ☐ ☐ ☐ ☐ ☐

c) the tutorial group productivity
☐ ☐ ☐ ☐ ☐ ☐ ☐ ☐ ☐ ☐

d) the usefulness of ELEUM
☐ ☐ ☐ ☐ ☐ ☐ ☐ ☐ ☐ ☐

15 *Suggestions for improvements (open ended question):*

Thank you for your cooperation!

Chapter 18

Faculty development

Marie-Louise Schreurs and Willem de Grave

Ever since the inception of the PBL programme in Maastricht, the Faculty of Health, Medicine and Life Sciences (FHML) has recognized that an educational institution can be no better than the teachers and administrators who work in it (Guskey, 2003). It is therefore essential to put effort into the professional development of faculty teachers. From the start of the medical faculty, the teachers have been required to attend workshops about the educational strategy of problem-based learning (PBL) and the role of the tutor in order to ensure an effective and sustainable implementation of PBL. These professional development activities were necessary because teachers came to the Maastricht programme with traditional views of education which they had to change to acquire different teaching skills and ensure the successful delivery of the PBL programme. Professional development at FHML has developed over the years into an extensive and consistent set of programmes for a wide range of teaching roles in the PBL system.

Theoretical considerations regarding faculty development

Research on the effectiveness of faculty development has identified several principles and characteristics of effective programmes. The FHML faculty development programme is guided explicitly and implicitly by several of these principles. The following description of theoretical considerations serves to create a framework for analysing the faculty development programme of FHML.

Faculty development for a PBL programme consists of planned activities to increase the professional competencies of staff for different teaching roles to guarantee sustainable implementation of PBL. These activities can focus on *individual* teachers, but also on *groups* of teachers and/or the *organization* (Sessa & London, 2006). Individual learning can be realized for new skills, knowledge, and attitudes. Korthagen et al. (2001) distinguishes several levels of individual learning, including changes in behaviour, knowledge, beliefs, motivation, mission, and identity. At group or team level, learning is directed at changing the communication between team members. At the organizational level, learning is concerned with the development of visions and strategies. The individual, group, and organization levels are highly interdependent. Consequently, faculty development activities can differ in their focus on as well as the interaction between the different levels. In reviews of effective faculty development it has been emphasized that activities should be focused not only on the individual level but also on the group and organizational level (Guskey, 2003; McLean et al., 2008; Steinert et al., 2006).

In several reviews of effective professional development, lists of characteristics or features are presented (Guskey, 2003; McLean et al., 2008; Steinert & Mann, 2006; Steinert et al., 2006). There is, however, limited evidence to underpin those lists. Furthermore, the characteristics are sometimes derived from research in contexts other than medical education (e.g., Guskey, 2000). Steinert et al. (2006) used the best evidence on medical education (BEME) approach to review the evidence for key features of effective faculty development in medical contexts. In order to create a framework for analysing the existing programme of faculty development in FHML the focus here will not lay on a very detailed list of characteristics but on more general topics.

Principles of faculty development

A first principle of effective faculty development is that the programme should be *theory-based*. This means that well-known principles of effective teaching and learning, such as principles based on theories of adult learning and experiential learning, and principles of instructional design, should be incorporated in the programme. An important guideline is: Teach what you preach.

Another characteristic of effective programmes is flexibility in the use of instructional methods for achieving the objectives. Four types of methods can be distinguished: training activities, coaching activities, work-based methods, and e-learning-based methods. They can be used singly or in different combinations. Traditionally, training activities have been the dominant method but, recently, the other three types of methods and combinations of them have come to the forefront.

A third principle of effective faculty development is that longitudinal programmes—often integrated with practice—are more effective in achieving real change. Important factors are application of what has been learned and support and feedback from colleagues and/or coaches in the work environment.

An important characteristic of effective programmes for faculty development is linkage with concrete innovations in curricula. The need for faculty development becomes more salient to teachers when they must take on new teaching roles in a renovated curriculum. Linking faculty development to innovations also supports the implementation of the innovation. A project-based approach to faculty development focused on innovations is often recommended.

A fifth principle of effective faculty development is flexibility not only with respect to the methods used but also with respect to teachers' differing knowledge and experience levels. The focus of these activities can be on novice, beginning, and more experienced teachers in relation to different roles in the educational system. In order to adapt a programme to teachers' needs, faculty development activities should be aligned with a continuous faculty evaluation programme.

A sixth condition for an effective programme is that the teachers of the programme are well trained and effective in delivering the programme. So there should be a programme for the training and coaching of the trainers as well. Staff developers can be a select group, but they can also be recruited from a broader group of staff with good teaching records.

A final principle of effective faculty development programmes is a systematic approach in designing such programmes, starting from needs assessment and moving on to formulating goals, implementation, final implementation, and evaluation and feedback (McLeod et al., 2008). With regard to the design process, Steinert and Mann (2006) emphasize the importance of understanding the organization and the organizational culture and incorporating principles of adult learning. McLeod et al. (2008) draw attention to fostering a sense of ownership of faculty development in the participating staff members by involving them in the planning of activities.

The above principles and characteristics serve as a framework for analysis of the experiences of the FHML faculty development programme.

Implementation of the faculty development programme

Over the years, different aspects have influenced the development of the FHML faculty development programme. During the past thirty years the programme has evolved along four lines:

1 Because the medical faculty of Maastricht started out with a radically new educational approach (PBL), preparation and training of all teachers was required. All staff members had to become

acquainted with the concepts and educational practices of PBL. Faculty development aimed to familiarize teachers with the new roles and tasks, like the role of the tutor. The main focus was the individual level of new teachers in mandatory workshops.

2 After several years, more diverse roles of teachers came to be addressed, such as the roles of examiner, information provider (lecturer and teacher in practical or clinical settings), facilitator (tutor), role model, curriculum planner, unit organizer, and resource developer (Harden & Crosby, 2000). Workshops were offered on problem design and unit design, the lecturer in PBL, and the design of skill training programmes. These faculty development programmes were also mainly directed at the individual level to improve the skills of individual teachers but also at the team level, albeit to a limited extent only (Schreurs et al., 1999).

3 In the beginning, attention was primarily focused on the Bachelor phase. Today, faculty development is also targeted at the Master phase and postgraduate clinical training. Different types of students and diverse educational environments ask for different instructional formats. In this respect there has been a change in emphasis from the individual level to the team and organizational level.

4 During the early years of Maastricht University, faculty development focused mainly on the design of the new curricula of medicine and health sciences. After some time there arose a need for curriculum change, which could benefit from support by faculty development activities. Learning about workplace learning was integrated with concurrent curriculum development activities. Programme groups designed a new curriculum and at the same time were learning about new approaches to curriculum design. More recently, an organizational level approach to faculty development was realized (Moust et al., 2005).

Nowadays, faculty development activities serve the needs of novice, advanced, and expert teachers. The short tracks (workshops), and longitudinal programmes are designed to support the diversity of tasks of FHML teachers: teaching, coordinating, and leadership roles. The faculty development programme focuses on different levels of professionalism as described by McLean et al. (2008). For an overview of the faculty development programme in the 2009-10 academic year see Table 18.1.

The faculty development continuum contains the following elements:

Introduction to PBL and tutor training

Aim: Orienting new staff members to the educational culture of the faculty.
For whom: Mandatory for all new staff members.
Goals: To learn about the underlying principles of PBL and the basic skills for the tutor role.
Instructional methods: Interactive training in small groups of six to ten participants.

The workshops are based on evidence from various sources on effective tutoring and the functioning of tutorial groups (e.g., Dolmans et al., 2002).

Workshops in discrete skills

Aim: To meet the specific needs of individual teachers, a wide range of optional courses is offered. Workshops can also be organized on demand and tailored to a specific group.
For whom: Staff with educational tasks who need specific skills to optimize their performance.
Instructional methods: Short workshops in small groups. The methods also depend on the content of the training.
Themes: The topics offered include setting up and guiding thesis groups, different instructional formats within PBL, unit and problem design within PBL, mentor training, interactive lecturing,

Table 18.1 Faculty development programme 2009–2010

Type of activity, title	Target group	Characteristics	Duration
Short tracks aimed at educational development			
Writing unit books and constructing problems	Members of block planning groups	Theory, application, practice, discussion	4 sessions (16 hours)
Test construction	Teachers who have a role in or are interested in assessment	Theory, application, practice, discussion	2 sessions (8 hours)
Interactive lecturing	Teachers who want to improve their lectures	Theory, application, practice, peer feedback	2 sessions (8 hours)
Alternative methods for PBL	All faculty	Theory, application, practice	2 sessions (8 hours)
Short tracks aimed at teaching and tutoring			
Introduction to PBL and tutoring	All new staff members	Theory, practice, peer feedback	4 days (32 hours)
Drama techniques for lectures and presentations	All staff members	Introduction, practice, role play	2 sessions (8 hours)
Guiding thesis circles	Thesis supervisors	Introduction, practice, work place learning	1 session (4 hours)
Short tracks aimed at teaching and tutoring in the medical curriculum			
Consultation and reflection workshops	Those who perform this role	Introduction, exchange of experiences, consultation	
Cluster coaches in year 3	Those who perform this role	Introduction to the role of the coach	1 hour
Conducting admission interviews	Those who perform this role	Theory and practice of interviewing	2 sessions (6 hours)
Mentoring in year 1 and 5	Those who perform this role	Introduction and practice	2 hour sessions
Assessing professional behaviour	Those who perform this role	Introduction and peer feedback	1 hour introduction, 2 hours peer feedback
Basic training in clinical teaching	Trainers of postgraduate trainees in hospitals	Introduction and practice	1 day (8 hours)
Basic training in workplace assessment	Clinical trainers of postgraduate trainees and students in clerkships	Introduction and practice	1 day (8 hours)
Workplace assessment: 360 degree feedback	Trainers of postgraduate trainees in hospitals	Introduction and practice	1 session of 4 hours
Portfolio	Those who guide students in portfolio learning	Introduction and practice	1 session of 2 hours

Table 18.1 (*continued*) Faculty development programme 2009–2010

Type of activity, title	Target group	Characteristics	Duration
Mini clinical evaluation exercise	Trainers of postgraduate trainees in hospitals	Introduction and practice	1 session of 4 hours
Aimed at evaluating education			
Internal quality improvement	Particularly for members of block planning groups	Introduction, practice and discussion	1 session of 4 hours
Longitudinal tracks			
BTQ track (Basic Teaching Qualification) ◆ Pre-defined track ◆ Demand driven track	All those who perform teaching tasks	Workplace learning Training Coaching Reflection Portfolio learning	185 hours during one year
BTQ coach training	Coaches of BTQ participants	Workplace learning, training and reflection	Workplace learning, training and reflection
Master of Health Professions Education	Staff members who are interested in scholarship in health professions education	Workplace learning, training	2 year part-time course, distance learning and on-campus learning
Tracks tailored to individuals or special groups			
Tracks to meet special wishes of teams of teachers for curriculum innovation projects	Those involved in curriculum innovation projects	Workplace learning, training, and coaching	Varying duration

basic clinical teaching skills, introduction to unit examinations, coaching, individual guidance of learning, lecturing, drama skills, portfolio learning, mind mapping, construction of assessment instruments, and tailor-made courses.

The basic teaching qualification (BTQ)

Aim: Professionalizing teaching to ensure that individual staff members are equipped with the necessary competencies in teaching, developing, implementing, and evaluating the education programme. This will help to ensure that all staff with teaching responsibilities meets a number of basic criteria that are prerequisite for good teaching.

For whom: Staff with educational tasks.

Goals/objectives: The BTQ of Maastricht University covers six teaching-related competencies: subject-related aspects, development of teaching, teaching delivery, assessment and testing, self-reflection, and cooperation. After successful completion of the BTQ programme teachers receive a nationally recognized certificate.

Instructional methods: The full BTQ programme consists of a longitudinal programme of 185 hours spread over a period of one to two years. The programme comprises a combination of formal and informal learning and training activities, portfolio learning, workplace learning, and coaching. The programme is delivered in two formats: a supply- and a demand-driven track. The former consists of a pre-defined programme and the latter allows participants to plan activities in line with their educational needs and existing competencies.

The coach in the workplace acts as a facilitator and provides on-the-job supervision.

The portfolio is discussed individually and forms the basis of the final assessment.

The Master of Health Professions Education (MHPE) programme

Aim: Developing educational scholarship in the health professions domain.

For whom: For professionals with a Bachelor degree in the health professions domain who wish to pursue a career in health professions education.

Goal: The acquisition of knowledge and skills with relevance to innovative health professional education. The theme of the programme is the competencies required of an educationalist in the health professions domain.

Instructional methods: Two-year half-time programme, mostly distance based. Participants spend a maximum of three short full-time periods in Maastricht. The programme consists of a modular curriculum with units lasting around eight weeks.

Advanced teaching qualification

Aim: To provide a teaching qualification for staff in leadership roles in education. This course builds on the BTQ and supports more complex educational roles. It will be offered in the near future.

For whom: Staff members with leadership roles in education, such as programme directors and chairs of education committees.

Goal: Developing educational leadership by analysing problems and generating solutions for complex educational tasks, such as curriculum design, quality improvement, and organization and management of education.

Apart from the above-mentioned activities, support is increasingly supplied for curriculum innovations. If a specific educational programme is being renovated, faculty development supports the team engaged in developing the curriculum change. How to design an attractive programme and how to develop as an educator are motivating forces in this process. In this way faculty development is firmly embedded in the organization.

Discussion

The faculty development programme has undergone several changes. Also the mission of the faculty in relation to faculty development has changed. The main changes are:

1 Movement from one-dimensional courses for new staff members to a multidimensional training programme to serve staff members of all levels of expertise. There is a continuum of professional development opportunities ranging from skills workshops to longitudinal trajectories. The mission of the faculty is no longer restricted to providing staff with skills they are lacking but that are essential for the PBL programme, but it has extended to include the improvement of the quality of teaching staff and the promotion of continuing professional development. The concept of lifelong learning as an important attitude of staff is embedded in the entire programme. Not only FHML but also regional networks of affiliated hospitals are involved in these developments.

2 The programme uses a broad variety of instructional methods, such as workshops, case analysis, discussion, peer coaching, self-study, and workplace learning, to cater to teachers with different preferences for learning. The design of the programme is based on evidence from research about the effectiveness of PBL, tutorial groups, and the role of the tutor (see Chapter 6).

Currently, the focus of faculty development has shifted from individual to team and workplace learning. Adult learners use various ways of informal and formal learning to improve their teaching practice. Discussion and collaboration with colleagues is a strong method which is stimulated by the faculty development programme. Peer coaching is integrated with most of the training activities.

3 Educational innovation within PBL has become an opportunity for faculty development. Over the years, weaknesses in PBL have become apparent, for example students getting bored with using the same routine to handle problems year after year. Variations in PBL, such as more complex problems and PBL in small project groups, have been developed. These innovations are generally accompanied by curriculum changes. Involvement of staff members in innovations is encouraged to create ownership of and support for curriculum changes. Because today educational innovation is part of the mission of FHML, the focus of faculty development also encompasses the organizational level.

4 The principle of 'teach what you preach' is incorporated in the design of faculty development activities. For example, taking part in analysing a case in a mock tutorial group is a powerful learning experience during tutor workshops. Participants also learn from their trainers as models of teaching and from the training programme as an example of a design of a learning environment. Therefore, investment in the professional development of staff educators is also an important item on the faculty development agenda.

5 Faculty development is increasingly integrated in a system of quality improvement in several ways. Results of programme evaluation can reveal weaknesses in the curriculum and in individual staff members. This can be used as input for faculty development to address these weaknesses.

6 As faculty development activities have expanded over the years, a shortage of training staff has occurred. In order to cope with this scarcity, a 'train the trainers' programme has been developed. Senior staff members with training abilities are trained to educate their colleagues. This is done for training courses in basic clinical teaching skills in the affiliated hospitals. Also students with an affinity for teaching are trained as tutors for their peers. An advantage of this strategy is that participants can easily identify with these trainers, who are familiar with the participants' problems from recent personal experience.

7 The principles of adult learning are more and more integrated in the faculty development programme. Characteristics of adult learning are adapting to learners' needs through needs assessment, integrating learning with work, cooperating with colleagues in faculty development, more independent learning through e-learning facilities, and self-directed learning, for example by means of portfolio learning. Diverse learning methods adjusted to the needs of adult learners are combined in faculty development activities.

8 The shift in focus from the individual level to the organizational level means that nowadays staff educators must be more proactive to serve the faculty development needs of the organization. An active search for opportunities to improve the quality of staff involvement in innovations by offering supporting curriculum development activities has become an important part of the work.

Future developments

In the coming years, faculty development will focus on improvements in the programme.

More and more ICT developments will be incorporated in curricula, such as virtual learning environments and e-learning tools. Staff will need to be trained in the use of these tools and their implementation in the curriculum.

Another line of development is the integration of e-learning in faculty development activities, for example the use of a virtual learning environment by a training group and the use of an e-portfolio in longitudinal faculty development.

Furthermore, FHML staff members are encouraged to pursue a career in education. FHML aims to promote high-quality education not only by engaging teaching staff in educational research but also by encouraging them to pursue a career in education.

The movement towards longitudinal approaches to faculty development will continue. Staff members will be encouraged to plan more longitudinal activities, with training and learning interwoven with educational tasks.

More attention will be paid to public relation efforts. Apart from mailings and brochures, more web-based resources will be developed to promote the programme and bring it to the attention of potential participants.

Annotated literature

McLean, M., Cilliers, F., Van Wyk, J. (2008). Faculty development: yesterday, today and tomorrow. *Medical Teacher* **30**(6), 555–84.

This article provides a framework that may be used in designing tailored faculty development programmes. It describes a chronological evolution of faculty development in medical education from 1975 to the present. Major trends and driving forces are identified. Activities used in faculty development programmes should encourage experiential learning and reflection. Collaboration across medical disciplines, and, where possible, across professions should be encouraged.

Steinert, Y., Mann, K., Centeno, A., Dolmans, D. H., Spencer, J., Gelula, M., et al. (2006). A systematic review of faculty development initiatives designed to improve teaching effectiveness in medical education: BEME Guide no. 8. *Medical Teacher* **28**(6), 497–526.

This article reviews 53 papers to address the question: What are the effects of faculty development interventions on the knowledge, attitudes, and skills of teachers in medical education? The results are categorized by intervention type into the levels of Kirkpatrick: reaction, learning, behaviour, and results. Key features of effective faculty development are identified. The most important aspects that reinforce the effectiveness of faculty development are experiential learning, the value of feedback, importance of peers, and adherence to principles of adult learning.

References

Dolmans, D. H., Gijselaers, W. H., Moust, J. H., de Grave, W. S., Wolfhagen, I. H., and van der Vleuten, C. P. M. (2002). Trends in research on the tutor in problem-based learning: conclusions and implications for educational practice and research. *Medical Teacher* **24**, 173–80.

Guskey, T. R. (2000). *Evaluating professional development*. Thousand Oaks: Corwin.

Guskey, T. R. (2003). Analyzing lists of the characteristics of effective professional development to promote visionary leadership. *NASSP Bulletin* **87**(637), 4–20.

Harden, R. M., and Crosby, J. (2000). The good teacher is more than a lecturer. The twelve roles of the teacher. *Medical Teacher* **22**, 334–347.

Korthagen, F.A.J., Kessels, J., Koster, B, Lagerwerf, B., Wubbels, T. (2001). *Linking theory and practice: The pedagogy of realistic teacher education*. Mahwah, NY: Lawrence Erlbaum Associates.

McLean, M., Cilliers, F., Van Wyk, J. (2008). Faculty development: Yesterday, today and tomorrow. *Medical Teacher* **30**, 555–584.

McLeod, P.J., Steinert, Y., Nasmith L., Conochie L. (1997). Faculty development in Canadian medical schools: a 10-year update. *Canadian Medical Association Journal* **156**, 1419–1423.

McLeod, P.J., Steinert, Y., Snell, L. (2008). Use of retrospective pre/post assessments in faculty development. *Medical education* **n 42**, 543.

Moust, J. Roebertsen, H. Savelberg, H. & Rijk, de A. (2005). Revitalizing PBL groups: evaluating PBL with study teams. *Education for Health* **18**, 62–73.

Schreurs, M.L.J.J., Roebertsen, H. & Bouhuijs, P.A.J. (1999). Leading the horse to the water. Teacher training for all teachers in a faculty of Health Sciences. *International Journal of Academic Development* **4**, 115–123.

Sessa, V.I., London, M. (2006). Continuous learning in organizations: individual, group, and organizational perspectives. Lawrence Erlbaum asc.

Steinert, Y., Mann, K., Centeno, A., Dolmans, D. H., Spencer, J., Gelula, M., et al. (2006). A systematic review of faculty development initiatives designed to improve teaching effectiveness in medical education: BEME Guide no. 8. *Medical Teacher* **28**, 497–526.

Steinert, Y., and Mann, K. (2006). Faculty Development: Principles and Practices. *Journal of Veterinary Medical Education* **33**, 317.

Chapter 19

The institutionalization of student participation curriculum evaluation: From passionate volunteers to skilled student delegates

Fred Stevens, Marre Andrée Wiltens, and Krista Koetsenruijter

One of the most striking characteristics of the organization of the medical curriculum of the Faculty of Health, Medicine and Life Sciences (FHML) at Maastricht University is the strong and broad involvement of students in planning, evaluation, and decision-making in relation to the curriculum. Since the start of the faculty in 1974, student involvement has been consistently high. Students participate in curriculum planning groups, advisory committees and boards. In fact, participation extends to all levels of curriculum decision-making, from the educational shop floor to the faculty board.

Introduction

There are several reasons why student involvement in the organization of medical education is important. Firstly, students have first-hand experience of the curriculum and are therefore uniquely able to provide information for renewal and improvement (Slater, 1969). In addition, students are the consumers of education and as such their voice must be heard in order to preserve educational quality (Visser et al., 1998). Also, students are stakeholders in education and their participation is an important legitimization of the faculty's teaching efforts (Sallis, 1996). Finally, active involvement in decision-making with regard to the curriculum is a logical responsibility for students, especially in a problem-based curriculum, like that at Maastricht, which is based on the notion that students are active learners. Or, to put it differently, it is fully recognized that the participation of students as *competent*, *active*, and *constructive partners* is critical to improving the quality of education. Notwithstanding these evident reasons for student involvement, student participation in curriculum decision-making varies widely between universities, between faculties, and even between curricula within one faculty. This chapter focuses on student participation in the FHML medical curriculum.

Student participation at FHML

At FHML, student participation has been consistently high, even after changes in the Dutch law on university decision-making about ten years ago, which substantially curbed the influence of internal advisory bodies in Dutch institutions of higher education, thereby strengthening the decision-making power of university and faculty boards. Under the heading of modernization of university governance, university and faculty councils as well as various advisory committees lost democratic control of university policy as well as crucial parts of their influence on the decision-making by the boards. The effects were immediately noticeable. Many faculty members and students stopped voting in elections for representative bodies, as they felt it made little sense to participate without direct influence. More tensions and disagreements arose between the boards on one side and councils and committees on the other. For the first time, university councils, faculty councils, and advisory committees had vacant seats. Until very recently, the boards of several faculties of Maastricht University had difficulty recruiting faculty and/or student members. The growth of universities in student and staff numbers also contributed to the increased distance between governing boards and bodies representing the university shop floor.

But while a decrease in student participation has been an overall trend in Dutch universities, this has been much less marked at FHML. Medical students in particular have managed to maintain their influence. In fact, their impact on curriculum content and design has not diminished at all. Currently, student participation is flourishing as never before. The question is why this is the case. First, explanations can be found in theories of democracy. Next, there are explanations relating to the local educational culture at FHML. And then there is the way in which the students themselves have organized their participation. In the following sections these three explanations will be discussed.

Conditions for student participation

From a perspective on student involvement in which the faculty is viewed as a participatory democracy, there are at least three conditions that should be fulfilled: (a) consensus on aims, (b) absence of economic crises, and (c) level of education (Doorn, 1978; Philipsen, 1983; Visser et al., 1998). Firstly, for a democracy to be able to function there must be *consensus on aims*. When there are conflicting aims within an organization, democracy has little chance of success due to conflicts and power games. This can happen easily in faculties that offer a large variety of programmes. Medical schools offer only one core curriculum, which promotes agreement on aims, i.e., educating and training future generations of physicians. Within the medical curriculum of FHML consensus on aims is strong among faculty and students and there do not seem to be many seriously competing goals.

A second prerequisite is prosperity and the absence of economic crises. An organization struggling to survive tends to be less keen to embrace democracy. Or, to put it differently, when survival is the first priority, democratic principles must take a backseat. Dutch medical schools are rarely faced with serious financial problems. And even if there are such problems, budget cuts tend to have little impact on students, because the stakes are too high. Moreover, medicine is popular with students and every year there are many more applicants for it than students are allowed to study places. Annual admittance to medical schools is limited by government regulations and is currently set at 2,850 students spread over the eight faculties of medicine in the Netherlands. Medical schools are also relatively impervious to the effects of serious economic crises, as the demand for physicians remains consistently high even in times of economic hardship. Moreover, the government is generally quite generous in funding faculties of medicine, particularly as compared to many other faculties.

A third necessary and obvious condition is a minimum educational level of the participants in a well-functioning democracy (in this case the students) if they are to make a real impact on decision-making. It goes without saying that medical students are highly educated. This makes it easier and also more rewarding to involve them in faculty decision-making, to the advantage of all.

The institutionalization of student participation

At FHML, the above prerequisites are all fulfilled. However, this does not suffice to explain why student democracy and participation developed so well here. An additional explanation could be that student participation is highly institutionalized, in other words interwoven in the fabric of the institution, i.e., the system of norms that regulate the relations of individuals to each other and define what the relations between individuals ought to be. The institutionalization of student participation at FHML is firmly grounded in the orientation towards problem-based learning (PBL), which is characteristic of Maastricht University. Students' active involvement in the educational process in tutorial groups ameliorates the traditional hierarchical relationship of students and teachers and encourages students to speak up for themselves (Hofstede, 1986). The institutionalization of student participation at FHML dates back as far as the early 1970s, when the faculty was founded. At first there was individual involvement of students in curriculum planning groups, advisory committees, and boards. In the late 1990s, the students organized themselves in a rather loosely structured student council. The aim was to gain consumers (information) and provide feedback on the major topics addressed by various bodies within the faculty. Early in the new millennium a change took place. The organization of the student council became better structured, the domain of activities broadened, and student involvement in faculty policies intensified. The result was that the student council now operated more pro-actively. Student opinion spoke with one voice and was disseminated at all levels of the faculty. An evident consequence was that student opinions were valued more and had more impact. Obviously, there is also a strong positive connection between the institutionalization of student participation and the attention for PBL.

The organization of student participation

The student council consists of all the students who sit on a committee within the medical school. The specific tasks of the different committees are not elaborated here, as our focus is the overall student involvement. Figure 19.1 presents an overview of the committees and the student council. As shown in the left hand panel the student council consists of two bodies, the executive board and the advisory board, which include all students (or representatives) who take part in faculty activities. The work of the student council will be illustrated by describing the evaluation of education during the Bachelor phase. The delegate for the Bachelor phase represents all the Student Evaluation Committees (SECs) active in this phase (the first three years of the six-year curriculum). There is an SEC for each curriculum year, consisting of six to ten students who evaluate the quality of the curriculum in that year, unit by unit. SECs evaluate the quality of lectures, tutorial groups, lab practicals, and skillslab activities and, at the end of every curriculum unit, prepare a report that identifies the main issues for which improvement is required. After an SEC has discussed the strengths and weaknesses of a unit, one of the members writes a summary report, which is sent to the unit planning group and the student representative for the Bachelor phase. The student representative discusses the main topics of the report in the executive board of the student council, and then communicates this to the Bachelor curriculum coordinator and the education management team of the faculty. In this way, major topics that emerge from the discussions in the executive student board are also put on the agenda of the faculty management team. The process just described constitutes a quality circle (Figure 19.2) which is primarily conducted by students and parallels the quality circles run by the faculty. The student quality circle relates to all levels of the faculty, because of the involvement of the executive student board. Each SEC also monitors whether recommendations for improvement are addressed. The above example shows the importance of the student council and illustrates how powerful student influence can be, firstly by disseminating, next to the faculty's own formal quality circle(s), a consumer's view on

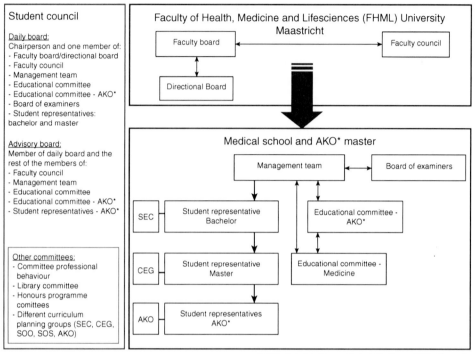

Figure 19.1 The structure of the student council (left); the different committees and their mutual connections (right).

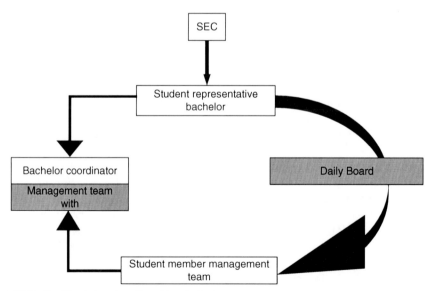

Figure 19.2 Quality circle primarily set by students.

the quality of the curriculum; secondly, by using a *bottom up* approach in the SEC's reporting to unit planning groups, as well as a *top down* approach by the student representative's reporting to the faculty's education management team.

The overall aim of the student council is to represent the students in faculty bodies involved in decision-making in education. One of the strengths of the structure of student participation is that students can express one collective opinion and, more importantly, speak with one voice about issues discussed in the different committees. An additional effect is that faculty members actively ask student representatives about students' experiences in day-to-day medical education. The members of the student council feel not only highly appreciated; they also are keener to state and defend their opinions.

The executive student board discusses current issues within the faculty. Most of the time, these issues are prepared or followed up in the different committees of FHML. The initial discussion in the executive board enables students to simultaneously disseminate a collective opinion in all the committees. This strengthens the students' position in the discussions. Additionally, the students are able to act proactively on issues relating to teaching. The student advisory board meets monthly to brainstorm on 'hot topics', such as the implementation of PBL, assessment, (lack of) motivation, and professional behaviour. General surveys are organized when specific problems require the opinion of all the students. The advisory board opinion surveys and discussions with fellow students together create a good insight into the views of the (majority of the) students.

The student perspective on problem-based learning

PBL became a controversial topic on the agenda of the student council during the academic year 2007–8, when PBL came under severe criticism from students. Some students felt that the principles of PBL were no longer adhered to. Others thought that PBL was outdated and had outlived its usefulness. The daily board of the student council decided to survey all Bachelor students on their views of PBL. This yielded information on the advantages and disadvantages of PBL as experienced by the students. Although the survey did not pretend to gather valid and reliable data, the results gave a good impression of students' views of PBL at that time. In Table 19.1 the aims and the practice of PBL are presented in relation to the four advantages and disadvantages most frequently reported in the survey.

The table shows discrepancies between the aims and practice of PBL. The faculty designs an educational framework that is preferably based on scientific evidence. However, this 'perfect'

Table 19.1 Overview of aims and practice of PBL as experienced by students

PBL aims (the advantages)	Daily student practice (the disadvantages)
Interactive, creative, and practice-orientated education, use of different sources of information.	Students focus on the standard (recommended) literature and the Internet, preferably in their native language.
Discussing ideas and notions results in more knowledge and better recall.	Free riders cause regression towards the mean in tutorial groups. 'Seven jump' is no more than a ritual.
Self-directed learning promotes the development of personal, individualized learning objectives.	Inadequate fit of personal learning objectives and assessment requirements.
Few contact hours, more student autonomy in time allocation.	Tutor involvement is decisive for the effectiveness of group process.

system does not always correspond with students' experiences. Bachelor students have first-hand experience of the successful implementation (the advantages) of the framework but most of the time they are confronted with the practical failures (disadvantages). During the Master phase this changes however and students increasingly report advantages of PBL during the Bachelor phase. A question that continues to fuel debate is therefore whether students just like to complain about PBL, or just are not aware of any positive experiences of PBL during the first three years.

Student experiences of tutorial groups

One of the major criticisms of PBL relates to the role and functioning of the tutor (Table 19.1). The variability in the quality and commitment of tutors leads to divergent student experiences, which give rise to negative comments. Because the tutor is of crucial importance to students in PBL, these issues will now be discussed in more detail.

One of the problems relates to the role of the tutor in guiding the group process. This role occasionally requires a tutor to intervene and stimulate students to properly follow the steps of the 'seven jump' (see elsewhere), which determine the process by which the group deals with the problems presented to them. It is the task of the tutor to motivate the students to engage in a proper brainstorming session and in a productive discussion of the information gathered by the students during the self-study step. To the dissatisfaction of some of the students this is not always achieved. Another, related, issue is the problem of free rider students, who shirk responsibility and profit from the work done by the other students. Students feel that tutors should actively deal with this problem but much of the time tutors fail to notice free rider behaviour to the frustration of the other students in the group. Another related issue is that, according to some students, some tutors are not strict enough and reluctant to confront students with negative behaviour in the group. This further frustrates the active students, because they see 'lazy' students getting away with unproductive behaviour without reprisal.

Implementation

As noted earlier, active involvement of students in the tutorial groups decreases the hierarchy between students and teachers and encourages students to speak up for themselves. In this particular case, aware of students' negative experiences with PBL, the advisory group of the student council met with the dean of FHML. Topics of discussion were students' perceptions of PBL, the bottlenecks in PBL, and measures to address these. Based on this discussion a letter was written setting out points requiring action, which was well received by the dean. Also, on the instigation of the student members, the education committee chose PBL as the theme of its annual *Education Afternoon*. During the Education Afternoon, pressing educational problems, this time PBL, are discussed by students and faculty staff to inform each other and exchange ideas for educational improvement. The meeting with the dean and the topic of the Education Afternoon are examples of the positive reception of student involvement at FHML. Students are the first to experience educational problems, such as the negative effects of variation in tutors. Initially, this problem received little attention from the faculty. However, in all the committees of the faculty, the students simultaneously started a discussion on the role and importance of the tutor. They kept hammering at this issue, until faculty members were convinced that something needed to be done. Currently, a process is ongoing at FHML to revitalize the role of the tutor in PBL.

Remuneration of students

As described earlier, students play a key role in evaluating and improving the quality of medical education at FHML. Students receive remuneration for several student membership roles. One of

Table 19.2 Remunerated students in different council and education roles

Committee	Number of students	Weight of role based on hours spent
Chair, student council	1	100[b]
Student advisor of FHML executive board[a]	1	50
Student member faculty council1	9	50
Student member management team[a]	2	50
Education committee 6-year curriculum/AKO[a]	6/3	40/30
Examination committee	1	20
Student representatives: Bachelor and Master phase	2	40
Curriculum planning groups (SEC, CEG, SOO, SOS, AKO)	22	5
Other forms of student participation (committee professional behaviour, library committee, honours programme planning committees)	~300	Variable

[a] Remunerated executive roles in official consultative and management bodies.

[b] To become a full-time function.

the reasons for this is to show the students that their efforts in improving the faculty's educational quality are valued. Another reason is to guarantee and improve the continuity of student participation. Every member of the student council (Figure 19.1) receives a scholarship or a fee, depending on the importance of the student role, the time investment, and statutory regulations. All memberships of students in formal faculty bodies, the FHML board (one member), the faculty council (nine members), the medical school management team (two members), and the education committee (six members), are rewarded by scholarships. The chair of the student council also receives a scholarship. All other student roles are rewarded by a small fee. An overview of roles and remunerations is given in Table 19.2.

Although remuneration is based on hours in function, this is only a fraction of the actual time investment. Evidently, the faculty's decision to financially compensate students for their participation is primarily an acknowledgement of and incentive to the crucial role of students in quality management. Nevertheless, it goes without saying that the majority of participating students are not motivated by extrinsic factors, such as financial compensation or their CV, but by intrinsic factors, like exerting influence and engaging in interesting and important work conducive to their future career.

Future developments

Over the years, the student council has become more institutionalized and, in the new millennium, more proactive as well. The latter resulted from an improved organizational structure and a willingness to act more professionally. Although professionalization has increased over the past few years, it remains an ongoing process. At the time of the writing of this chapter, the role of the chair of the student council was being changed from a part-time into a full-time function, which is expected to enhance guidance and professionalism. As a result of this change, the student council looks forward to taking more initiatives in discussing pressing educational problems and raising new ones. In parallel to students' efforts to improve teaching, FHML is engaged in a drive to promote faculty development of its teaching staff. Teaching staff are offered opportunities to learn how to teach, what is expected from them, and how to function as an effective tutor. Currently, FHML is in the process of renewing the medical curriculum. It goes without saying that students, as consumers and stakeholders, will play a key role in the curriculum redesign. Although student participation seems to be right on track, it is important not to sit back complacently but to persist in efforts to become more professional and effective. One of the main weaknesses of the student council is the lack of evidence for students' views and the representation of all students by only a few. Therefore, it is imperative to strive for better representation of the majority on the students and to give feedback on what has been achieved.

References

Doorn, J. A. A. (1978). Democratie. In: L. Rademaeker (ed.), *Sociologische encyclopedie [Sociological Encyclopedia]*. Utrecht/Antwerpen: Het Spectrum. Pp. 134–6.

Hofstede, G. (1986). Cultural differences in teaching and learning. *International Journal of Intercultural Relations* 10, 301–20.

Philipsen, H. (1983). Maatschappelijke aspecten van democratisering [Societal aspects of democracy]. In: F. C. B. van Wijmen (ed.), *Democratisering [Democracy]*. Alphen aan den Rijn/Brussel: Stafleu. Vol. 3, pp. 12–24.

Sallis, E. (1996). *Total quality management in education*. London: Kegan.

Slater, C. (1969). Student participation in curriculum planning and evaluation. *Journal of Medical Education* 44, 675–8.

Visser, K., Prince, K. J. A. H., Scherpbier, A. J. A. A., van der Vleuten, C. P. M., and Verwijnen, M. G. M. (1998). Student participation in educational management and organization. *Medical Teacher* 20, 451–4.

Chapter 20

Hybrid learning spaces: Learning resources and facilities for problem-based learning

Gaby Lutgens, Fons van den Eeckhout, and Jeroen ten Haaf

We live in a society in which we can hardly keep up with the growth in information and technological developments. Today's students are 'digital natives', who have grown up with technology. They enter higher education with aptitudes and expectations shaped by the use of the Internet, digital media, and portable communication technologies. In addition to regular students, we see more students who integrate educational routes with professional careers. For both groups, the university should create learning spaces that enhance student engagement and reflect the prevailing aspects of the virtual world, self-paced, independent, and social. The value of high-quality physical spaces and online solutions is increasing. The library has an important role here: to provide learning spaces in a 'social' context as well as a traditional 'scholarly' presence. Along with its services, resources, and technology, the university library invests in creating a physical and virtual agora and community for the twenty-first century.

Introduction

Maastricht University has always used problem-based learning (PBL) as the main educational approach and the whole organization is adapted accordingly. There are few lecture halls, but many rooms for tutorial group sessions, in which groups of ten to fifteen students collaboratively explore problem tasks. There is not just one teacher transferring knowledge and interacting with students, but as many tutors as there are tutorial groups.

An important ingredient of tutorial group sessions is the seven-jump process (Figure 20.1). Between two sessions, often scheduled three or four days apart, students engage in self-study and consult information sources or teachers in search of answers to the learning issues formulated in the tutorial group.

Unlike students in a traditional curriculum, PBL students are not obliged to use specific books or journals or to buy set books. In contrast, students are encouraged to search a variety of resources and come up with different information than the other students to ensure a lively discussion in the tutorial group in which problems are viewed from different perspectives. Therefore, students need to learn how to determine which information to search and which resources to use to gain useful insights into their learning issues.

Facilitation of students' self-study requires the availability of many titles on the same subject and even different kinds of information resources, some of which students can and cannot afford to buy.

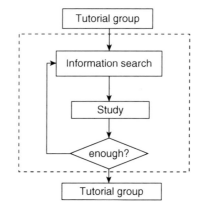

Figure 20.1 A schematic reproduction of the `Seven Jump´ with special attention to Step 6: What happens between the tutorial group meetings.

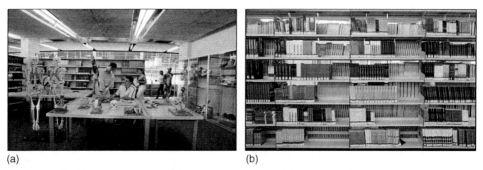

(a)   (b)

Figure 20.2 (a, b) An impression of the Study Landscape of the Faculty of Health, Medicine and Life Sciences.

The study landscape: a dedicated learning resource centre

In 1976, Maastricht University Library developed the concept of the Study Landscape (Van den Eeckhout, 1996) to respond to students' needs (Figure 20.2). It consists of a combination of study spaces and learning resources, supervised by skilled librarians and with generous opening hours (Box 20.1). The Study Landscape contains a variety of titles and types of resources, directly related to the curriculum. Text, pictures, models, diagrams, and moving images, all are present. To ensure just-in-time availability of information to all students, large numbers of titles (3–25 copies of each title) and programmes (selected by teaching staff) are bought by the library and all the necessary facilities are concentrated in one building. The materials are not on loan, so—if not on somebody's desk—are always available. In this way financial resources are used efficiently and, last but not least, the library provides high-quality and up-to-date resources and services.

Although the collection is inevitably limited, the large quantity of available resources forces students to choose which resources to study and which not to study. To put it in one sentence: the Study Landscape is where students (individually or in groups) can find information and equipment to read, view, and process selected information. The Study Landscape also contains computer workplaces, computer (class) rooms, scanners, and printers.[1]

---

[1] Since 2006, the University Library has centrally managed practically all on-campus student computer facilities. As well as scale benefits in terms of management and costs, overcrowding due to peak usage of the facilities by students of one faculty has occurred less frequently.

Box 20.1 Study Landscape around 1990
◆ Books, journals, videos and other resources
◆ Individual and group study places containing several facilities
◆ Information desk and information skills program

The Study Landscape is based on close collaboration between the library and teaching staff. In consultation with unit coordinators and discipline specialists learning resources are constantly being updated. As the collection grew, services were developed to help students find and use information.

In this chapter, the development of the Study Landscape over the past few decades is described: How does it offer access to all the information and tools for searching, using, sharing, and building knowledge in relation to teaching and learning at Maastricht University (the Faculty of Health, Medicine and Life Sciences (FHML) in particular)? What changes have occurred and are likely to occur in a future characterized by a knowledgeable society with growing needs for flexibility and mobility, and students that are 'digital natives'?

Where do we stand today?

Several processes have been initiated in response to the explosive growth of the amount of (digitally available) information and the introduction of educational technology within the university. For example, the university library has looked for tools to store, describe, and search the growing collection of resources not only within the local library but also in connected libraries. Within a period of a few decades, databases have become connected and search systems have become more powerful and easier to use. As users gained access to more and more resources and facilities, they and the library became interested in more ambitious services. One might think of a digital collection in addition to (and sometimes even instead of) 'hard copies', but also they gained access to statistical software and mail functionality. Less than a decade ago, the university started to implement a virtual learning environment (VLE[2]). At first the main aim was to organize face-to-face education and offer (links to) learning materials, but later group tools were introduced to promote interaction between students and teachers and to facilitate computer-supported collaborative learning. Today there are online booking facilities for resources and workspaces, tools to register for courses (e.g., on information literacy), e-reader services (digitized versions of books and articles) as an extension of the literature lists provided by teachers, and integration of the e-library, providing online access to all databases and services like dictionaries and online information desks (Table 20.1).

So, which resources and facilities have been created since 1990 (as described in the previous paragraph) to support teaching and learning? As teachers became aware of the possibilities of a digital collection and learned how to implement university library services within their courses to support the search and study of resources, it became increasingly desirable to connect the e-library with the VLE. Teachers use the VLE to describe and organize their courses, offer materials,

---

[2] Since 2003, all faculties of Maastricht University have used *EleUM* (the e-learning environment of Maastricht University), a set of tools connected to the Blackboard course management system, including other e-learning facilities, like online discussion and whiteboards, and software applications (office tools, statistical programs, multi-media equipment, video tools, and the like).

Table 20.1 Student facilities in the university library

		Location A	Location B
Computer rooms	> 20 computers	1	9[b]
	10 – 20 computers	5	11
	< 10 computers	3	5
Total number of computers[a]		315	567[a]
Study rooms	> 20 seats	3	3
	10 – 20 seats	10	3
	< 10 seats	31	14
Total number of seats (without a computer)		455	434
Total number of seats, with or without a computer		770	1001

The university library is situated in two locations. Location **A** is in the city centre, close to the faculties of Humanities and Sciences (FHS), Arts and Social Sciences (FASoS), School of Business and Economics (SBE), and Law (FL). Location **B** is outside the city centre, near the academic hospital and the Faculties of Health, Medicine and Life Sciences (FHML) and Psychology and Neuroscience (FPN). The figures represent the facilities in March 2009, when approximately 12,000 students were enrolled at Maastricht University.

The growing need for seats and facilities in the Study Landscapes and the substitution of digital media for many physical resources led to the use of the resulting vacant spaces to create additional physical study facilities, including computer workplaces. The diversification in type, number, and size of rooms (silent, discussion, computer, presentation rooms, etc.) was geared to student requirements.

[a] Not explicitly mentioned are outlets for laptops, since the wireless network makes logging in from laptops possible anywhere within the library building.

[b] At location **B** several computer facilities, managed by the library, have been realized outside but in the vicinity of the library, like Link, the Internet cafe. Until recently this facility created in the vicinity of physical resources like books and anatomic models, but outside the Study Landscape, met with the need of students to have their coats, bags, cell phones, food, and drinks within reach. Since the summer of 2009 it has been allowed to bring these into the library as well. These computer facilities are included in the table.

[c] A number of rooms also contain multimedia and audiovisual equipment.

such as tasks, e-readers, videos, and literature, and use the communication tools to monitor and coach their students, for instance during cooperation in knowledge building or project work. In order to prevent disturbance of information searches and study processes initiated from the course within the VLE, the e-library (containing catalogues, databases, and other online facilities) has been imported into the VLE. Students can seamlessly open catalogues or convert documents to PDF files while browsing their VLE courses. From practically any course they can access a course-based e-reader. For students, these tools and services are part of their learning environment. After starting up the VLE, they can access all that has been integrated or made accessible from the VLE: e-documents (syllabi, lecture notes), their portfolio, assignments (often linked to a plagiarism check), discussion and collaborative learning tools (like Polaris[3]), and web 2.0 functionality (wiki, blog, and podcasting tools).

---

[3] POLARIS is a tool especially developed for the Maastricht PBL environment to support students in searching for information, reporting on their findings, and collaboratively building a knowledge database in relation to the tasks (Ronteltap & Eurlings, 2001).

Ongoing communication with the faculties (often initiated by teachers using the VLE) has led to choices and developments in relation to the (traditional) library. The use of e-readers for instance has created a demand for more digital resources. Because students were spending more time in the VLE (downloading resources, submitting assignments, or interacting with peer students), more computer workplaces were created within the Study Landscape and a 'virtual student desktop' was added. Students who log in via the Internet enter an enriched desktop similar to that presented on campus. This desktop, named Student Desktop Anywhere, offers all the applications and resources available on campus. Furthermore, functionality accessible via the VLE and instructions on how to use them within the faculties have been integrated into the skills programme on information literacy in the introductory courses at the start of the academic year and in self-instruction modules and tutorials. And, in addition to the information desks at the library locations, a virtual help desk has been set up. In other words: the Study Landscape has become a hybrid learning space.

The overview presented above describes the facilities in today's Study Landscape. A hybrid environment has been created in which physical and digital facilities and resources are integrated and connections made with other internet facilities and resources, such as the institutional VLE and applications to support learning processes in and from the student desktop (Box 20.2).

The hybrid learning space has become an environment in which campus facilities (physical resources, facilities, and workplaces), electronic facilities (the VLE and the e-Library), and home facilities (personal laptops and computers, and the student desktop) are available and attuned to each other. Students can choose to use facilities on campus or anywhere else. Obviously, this changes where students choose to work. There is no need for them to come to the library to search and use learning materials or work on assignments. Interestingly, recent surveys of students' opinions about the facilities on and off campus show that the Study Landscape is still the place to be: 95% of the students attend the university library. Regular student evaluations are used as a 'thermometer' of the organization, to map the expectations, satisfaction, and wishes of students. They show that the library is highly appreciated by its users. See also the Flycatcher boxes in Figure 20.3.

Where are we heading?

With the introduction of the Bachelor–Master programmes and the adoption of the principle of lifelong learning, the university is focusing increasingly on student mobility and (part-time) professionals who (re)attend higher education. From the perspective of the FHML one can think of

---

Box 20.2 The hybrid learning space around 2009

Books, journals, videos, CD-ROMs, etc		e-books and e-journals, resources on the Internet
Computers at the university Wireless network for laptops	Individual and group study places	Virtual student desktop[a] e-Library VLE
Information desk Information skills programme		Virtual desk Self-instruction modules

[a] Containing applications like Microsoft Office, SPSS, concept mapping tools, etc.

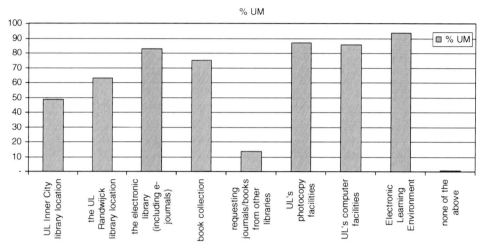

Figure 20.3 Use of different education facilities. In 2007 Flycatcher (an external agency that monitors all educational facilities at Maastricht University on a regular basis) sent a questionnaire to 1186 students. A total of 780 students completed the questionnaire (response rate 67%). The figures represent the number of respondents (in percentages) making use of the facilities. The monitor also surveys user opinions on facilities and services managed by the university library. In this box relevant data in relation to the (Virtual) Study Landscape are presented. The complete monitor consists of general satisfaction surveys, complemented by in-depth surveys on specific areas. Students indicated which university library facilities, both the physical and electronic, they used at least once in the past 12 months.

blended[44] master programmes—like that in Health Services Innovations—postgraduate courses, and the distance Master of Health Professions Education. Programmes like these increase the need for part-time or online curricula, digital resources, and online education and learning tools. Here lies a challenge. Will the university be able to maintain a 'hybrid learning space' in which students can use electronic and physical learning resources and facilities, both individually and collaboratively, and in which all (electronic and physical) facilities are combined to support teaching and learning processes?

The challenge lies in selecting, adapting, and maintaining a coherent set of tools and systems to aggregate a virtual teaching and learning environment closely connected to activities and physical resources offered on campus. Crucial is a well-functioning infrastructure, on campus, *en route* between campus and home or work (for instance on the train), and *at home* (or any other study location). Also strict requirements must be set for hardware both on and off campus. In order to facilitate optimal use of all the (online) learning resources, support for helping students and teachers organize their home infrastructure, access and use the university network and tools, and become skilled in implementing the available tools in teaching and learning processes must be provided. This requires information on how to access and use new tools as well as didactic support to achieve and maintain information literacy: how to use wikis, weblogs, and other web 2.0 facilities for teaching and learning. Information is also needed on how to make use of

---

4 'Blended' in this context refers to courses mixing face-to-face activities with online interaction, whereas 'distance' refers to situations in which students hardly meet (for instance, only for an introductory programme and closing ceremony).

tools to detect plagiarism in an environment of more and more digital information sources and digital submission of papers and assignments, but also on how to create a digital library for easy publication within the VLE and e-book readers, or how to use tools for collaborative knowledge building about multidisciplinary topics by students who meet face to face only rarely, if ever. Therefore, the hybrid learning space should incorporate online support services for all the above-mentioned activities. It does not matter whether the answer to a problem is provided by a person or generated through an intelligent 'question and answer system', as long as it is a quick and adequate answer. The (virtual) support desk could offer information and services from teachers, staff development teams, information specialists, system experts, or student service centres. But what does this imply for the traditional Study Landscape or library? Traditionally, the academic library was thought of as the centre of the academic community. Today, the academic library is extending its reach to build relationships outside the library. It is increasingly important to pursue partnerships with faculty, staff, students, and communities that promote programmes focusing not only on literacy, but also on cultural awareness and diversity. Despite the addition of numerous online resources and facilities, students keep asking for more and better study places at the university. And just as faculties invest in wireless networks in lounge-like meeting places, the Study Landscape is being equipped with flexible study places. Savin-Baden (2008) describes the role of different types of study places in her book on learning spaces. There are diverse forms of spaces (whether physical or virtual) within the life of an academic where opportunities to reflect and critique their own learning position occur. Hybrid learning spaces can be interpreted not only as a mix of physical and virtual facilities, but also as an environment in which study (or work) flows seamlessly over into leisure time. A hybrid environment in the latter sense enables students to mix study and social activities (receive instant messages from the home front or check their Facebook page while on campus to meet with peer students). Students appreciate it when the Study Landscape offers this functionality as well. Computer rooms or silent spaces near the physical book collection where they can study, but also a place where they can feel at home and free to discuss learning tasks but also socialize over a nice cup of coffee and flop into a comfortable chair to phone their boyfriend while, nearby, students are being supported in the use of a specific database. Students and faculty see the library as important and unique, providing learning spaces in an environment that offers a 'social' context as well as a more traditional 'scholarly' presence. Along with its services, resources, and technology, the library can be a physical and virtual agora and commons for the twenty-first century (Smith, 2005).

In order to achieve this both aspects need to be developed: a rich and at the same time convivial learning space (see also 'The Learning Grid, offering a mix of learning opportunities' described by Bell, 2007) combined with more and better connected online facilities.

Discussion and future developments

The university library is traditionally responsible for acquiring, storing, maintaining, and distributing resources for research, learning, and teaching. In addition, the library at Maastricht University maintains the VLE and several connected applications. The library therefore is responsible for creating and maintaining the hybrid learning spaces. As a user-oriented organization, the university library focuses on the needs of those involved in teaching and learning processes. Since e-learning develops rapidly, close cooperation is needed between the faculty and the library in order to optimally facilitate the changing teaching and learning activities. It is the task of the library to detect needs and initiate services: from increasing server capacity to accommodating the growing amount of multimedia documents and devices, to having students and staff annotate resources in the (digital) collection, extending the opening hours of the Study Landscape, and offering online services 24/7. In line with these developments, the university library encourages students to function as a feedback group to help the library in adapting its facilities to their wishes. Students might even be invited to take responsibility for maintaining facilities and supporting users within the Study Landscape. So in addition to giving their opinions on physical and online services within the hybrid learning spaces (as is done by Flycatcher or evaluation forms of workshops and other services), students might also support other users of services and resources. One should not be surprised to see a student offering help to a colleague who looks puzzled while searching a database or when students invite their teacher to come to the common room in the Study Landscape to elaborate on a topic of the lecture she gave the day before. It goes without saying that it is important to build upon evidence-based stories of success in implementing online solutions within teaching and learning scenarios. It is here that the faculty and the library can start to explore new opportunities.

Annotated literature

Bell, A. (2007). *Convivial spaces, convivial services: space re-design and its potential impact on the future of academic libraries*. University of Warwick, UK.

Prensky (2001) stated that 'Today's students are no longer the people our educational system was designed to teach.' It can, perhaps, be equally argued that today's students are no longer the people our traditional library spaces were designed to support. Many libraries are currently investing heavily in new learning spaces. What is less clear is how far such opportunities are being used to develop strategic service innovations that both anticipate and support emerging user needs to enhance the student experience. At the same time far less attention has, to date, focused on how physical space re-design and associated service innovations can support the teaching and research experience.

Savin-Baden, M. (2008). *Learning spaces: creating opportunities fro knowledge creation in academic life*. Maidenhead, UK.

Maggi Savin-Baden is Professor of Higher Education Research at Coventry University and Director of the Learning Innovation Group. She has published six books on PBL; this book is number seven. It is timely as it seeks to reclaim universities as places of learning. The ability to have or to find space in academic life is becoming increasingly difficult as we are increasingly consumed by teaching and bidding, overwhelmed by emails and underwhelmed by long arduous meetings. This book explores the concept of learning spaces, the idea that there are diverse forms of spaces within the life and world of the academic where opportunities to reflect and critique their own unique learning position occur.

References

Bell, A. (2007). *Convivial spaces, convivial services: space re-design and its potential impact on the future of academic libraries*. University of Warwick, UK.

Van den Eeckhout, F. (1996). Study Landscape: a learning resource centre for PBL. *Health Libraries Review* **13(1)**, 49–55.

Ronteltap, C. F. M., and Eurelings, A. M. C. (2001). *Activity and interaction of students in an electronic learnnig environment for problem-based learning*. Paper presented at American Educational Research Association, Annual Meeting, Seattle, April 10–14.

Savin-Baden, M. (2008). *Learning spaces: creating opportunities for knowledge creation in academic life*. Maidenhead, UK: McGraw-Hill.

Smith, K. (2005). *Library as place: rethinking roles, rethinking space*. Council on Library Resources.

Chapter 21

Assessment in problem-based learning

Lambert Schuwirth and Cees van der Vleuten

An assessment programme should be in line with the education programme (Biggs, 1996). This concept of constructive alignment is of vital importance because whenever conflicts arise between assessment and the education programme, it is typically the assessment programme that plays the dominant role in determining students' learning activities (Frederiksen, 1984). It is only logical then to conclude that a typical assessment programme for a problem-based learning (PBL) curriculum differs from that for a traditional curriculum. Although this does not mean that there are many specific assessment instruments for PBL, it does imply that the assessment programme must support the central concepts of PBL, such as contextual learning, constructive learning, and collaborative learning.

Design of the programme

History

Maastricht medical school was one of the first schools in Europe to introduce a curriculum based on the principles of PBL. Since at the time there was only limited experience with assessment in a PBL context, inevitably, the assessment system had to be developed from scratch. Initially, the main feature of the assessment programme was the so-called unit test, consisting almost entirely of true–false items and relating directly to the content of the different units. However, it soon emerged that the effect of these tests on students' learning behaviour ran contrary to the desired aim of promoting self-directed learning, a core characteristic of PBL. For, instead of formulating individual learning goals, students were mainly focused on what they believed was going to be in the test. When this came to light, a remedy was sought and found in the concept of progress testing, which will be discussed briefly later in this chapter and more extensively elsewhere in the next chapter. The central feature of progress testing is that students cannot revise specifically for a test. Instead, a regular study pattern guided by individual learning goals is more likely to be successful. After the introduction of progress testing, the unit tests became purely formative in nature. However, in response to criticism from various quarters that the assessment programme was too mild, in the mid-1980s the unit tests were made summative again.

The prevailing concept of medical competence in the 1980s was that of a combination of knowledge, skills, attitudes, and problem-solving ability. So, at that time a series of new independent assessment instruments (Objective Structured Clinical Examination (OSCE) for skills, case-based testing for clinical reasoning and feedback groups for attitudes) were developed to fit this concept. Since then the conceptualization of medical competence has changed, resulting in the realization that a reductionist approach—one single best instrument for each component—cannot be effective. Nevertheless the main problem remained unchanged, namely the persistent mismatch between the assessment philosophy (reductionist) and the educational strategy (integrative), with detrimental effects on student learning behaviour. In an effort to resolve this, it was decided to reorganize the assessment programme to better match the education goals.

The guiding principles for the designers of this new programme were five questions: why, what, when, who, and how.

Why: the purposes of the assessment programme

The general purpose of the assessment programme in a PBL curriculum is somewhat different from that in a traditional programme or of a licensing body. For licensing bodies the main purpose is to discriminate between competent and non-competent candidates, while in traditional educational programmes it is to determine whether students have mastered the subject matter to a sufficient degree. In a PBL curriculum, however, where self-directed learning is central, assessment has another crucial role, namely to make students aware of their weaknesses and strengths. Simply informing students whether they have passed or failed a test will not achieve this, because it offers students no clues as to how to improve their self-directed learning.

For the Maastricht PBL programme, steering the learning of students in the desired direction was defined as the main purpose of the assessment programme. Although the impact of assessment on student learning is not a particularly well-researched area of education, there is evidence that assessment drives the learning of students through its content, its format, its scheduling, and the regulatory structure of the assessment programme (Frederiksen, 1984).

Another, related, goal of assessment is to provide information to the medical faculty about the quality of the education programme. Where individually identified strengths and weaknesses can steer the learning of individual students, signs of common areas of weakness or misconceptions can provide valuable information about the quality of the education programme as a whole. This kind of information from assessment outcomes can and should be harnessed to ensure continuous improvement of the quality of education.

Of course the third important goal of assessment is to ensure the quality of graduates as competent workers in the healthcare system.

What is assessed?

It seems obvious to state that assessment must ensure the quality of graduates. However, the operational definition of quality is less obvious but nonetheless prerequisite for achieving this quality goal. A simple but helpful model in this respect is Miller's pyramid (Miller, 1990). In this—well-known—model four layers are distinguished, indicating different scope and depth of competencies. The bottom layer (the basis) is labelled 'knows', the second 'knows how', the third 'shows how', and the top 'does'. For the PBL assessment programme, the model was used to make two choices. First of all, it was decided to aim, wherever possible, at including the highest possible layers of the pyramid in assessments. In PBL, where much of the learning takes place in the context of cases or problems, assessment cannot be limited to the bottom layer but should incorporate at least the 'knows how' level. The second choice was to ensure optimum coverage of all the layers of the pyramid. So, the bottom layer must never be neglected, not even in the most senior years.

Where Miller's pyramid was helpful in determining the 'scope and depth' of the assessment of competencies, the competency profiles described in the national blueprint for all Dutch medical curricula (Metze et al., 2001) were used to define the specific competencies. The blueprint distinguishes four roles:

+ Medical expert;
+ Worker in the healthcare system;
+ Scholar; and
+ Person.

The individual competencies, determined for each of these roles, are central to the assessment programme throughout the six years of the curriculum, although more explicitly so in the senior years.

When: the timing of assessment

If an assessment programme is to provide rich information about students' strengths and weaknesses in relation to the four roles (at different levels of Miller's pyramid), it must be comprehensive. An important implication of this is that there should be as many assessment moments as possible, although not all of these need to be decision moments. Decisions must be based on the aggregate information from various assessment moments, the guiding principle being that the higher the stakes of a decision, the more extensive information is needed from different assessments to underpin it. The culmination of this principle would be continuous assessment. If the outcomes of the curriculum are to be described in terms of ever-evolving competencies, it is only logical to use continuous or longitudinal assessment as much as possible. In order to achieve this, it is crucial that several elements should be continuous or longitudinal and that the end results of and feedback derived from one education phase should serve as the starting point for student learning in the next phase.

Who is involved in assessment?

In the PBL education setting in which students are more actively involved in and more responsible for their own learning (self-directed learning), the faculty wanted to design a feasible assessment system in which students had more responsibility for their own assessment. The main focus of students' responsibility was their use of the feedback from assessments to guide their learning. Therefore a central role was assigned to a mentor for each student, who reviews the student's progress periodically (using a portfolio).

How is assessment to be set up?

It is especially important for continuous assessment that students should take more responsibility for their own assessment. Consequently, students need to be made aware of the value of feedback from assessments and how to use it in directing their own learning. This is by no means easy to achieve considering that most students have been educated in more traditional curricula with traditional assessment programmes. In such programmes a 'pass' on a test means that a circumscribed part of training is finished and requires no further attention. Contrary to this concept, PBL or otherwise competency-based curricula strongly emphasize the benefits to be gained by students from carefully analysing their test performances. Another important decision in designing the assessment programme was to aim for more authenticity. Although many programmes rely exclusively on highly structured examinations, such as structured orals and multiple-choice tests, this type of assessment is clearly not very compatible with the basic PBL concepts of contextual and constructive learning.

Description of the FHML programme

Figure 21.1 shows the programme for year 1, but the basic design is similar for the first five of the six years of the medical curriculum.

The assessment programme contains a modular and a longitudinal component. In the figure the different units are shown below the horizontal line and the longitudinal parts above the line. The units in the first two years are commonly referred to as blocks and comprise standard PBL

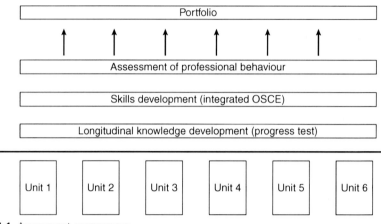

Figure 21.1 Assessment programme.

(paper case) sessions; in year 3 the units are referred to as clusters and paper cases are replaced by real patients; the units in years 4 and 5 are clinical clerkships.

In their sixth and final year students undertake a clinical and a research attachment of eighteen weeks each. During the clinical attachment, students work as junior house officers in a discipline of their choosing. Each student has a clinical supervisor who guides, mentors, and evaluates their performance. A similar setup is used for the research attachment, where students participate in an ongoing research project or devise their own research project within the framework of a research school. One of the senior researchers acts as mentor and evaluator.

Unit-based assessment

The faculty wanted to allow for optimal flexibility in unit design and the same objective was pursued for unit-based assessments. Consequently, no specific format is prescribed, although the planning group of each unit must draw up a plan, detailing how assessment will be designed, organized, and implemented. This plan is submitted to the certifying committee, which can propose amendments. Additionally, the committee examines whether the plan meets the quality criteria for fair assessment (reliability, validity, educational impact, cost-efficiency, and acceptability) (Van der Vleuten, 1996) and complies with the rules and regulations of the faculty. Various assessment forms are possible: end-of-unit tests (open-ended and multiple-choice test types), projects, assignments, continuous assessment, etc. The guiding principle for all unit-based assessments is that it should be designed to steer student learning behaviour in the desired direction.

A similar approach was taken for years 3–5. In the third year, students rotate through four ten-week clusters, each focused on one of four domains: abdomen, circulation and lungs, psycho-medical problems and mental healthcare, and locomotor apparatus. Real patient encounters serve as 'PBL cases'. Students conduct a patient consultation, derive learning goals from that (focused on the connections between basic science and clinical observations), study these goals, and report their findings to the group. For each cluster the final goals are formulated in terms of four competency domains, defined as the four roles described above (medical expert, scholar, worker in the healthcare system, and person). The assessment programme must provide information on the progress made in each of these roles. In order to pass a cluster, students must show satisfactory performance in each of the four roles.

Assessment during the clinical clerkships in years 4 and 5 follows the same pattern.

Progress testing

The concept of progress testing is discussed in more detail in the next chapter, but a brief description is given here. The progress test is a comprehensive knowledge-based test covering the whole domain of functional medical knowledge. All medical students (all six year classes) sit four progress tests in the course of the academic year. Each test is the same for all six year classes and consists of two hundred multiple-choice items. The scores on each test are converted to a qualification (good, satisfactory, or unsatisfactory) based on a year class specific pass-fail score, and the combination of qualifications at the end of the year determines whether a student receives a pass or a fail. Progress testing was originally developed to avoid test-driven learning as this was considered ill fitting for a self-directed PBL learning environment (Van der Vleuten et al., 1996). Progress testing is a reliable and valid approach to assess the growth of medical knowledge. As such, it is an important element of the assessment programme. Because knowledge is sufficiently tested by the progress tests, considerable latitude can be allowed to unit planning groups to use a variety of and perhaps less knowledge-orientated assessment formats.

Skills assessment

The medical curriculum includes a longitudinal skills programme. In all units students are offered a series of training sessions in history taking, physical examination, and therapeutic and laboratory skills. At the end of years 1, 2, 3, and 5, all students take a station-based examination, a so-called Objective Structured Clinical Examination (Harden & Gleeson, 1979). Students rotate through a series of rooms. In each room they must perform a task (e.g., perform an abdominal examination) on a manikin or a simulated patient while an examiner judges their performance using a rating scale (rather than a checklist) (Regehr et al., 1998). While performing a skill students must explain what they are doing, why they are doing that, and what basic science principles are involved. Also, students must explain their findings and the implications for diagnosis and management. In the first year the assignments are quite straightforward and focused on skill performance, but in the more senior years the problems become increasingly complicated. Although some time of this rather expensive method is now used to ask (skill-related) knowledge, which could be done cheaper in a written test, the integration of skills and underlying knowledge are seen as essential for a PBL environment. Therefore, it was decided to integrate them into one assessment method. This is often referred to as ISCE (integrated structured clinical examination). The emphasis on integration is based on experiences with prior OSCEs, which focused exclusively on skill performance. Typically, students prepared by memorizing the required procedures without understanding why they performed them. By integrating skills and underlying knowledge a more in-depth understanding of the physical examination is assessed.

Professional behaviour

The assessment of professional behaviour is an essential component of the assessment programme. There is a vast literature on how to define professional behaviour or professionalism. One stream defines it as a trait or characteristic (Arnold et al., 1998), while others define it in terms of observable and therefore assessable behaviour (Project team Consilium Abeundi, 2005). The medical faculty decided to follow the second stream, defining professional behaviour as observable behaviour. This implies that assessment should be based on repeated and prolonged observation of behaviour and not on a one-off examination. A second decision was to set up the assessment in such a way that it encourages all medical students to improve their professional behaviour instead of being primarily concerned with filtering out any 'bad apples'.

On two occasions in each unit, professional behaviour forms are completed by the tutor and all the students in the group for each of the students, including themselves. The first assessment—partway through the unit—is formative; the second—at the end of the unit—is summative. The assessment form is subdivided into three aspects: dealing with tasks, dealing with others, and dealing with oneself. Although a judgement is made whether professional behaviour with regard to these three aspects is satisfactory, the main function of the form is to stimulate all parties to provide (written) feedback on what is going well and which aspects need improvement. Ideally, students use suggestions for improvement to formulate targeted learning goals. Despite the highly informative nature of the form and the attention to narrative feedback, all unsatisfactory outcomes are recorded. Whenever a student's performance is judged as unsatisfactory, the student is invited for an interview with the committee on professional behaviour to explain that result and propose plans for improvement. If necessary, a student counsellor is involved as well. If an unsatisfactory result is a one-off situation, it has no consequences for the final judgement of professional behaviour, but a pattern of unprofessional behaviour will likely translate to an unsatisfactory result at the end of the year. The effect of this procedure is that a dossier is compiled documenting any remedial action taken as well as the outcomes.

There are two major benefits from this procedure. The compiled dossier has legal trustworthiness and the decision to fail a student is not based on a single 'subjective' judgement but on the opinions of several faculty members. Obviously, this enhances the reliability of the decision but it also enables faculty to share the responsibility for such a decision. In this way no single teacher will feel that he or she is solely responsible for a negative judgement of a student. When teachers feel the responsibility for a negative judgement is theirs only, they may be hesitant to pronounce it.

Portfolio

In the assessment programme the portfolio is not used to assess reflection as such, but to monitor students' progress in the four roles mentioned earlier (medical expert, scholar, worker in the healthcare system, and person). Students include in their portfolio an analysis of their strengths and weaknesses based on all their assessments and incidental feedback. This analysis must be accompanied by learning goals, which must be SMART (specific, measurable, attainable, realistic, and timely) and follow directly from the identified weaknesses. Analyses must be supported by 'evidence', such as assessment outcomes and written feedback.

Several times a year students discuss their portfolio with their mentor, who gives detailed feedback. The minutes of these discussions are included in the portfolio. At the end of the year the mentor gives a recommendation as to whether the portfolio is satisfactory. By signing the recommendation students indicate their agreement. If they do not agree, they present their own view in writing. Next, all portfolios are judged by independent mentors (one for each portfolio). If there is concordance between the judgements of the independent mentor, the student's mentor, and the student, the assessment is completed. If there is disagreement, additional judges evaluate the portfolio. A key principle informing this assessment process is that judgements may be subjective but that does not imply they are unreliable. Although some institutes 'scaffold' individual judgements by using more structured and more detailed scoring rubrics, the medical faculty deliberately decided against this. Portfolio judgements are inherently subjective and the use of structured rubrics only increases the risk of trivializing the assessment by reducing it to ticking items on a list. Nonetheless, the pass-fail decision must be reliable and defensible. That is why more judgements are added in cases of uncertainty (too much dissent) about the decision.

In essence the role of portfolios in the assessment programme is to encourage students to take more responsibility for their own learning. In this respect the portfolio has a central role in year 6.

During this year students undertake a clinical and a research attachment of eighteen weeks each, during which they construct a portfolio in line with the CanMEDS competencies. The portfolio contains a personal development plan, outcomes of formal assessments (360 degree feedback, miniCEX, Critically Appraised Topics), minutes of progress appraisals, and any additional materials that contribute to the demonstration of progress in the seven competency domains. In the final assessment of the portfolio, the student's mentor recommends the qualification (honours, pass, fail) and a second judgement is given by the attachment coordinator. If there is disagreement, a full committee review the portfolio. Together with the progress tests, the portfolios of the two attachments constitute the complete assessment programme for year 6.

Issues of practical implementation

In any assessment programme, differences between the programme-on-paper and the programme-in-action are inevitable. Some of the most salient discrepancies will be described here. Although originally considerable latitude was allowed to planning groups in designing the assessment programmes for their own units, a routine has evolved in which assessment of virtually all units in the first two years consists of a multiple-choice end-of-unit test and one assignment. The weighting of these two formats is set at 20% for the assignment and 80% for the test. The use of the latter is not underpinned by unit content but solely attributable to the size of the current year classes (over 340 students). With these numbers of students, open-ended questions, oral examinations, etc., are just not feasible. Uniform weighting of the different test components for all units was also due to logistical reasons. On the other hand, the assignments generally provide good coverage of unit content and offer a good forum for feedback.

Costs, logistics, and acceptability have proven to be major issues in relation to the longitudinal assessment components. With six year classes of over three hundred students each, a large group of mentors is needed to supervise all portfolios. Inevitably, there is substantial variety in the quality of mentors and their interaction with students. As in any organization, negative experiences are expressed most vociferously and tend to dominate the general opinion about this 'subjective' assessment. Despite extensive training, peer feedback meetings of mentors, and clearly written instructions and guidelines for mentors, this issue remains unresolved. The issue of variety in judgements is an even more powerful impediment to the successful implementation of the assessment of professional behaviour. There is considerable variety in the quality of the assessment and feedback provided by tutors and in tutors' efforts to persuade student to take this assessment seriously. Again it is the less than positive experiences that seem to dominate the general picture at the expense of the positive examples. Nevertheless, both assessment components have 'survived' so far and are continuing to develop, gradually bringing about a cultural change.

The costs associated with any judgement-based assessment system that requires the provision of feedback are obviously quite high. A reduction in the administrative costs of the assessment of professional behaviour has been accomplished by reporting and archiving only unsatisfactory judgements. This comes at a price though. The main purpose of this assessment is to improve all students' professional behaviour, but the administrative organization now in fact suggests that the only aim is to track down the bad apples.

Acceptability issues have prevented a truly longitudinal approach for the four competency roles over years 3 through 5. It would have been logical for students to carry over their assessment outcomes from a previous unit to the next one to foster continuous improvement and evaluate whether their learning issues are being achieved. Unfortunately, experience has taught that fear of double jeopardy and fear that a poor result in a previous unit will depress subsequent judgements is a major impediment to the implementation of truly longitudinal assessment.

Epilogue

The question now remains whether this programme is well tailored to a PBL curriculum. The programme is designed to foster continuous learning and avoid cramming. Therefore longitudinal assessment makes up a large proportion of the programme. You cannot dress up for a one-off assessment of professional behaviour nor can you pass the progress test by cramming for one test. The assignments of the unit-based assessments and the integration of skill-related knowledge in the OSCEs are examples of how integration and contextual learning are incorporated into the assessment. Though the end-of-unit examinations are multiple-choice questions (MCQ)-based, the MCQs are framed within the context of short cases and vignettes whenever possible, thereby stimulating students to relate knowledge to authentic contexts. Feedback on working with others in the assessment of professional behaviour is an example of how assessment can encourage collaborative learning.

A final glance into the future suggests that there is a good chance that this 'new' programme will become obsolete very soon. The emergence of new theories on medical competence, the widespread attention to non-cognitive aspects of medical competence (such as professionalism, scholarship, and communication) and especially the widely held notion of competencies instead of traits are likely to necessitate a complete rethink of the assessment programme. The ideas of programmatic assessment and the reappraisal of the role of human judgement in assessment will probably require an even higher level of integration. For example, the current approaches of using a compensatory model for test results within instruments (e.g., a station on communication skills and a station on abdominal examination in an OSCE) and a conjunctive model (no compensation between a station score on communication skills and judgements on this criterion in a mini-CEX) for results of different instruments need to be challenged from a competencies-based viewpoint. This being said, extensive research in this area will be needed if successful implementation of programmatic assessment is to become reality.

Annotated literature

Van der Vleuten, C. P. M., and Schuwirth, L. W. T. (2005). Assessing professional competence: from methods to programmes. *Medical Education* **39(3)**, 309–17.

This paper describes ideas on programmatic assessment. It makes the case that individual assessment methods are never perfect. Not only is the value of each *individual* instrument a trade–off between several characteristics, a careful combination of instruments is needed to capture medical competence as a whole.

Driessen, E., van der Vleuten, C. P. M., Schuwirth, L. W. T., van Tartwijk, J., and Vermunt, J. (2005). The use of qualitative research criteria for portfolio assessment as an alternative to reliability evaluation: a case study. *Medical Education* **39(2)**, 214–20.

This paper describes an organizational framework for the summative assessment of portfolios. The methods described are not based on psychometric principles but demonstrate rigour, validity, and reliability based on processes derived from qualitative research methodology.

Regehr, G., and Norman, G. R. (1996). Issues in cognitive psychology: Implications for professional education. *Academic Medicine* **71(9)**, 988–1001.

This is a must-read for all those involved in teaching and assessment, especially when medical problem solving is involved. It discusses the most important findings in cognitive psychology on the development of expertise and learning, and relates them to educational practice. In this way it provides the scientific underpinnings of modern educational approaches.

Frank, J. R. (n.d.) (ed.). The CanMEDS 2005 Physician Competency Framework. Available at http://rcpsc. medical.org/canmeds/CanMEDS2005/CanMEDS2005_e.pdf. Accessed 5 June 2009.

On this website the CanMEDS framework is described. This is one example of a redefinition of medical competence in terms of competency domains. The competency domains are described as seven roles: the professional, communicator, collaborator, manager, health advocate, and scholar as well as the medical expert. All the domains are necessary but not sufficient prerequisites for the domain of the medical expert.

References

Arnold, E. L., Blank, L. L., Race, K. E. H., and Cipparrone, N. (1998). Can professionalism be measured? The development of a scale for use in the medical environment. *Academic Medicine* **73**(10), 1119–21.

Biggs, J. (1996). Enhancing teaching through constructive alignment. *Higher Education* **32**, 347–64.

Frederiksen, N. (1984). The real test bias: Influences of testing on teaching and learning. *American Psychologist* **39**(3), 193–202.

Harden, R. M., and Gleeson, F. A. (1979). Assessment of clinical competence using an objective structured clinical examination (OSCE). *Medical Education* **13**(1), 41–54.

Metz, J. C. M., Verbeek-Weel, A. M. M., and Huisjes, H. J. (Eds). Raamplan 2001 Artsopleiding [Dutch blueprint medical curricula], Mediagroep Nijmegen, Nijmegen, the Netherlands.

Miller, G. E. (1990). The assessment of clinical skills/competence/performance. *Academic Medicine* **65**(9), S63–7.

Project team Consilium Abeundi. (2005). *Professional behaviour: teaching, assessing and coaching students.* Maastricht: Unviersitaire Pers Maastricht.

Regehr, G., MacRae, H., Reznick, R., and Szalay, D. (1998). Comparing the psychometric properties of checklists and global rating scales for assessing performance on an OSCE-format examination. *Academic Medicine* **73**(9), 993–7.

Van der Vleuten, C. P. M. (1996). The assessment of professional competence: developments, research and practical implications. *Advances in Health Science Education* **1**(1), 41–67.

Van der Vleuten, C. P. M., Verwijnen, G. M., and Wijnen, W. H. F. W. (1996). Fifteen years of experience with progress testing in a problem-based learning curriculum. *Medical Teacher* **18**(2), 103–10.

Chapter 22

Progress testing

Arno Muijtjens and Wynand Wijnen

Education is aimed at improving skills, knowledge, and competencies. To determine whether and to what extent this aim is achieved, improvement must be measured. This requires repeated measurement of the progress of students in the domain of interest. The progress test, which is currently used in five faculties of medicine in the Netherlands, is an example of such a procedure. It makes it possible to measure the growth of students' knowledge by repeated administration of different but comparable tests covering the complete domain of medical knowledge. By its nature the progress test is directed at the end objectives of the curriculum, that is, the knowledge students should possess when they graduate. With these characteristics the progress test fits the principles of student-centred and student-directed learning which are central to problem-based learning (PBL). Moreover, it allows joint construction and use by different universities that have different curricula but share the same end objectives. A progress test is a rich source of information about students' knowledge growth in all medical sub-domains: it provides feedback for individual students on the strengths and weaknesses of their individual knowledge development and also feedback for teaching staff on the average knowledge growth achieved by their curriculum. Progress testing is thus a valuable tool for monitoring knowledge growth and improving students' individual learning as well as the quality of the curriculum.

Introduction

A progress test is a comprehensive test covering the cognitive objectives of an educational programme. It resembles a final exam, but, unlike a final exam, it is taken not only by students who are about to graduate but by all students of all year groups. Differences in students' knowledge levels are indicated by the level of their test scores: the average scores of more senior students are expected to be higher than those of students in the earlier years.

If progress tests are to monitor progress in knowledge, repeated test results are needed of all students at different stages of the programme. Although a different test must be used at each measurement occasion to avoid undesirable effects of question recognition by students, ideally, each test covers the same knowledge domain at the same level of difficulty. For individual students the score is expected to increase in successive tests due to their incremental knowledge gains in the course of the educational programme. Thus progress testing enables assessment, at successive points in the curriculum, of the extent to which a student has reached the end objectives, in other words the (lack of) growth in knowledge over a period of time.

The focus of the test on the end objectives of the curriculum and the associated comprehensiveness of the test make it virtually impossible for students to prepare specifically for the test in its entirety. As a consequence, test-oriented learning is discouraged and continuous studying promoted. On the other hand, a student may very well be stimulated by progress test results to do more work on certain themes, when test results reveal weaknesses in knowledge (Verwijnen et al., 1982; Wijnen, 1991).

The role of the teacher in progress testing

The comprehensiveness of the progress test also has consequences for the assessor role of teachers. In discipline-based assessment, teachers are generally responsible for teaching and assessing course content. Often the whole assessment process is conducted by teachers, starting with test design, followed by item construction, standard setting, test administration, marking and scoring, quality control of the questions, and finally calculation of test results and feedback. However, since progress tests cover all the relevant disciplines, most of the assessment tasks must be transferred to a central level, although individual teachers remain responsible for the construction of the building blocks of the test—the questions about their specific subjects.

From end-of-unit test to progress tests

When the Maastricht Faculty of Medicine was established in the 1970s and immediately introduced a problem-based curriculum, it soon emerged that assessment was not in alignment with the education objectives. A key principle of problem-based learning (PBL) is to promote self-directed discovery learning in tutorial groups which engage in integrative analysis of several aspects of a presented medical problem. This approach differs fundamentally from the discipline-oriented approach that is customary in traditional curricula. To the dismay of the teachers of the new PBL medical curriculum, however, the tests at the end of each six-week educational unit were found to stimulate test-directed learning and preparation. The tests discouraged individual learning trajectories and stimulated rote memorization at the expense of in-depth insight, understanding, and lasting functional knowledge. The solution was sought in severing the direct connection between courses and assessment. Eventually, this resulted in the Maastricht progress test (Van der Vleuten et al., 1996; Wijnen 1977, 1991).

The interuniversity progress test (IPT) in medicine in the Netherlands

Since 1999, progress tests have been jointly constructed and concurrently administered by the medical faculties of the universities of Groningen, Nijmegen, and Maastricht (Van der Vleuten et al., 2004). The progress test was accorded comparable status in the examination regulations of each of the collaborating universities. In September 2006, the medical faculty of Leiden University joined the consortium, and in September 2007, the medical faculty of one of the Amsterdam universities (VU) started to administer the joint progress test to its medical students, as a preliminary step towards full participation (including participation in test construction) after gaining sufficient experience with the process. Thus five of the eight medical faculties in the Netherlands participate in the IPT.

Blueprint

Every year four tests are jointly produced and administered simultaneously in September, December, March, and May, respectively to approximately 7500 undergraduate medical students in the six-year curricula of the five collaborating medical schools. Each test consists of 200 multiple-choice questions (MCQs; single answer correct type) selected in accordance with a blueprint-based on disciplines and categories (Table 22.1). The questions assess knowledge at graduation level and consist of an introductory text (stem) followed by a question with two to five alternative answer options. The number of options is allowed to vary to prevent unlikely alternatives that are ineffective because they are easily recognized as incorrect even by students who know nothing about the subject. In addition to the alternative answers, a *don't know* option is provided.

Each question relates to a certain category (e.g., respiratory system, mental healthcare) and discipline (e.g., biochemistry, paediatrics). When all categories are crossed with all disciplines, a matrix is obtained (Table 22.1) which serves as a blueprint for each newly constructed instance of the progress test. In this way it is ensured that successive tests are comparable with respect to content. The number of questions per discipline and category is prescribed by the blueprint and reflects the frequency of occurrence and the importance of the categories and disciplines in relation to the end objectives of the curriculum.

Table 22.1 Blueprint of the interuniversity progress test

Disc	Clus	Category																	Total
		01	02	03	04	05	06	07	08	09	10	11	12	13	14	15	16	17	
AN	BS	2	1	2		1	1	1			1	1	1			1			12
BC	BS	1	1	1			1	1			1	1	1	1					9
CH	CK	1	1	3			1	1	1		2	4	1				2		17
DE	CK								5										5
EP	MI														7				7
FA	BS	1	1	1			1	1			1	1		1					8
FY	BS	1	1	1		1	2	1			1	1	1						10
GY	CK				4		2						1			1	2		10
HG	CK	1	1	1	1	1	1		1	1	1	1	1			1	7	1	20
IN	CK	6	1	2			6	1	2		3	3	1	1		1	1	1	29
KG	CK	1	1			1	1	1			1	1	1			1	1	1	11
KN	CK	1											3						4
MC	BS		1		2		1							4					8
ME	MI			2					4						2		1		9
NE	CK		1										5			1			7
OH	CK												2			1	1		4
PA	BS	1	1	1		1	1		1		1	1	1	1					10
PS	MI				9					5			1			1			16
SG	MI									2							2		4
Total		16	10	13	12	11	15	10	10	12	12	14	19	9	9	7	15	6	200

The numbers in the cells indicate the numbers of test items for combinations of discipline and category. The numbers in the margins are the numbers of items per discipline (rows) and per category (columns). The Clus column indicates the three clusters of disciplines (Disc).

Continued

Table 22.1 (*continued*) Blueprint of the interuniversity progress test

Disc	Discipline	Cat	Category	Clus	Cluster of disciplines	Size
AN	Anatomy	01	Respiratory System	BS	Basic Science	57
BC	Biochemistry	02	Blood and Lymph System	MI	Behavioural/ Miscellaneous	36
CH	Surgery	03	Musculoskeletal System	CK	Clinical knowledge	107
DE	Dermatology	04	Mental Health Care			
EP	Epidemiology	05	Reproductive System			
FA	Pharmacology	06	Cardiovascular System			
FY	Physiology	07	Hormones and Metabolism			
GY	Obstetrics and Gynaecology	08	Dermis and Connective Tissue			
HG	Family medicine	09	Personal and Social Aspects			
IN	Internal medicine	10	Digestive System			
KG	Paediatrics	11	Kidneys and Urinary System			
KN	Ear, Nose, Throat	12	Nervous System and Senses			
MC	Clinical Genetics	13	Molecular and Cellular Aspects			
ME	Metamedical Sciences	14	Epistemology and Methodology			
NE	Neurology	15	Stages of Life			
OH	Ophthalmology	16	Knowledge of Skills			
PA	Pathology	17	Preventative Health Care			
PS	Psychology and Psychiatry					
SG	Surgery					

Construction of questions

Questions are constructed by teachers of all the departments (disciplines) of the participating medical faculties (Figure 22.1). Each faculty appoints a test review committee, composed of a chair and five faculty members from basic science and clinical disciplines. The committees review all items produced by the staff of their faculty. When a question is not approved by the test review committee it is returned to the teacher who constructed it, with comments. The teacher can revise the question—possibly after discussion with the test review committee—or decide to withdraw it. Approved questions are stored in a central item bank, which also contains questions used in earlier instantiations of the progress test. Questions are only reused after reassessment by the review committee. Advances in medical knowledge may require modification of an answer key or another aspect of a question, or even withdrawal of a question from the item bank.

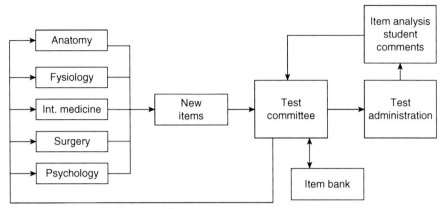

Figure 22.1 The quality control cycle of the interuniversity progress test.

From 1977 until 2005, progress tests were composed of 250 true–false questions (TFQs). Since September 2005, the interuniversity progress test (IPT) has been composed of 200 MCQs. The motivation for changing to MCQs was twofold: compared to TFQs, MCQs yield more reliable scores and a smaller chance of guessing the correct answer. Moreover, MCQs offer more flexibility in constructing questions for a diversity of subjects.

Construction of the test

The teachers who construct the questions determine the final form of the questions eligible for inclusion in a test, but the set of questions used for a test is selected by the central review committee, which makes sure that the test is consistent with the blueprint and checks for unwanted relationships between questions, such as when the stem of question X provides information about the answer to question Y. Also, the committee strives for a constant level of difficulty of consecutive tests.

Quality control

Items are stored in the item bank together with a reference to a book from the faculty's recommended literature list that contains the answer to the question (page indicated). After each test students are allowed to keep the test booklet that includes all the test questions and they receive a form with the corresponding answer keys and references to the literature. Using this information, students can calculate their scores, check wrong answers, and consult the literature to see why they failed certain questions. If students encounter an inconsistency, e.g., conflicting information in different books, they can report this to the test review committee. Based on the students' comments, the committee investigates whether the answer key of certain questions should be changed or whether certain questions should be removed from the test altogether. Also, after each test, an item analysis is carried out to calculate several psychometric parameters for each question: the percentages correct, incorrect, and don't know answers, and item-test correlation. These parameters are used to detect whether the questions are of sufficient quality. For example, a high percentage of don't know answers (among six-year-students) may be indicative of a lack of relevance or poor wording, and a high percentage of incorrect answers may indicate misleading wording, controversy in the literature, or an incorrect answer key. A negative item-test correlation implies that the better students were more likely to give an incorrect answer, while the weaker students were more likely to answer correctly, suggesting that the question does not discriminate between students in the right direction. Questions with suspicious values for any of the item parameters (percentage correct below 30%, item-test correlation below -0.1) and questions that require investigation by the test review committee based on students' comments are scrutinized by the test review committee. The committee then decides whether to maintain or withdraw questions from the test or to change answer keys. At this stage of the process, the final version of the test is established. Next, the definitive results are calculated and reported to students, teachers, and the faculty's education office. In the pre-test review phase on average more than 80% of the submitted questions are found to be flawed (97% showing a wording/phrasing/technical problem and 56% a content problem). In the post-test review phase on average 5% of the questions are dropped.

As the students are allowed to keep the test booklet and the answer keys after the test, the item bank cannot be considered a secret. To reduce the chance of students giving correct answers because they recognize reused questions, the questions are locked for reuse for a period of three years.

Scoring and test results

The scoring method rewards a correct answer with one credit point, an incorrect answer with a penalty equal to 1/(number of alternatives − 1), and a don't know answer with neither credit nor penalty. This method is known as formula scoring and aims to encourage students to select the don't know option rather than guess the answer if they have no knowledge about the subject of a question (Diamond & Evans, 1973; Rowley & Traub, 1977). A student's test result is obtained by subtracting the sum of the penalties from the sum of the credit points. The resulting figure is divided by the total number of questions and multiplied by 100 to yield the test score expressed as a percentage of the maximum attainable score. The resulting score is compared to a pass-fail standard to decide whether the test result is satisfactory. Standard setting is discussed in detail in the next section.

Figure 22.2 shows a summary of progress test results based on the scores obtained at the university of Maastricht during ten curriculum years (1989/90–1998/9). With four tests

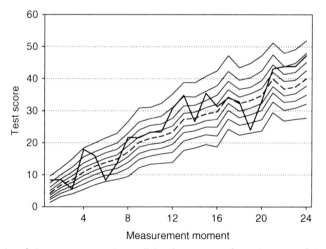

Figure 22.2 Results of the progress test in medicine (percentage formula score of the total test) obtained at the university of Maastricht in ten curriculum years, 1989/90 to 1998/9.

per year in a six-year education programme, there are 24 consecutive measurement moments. Per measurement moment, for the set of scores of the ten tests, the score level was derived below which 10% of the students' scores were located. The obtained sequence of points was connected by straight line segments to give the lower curve in the graph. Similar curves were obtained for score levels delimiting 20%, 30%, and so forth, up to 90% of the scores. The resulting bundle of curves indicates the outer boundaries of the score distribution (the width of the distribution). The location of the centre of the distribution is indicated by the fifth curve (broken line) which corresponds to the 50-50 point, the so-called median score. The curve indicates the average knowledge growth achieved during the six-year programme by the observed ten cohorts of students. At the first measurement moment, the average score is 3% increasing to 40% at measurement moment 24. Clearly, the width of the score distribution increases with each measurement moment: the standard deviation is 3% at measurement moment 1 and 9% at measurement moment 24.

A score of 40% at the end of a six-year programme may seem low at first, but, this impression changes when the effect of the penalty for incorrect answers is taken into account. Suppose a test consists of only true-false questions and there are no 'don't know' answer options; then a formula score of 40% corresponds with a correct score of 70%.

The graph also shows an example of a curve for an individual student (bold line): this curve also represents growth of knowledge, but the pattern is more irregular than that of the central curve of the average growth. The irregularities of the individual curve illustrate the shortcomings of knowledge measurements. The test score is (hopefully) largely determined by what the test aims to measure: the student's level of knowledge. However, the score will also be affected by confounding factors: a student may have more knowledge about the questions in a particular test or a student may have 'a bad day', etc. In general, confounding factors vary from one test to the next and therefore cause irregularity in the pattern of a sequence of measurements.

Setting standards

During the first two decades of the progress test, a relative standard, known as the Wijnen standard (Wijnen, 1971), was used. The basic assumption underlying this standard is that the level and learning efforts of the average student are sufficient to successfully complete the education programme. Therefore, the average score of a group of students is used as the reference point for pass-fail decisions. In addition, the procedure takes into account that each test score is affected by measurement error, which may cause a student's score to be lower than the average score even though that student's true knowledge level may not be lower. To adjust for this unfairness, Wijnen applies an uncertainty interval corresponding to the 95% confidence interval and lowers the pass-fail standard accordingly to two times the standard error of measurement below the average score. Because the reliability of the progress test is usually approximately 0.75, the Wijnen standard is one standard deviation (of score distribution of a cohort of students) below the average score. Since the standard of the test is derived from the distribution of the scores of the students who have taken the test, the Wijnen standard is also called a relative standard.

Each standard setting method has its drawbacks. With a relative standard the major drawbacks are the standard is not known in advance, a certain fraction of the participating students always fails, the standard can be influenced by the students, and the standard is not appropriate for heterogeneous groups of students. To overcome these drawbacks, starting in 1995, an alternative standard setting method was developed. With this method, the standard is obtained before test administration by applying the Wijnen procedure to the distribution of the scores of a series of previous progress tests (Muijtjens et al., 1998). However, in 2005, when the question format was changed from true-false to multiple choice, it was considered inappropriate to continue to use a standard setting procedure based on historical data. Therefore, it was decided to return to the Wijnen standard but with a slight modification to reduce the influence of a single year group. In this procedure the Wijnen standard is initially calculated for each of the six year groups. For the resulting six points (using year group as the *x* axis) a quadratic curve is fitted and, for each year group, the corresponding value on the fitted curve is used as the pass-fail standard.

Feedback

In addition to the test results in terms of the total score and the corresponding qualification (pass-fail), students and staff also receive detailed feedback on the knowledge levels in sub-domains. The recently developed Progress test Feedback (ProF) system enables students and staff of the five cooperating Dutch medical faculties to find longitudinal and predictive feedback on the web (Muijtjens et al., 2010; Timmermans et al., 2009). The feedback is query-based and graphically oriented, as illustrated in Figure 22.3. The upper left panel shows the scores on the progress test of May 2009 of a third-year student for each of the seventeen categories (indicated by dots). For reference, the bars indicate the score distribution per category for the peer group of third-year students. The left boundary of the first bar indicates the fifth percentile, i.e., 5% of the peer group scored below this boundary. Similarly, the right boundaries of the other bars indicate the fifteenth, seventieth, and ninety-fifth percentiles, respectively, of the peer score distribution. The fifteenth and seventieth percentiles correspond to the pass-fail and the good-pass standards, respectively, which are used to qualify the progress test results of individual students. The vertical line in the second bar indicates the position of the median score, the 50–50 point, representing the 'average score' of the peer group.

The upper right panel of Figure 22.3 shows the pattern of the third-year student's test scores for twelve successive progress tests (three curricular years, four tests per year). The observed scores are indicated by circles, and the pattern is represented by the lines connecting the scores. Similar to the single test results in the upper left panel, the areas indicate the percentiles of the peer group score distribution for the measurement moments. The pattern continues beyond the last observation (measurement moment 12) for another two measurement moments (13 and 14). These are predicted scores indicating the expected future results for this student, and the accompanying lines indicate the 95% confidence interval of the prediction.

The lower right panel is a similar representation of the same student's longitudinal score pattern for the subtests of the category *Cardiovascular system*. However, in this case a noise-reducing presentation of the knowledge development is used: the observed scores in consecutive tests are accumulated, resulting in a smoother pattern (Muijtjens et al., 2009). Each point of the pattern indicates *the average score obtained on all tests up to and including that moment*. The cumulative score is an attractive option, particularly for scores on subtests, because the observed score patterns for subtests are less reliable and often show irregular, noisy patterns due to the smaller number of questions.

By inspecting these data students can detect their stronger and weaker sub-domains and use this information to direct their study efforts. The average scores per year group provide teachers and education management with information about the extent to which certain education goals are being met. This information can be used to adjust education policy and/or the education programme.

Achievements

In addition to discouraging test-oriented learning, progress testing has several other attractive features (Van der Vleuten et al., 1996) (see Box 22.1). Because the progress test is aimed at the end

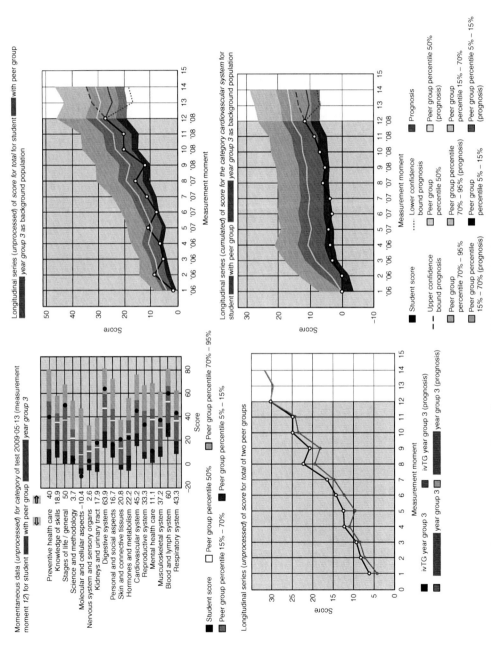

Figure 22.3 Feedback generated by the ProF system for staff and students of the interuniversity progress test.

Box 22.1 Advantages and disadvantages of progress testing

Advantages of progress testing:

- ◆ Test-directed learning behaviour is discouraged

Due to the comprehensive domain covered by the test, it is virtually impossible for students to specifically prepare for the test in its entirety. As a result, test-driven learning is discouraged and continuous learning is stimulated.

- ◆ Every individual learning activity that is relevant for the end objectives is rewarded.

The test is aimed at the end objectives, so essentially all relevant study activities are rewarded.

- ◆ The instrument is aimed at measuring functional, lasting knowledge.

The comprehensiveness of the instrument means that rote memorization of isolated facts does not help to obtain satisfactory test results, whereas functional lasting knowledge does help to achieve good test results. After all, at a later stage of the curriculum, a student should still be able to correctly answer questions about basic knowledge learned at an earlier stage of the curriculum.

- ◆ The same knowledge is repeatedly tested, which increases the reliability.

Basically each progress test is a repeated, independent test of the same domain (or set of domains). The cumulative test results therefore reliably represent the level of knowledge in that domain.

- ◆ Additional re-examinations are not required

Essentially the content of each progress test is comparable to the content of any preceding progress test, so by its very nature each progress test can be considered a re-test of the preceding test.

- ◆ Early detection of excellent students.

Because students are tested at graduation level throughout the whole programme, it is possible at an early stage to detect students whose knowledge level, compared to that of their peers, is closer to the end objectives. This information can be used to offer these excellent students an adjusted programme.

- ◆ The test results are a rich source of information for students as well as teachers.

The test results provide information on the level and growth of knowledge of students in all domains of the end objectives. The information reveals strengths and weaknesses in individual domains. At the individual level this information can stimulate students to (re)study certain themes, and at the level of groups of students it can help teachers to improve the curriculum.

- ◆ The test offers many opportunities for research

The dataset obtained from progress tests has several features that are attractive from a research point of view: the data represent a combination of cross-sectional and longitudinal design, with measurements of different (groups of) individuals at the same time as well as repeated measures within individuals.

- ◆ The test is curriculum-independent.

The progress test is curriculum independent as it is aimed at the end objectives of a curriculum and not the specific (sequence of) components of one curriculum designed to reach the

Box 22.1 **Advantages and disadvantages of progress testing** (continued)

end objectives. This offers opportunities for institutions that share the same end objectives (but have different curricula to reach them), to jointly construct, administer, and process progress tests.

Drawbacks of progress testing:

+ The reliability of the test is low for first-year students.

In general, only a small fraction of the questions can be answered by first-year students, so the effective length of the test for these students is limited. As a consequence, first year scores are less reliable than the scores obtained in later years.

+ Profile scores (subtest scores) are unreliable.

Because the test is comprehensive it is composed of questions about many different subjects. Thus there are only a few questions per subject and, hence, the reliability of the corresponding subtest scores is low.

+ The test requires a relatively long testing time.

To be sufficiently reliable the test must contain many questions and thus the required testing time is relatively long. To achieve a reliability of 0.80 with six-year students about 200 multiple-choice questions are required. Four hours of testing time are generally sufficient for the students to answer all the questions.

+ It is difficult to construct a progress test on the basis of less efficient question formats.

For a comprehensive test like the progress test efficient question formats like true–false or multiple-choice questions are indicated because less efficient formats would result in unacceptable testing times and processing efforts. However, this restriction is not too troublesome because generally the questions' content rather than their format defines what is measured by a test (Norman et al., 1987, 1996).

objectives of the complete education programme (and not the specific content of individual modules) it is possible to measure the level and growth of knowledge of students even when they follow different individual learning paths. The total test score for each of these students indicates to what extent the end objectives have been reached.

The pattern of the total test scores of a series of consecutive tests indicates the progress in knowledge in relation to the end objectives. This feature of progress testing has further implications. When groups of students attending different curricula (at different universities) take the same progress tests, the test results can be used as a common instrument to measure the knowledge growth of all the students, provided the curricula share the same end objectives. This means that the progress test is a suitable instrument for comparing the effects of different curricula on knowledge acquisition. Moreover, the average knowledge growth for all the students at the collaborating institutions can be used as a benchmark (Muijtjens et al., 2008a). Comparing the average knowledge growth of students at a single university with the benchmark indicates the relative success of that university's curriculum with regard to the end objectives (Muijtjens et al., 2008a, b; Verhoeven et al., 1998, 2005).

Progress test results not only show knowledge growth at an aggregated level but also at individual student level. The growth patterns at an aggregated level (e.g., the average knowledge growth from 1993 until 1999 for the cohort starting in 1993) provide information about the effects of the education programme. Individual growth patterns (Figure 22.3) can provide information on progress or lack of it even early on in a student's development. A student may initially obtain high scores, but subsequently show no further growth in knowledge. That student may still obtain satisfactory scores, but he/she has a high risk of dropping below the pass-fail standard in the near future. This can be foreseen (and possibly remediated) at an early stage by inspecting individual growth patterns.

Requirements

Progress testing can be developed and applied for many subject areas, provided a number of conditions are fulfilled:

- The (core) content corresponding to the end objectives must be clearly defined;
- Among the education staff there should be a sufficient level of consensus with regard to all the subjects that are considered to constitute the functional knowledge relevant for the end objectives;
- Training should be sufficiently homogeneous: rigorous specializations (in particular if initiated at the earlier stages of the programme) seriously impede successful implementation of progress testing;
- The institution must be willing to invest in setting up a central test organization to coordinate and safeguard the quality of the preparation and implementation of the progress test procedure. It should be noted that a central organization provides opportunities for improving quality as well as efficiency and relieves teachers of administrative and logistical tasks (Van der Vleuten et al., 1996);
- A central test committee is required to manage the test construction process and assure the quality of tests; and
- Successful implementation of the progress test procedure depends on acceptance by staff and students.

To end with

The central review and construction of the progress test obviously requires a substantial investment, partly due to the costs of improved quality control of the questions and the multidisciplinary character of the test. However, the centralized test organization enables teachers to focus on the content aspects of the test rather than the logistics and it should also be noted in this respect that with discipline-oriented testing the costs often are less clearly visible, because of the distributed character of the work involved in test development and administration as well as in calculation, registration, and distribution of test results.

Whether a progress test is appropriate for a programme of the Bachelor–Master model depends on the extent to which the above-mentioned conditions are met. Bachelor programmes are generally sufficiently homogeneous for enabling effective progress testing. For Master programmes, which often consist of several diverging specializations, progress testing might be less appropriate.

A progress test assesses knowledge. In addition to knowledge, other competencies, such as skills, problem-solving ability, and professional behaviour, are essential to the development of professional competence. In order to assess all these aspects, other instruments must be used in addition to the progress test. Therefore assessment programmes should be composed of a set of instruments and procedures to cover all these aspects. As part of such an assessment programme, a progress test offers an excellent opportunity for equipping an education programme with a non-interfering knowledge test.

The future of progress testing

Interinstitutional collaboration to jointly construct and implement assessment tools is advantageous because it improves efficiency and stimulates quality assurance. Several recent initiatives have been successfully maintained (Byrne et al., 2004; Prideaux et al., 2002; van der Vleuten et al., 2004). With interinstitutional progress testing, however, there is a substantial increase in the numbers of students taking the same test simultaneously, which requires increasing logistical efforts. This problem may be resolved by developing a calibrated item bank and constructing multiple equivalent forms of the test to be taken by several batches of students, or, even better, by developing a procedure for computerized adaptive testing (Wainer, 2000). In the latter setup a student sitting at a computer is presented with a sequence of questions aimed at estimating the student's level of knowledge in a certain domain. Each subsequent question is adapted to the estimate of the student's knowledge level at that point; i.e., the questions are selected to be neither too easy nor too difficult for the student in order to provide optimum information on the student's knowledge level. Because the test is adapted to individual students, a reliable indication of a student's level of knowledge can be obtained with substantially fewer questions than required for a (written) test for all students. An individualized adaptive test which can be taken at any moment is also more in line with the student-centred and self-directed character of PBL. These potential benefits of computerized adaptive testing in a PBL setting make it worthwhile to investigate developments of the progress test in this direction.

Annotated literature

Wijnen, W. H. F. W. (1991). The rationale of a school-based centralized examination system. In:
   A. J. M. Luyten (ed.), *Issues in public examinations*. Utrecht: Lemma. Pp. 149–60.
The author, one of the founding fathers of the PBL curriculum and the progress test at the medical faculty of Maastricht University, describes developments when PBL was implemented right from the start in the 1970s. The end-of-unit tests that were used initially were found to negatively impact on the instructional objectives of PBL. Progress testing substantially helped resolve this problem.

Van der Vleuten, C. P. M., Verwijnen, G. M., and Wijnen, W. H. F. W. (1996). Fifteen years of experience
   with progress testing in a problem-based learning curriculum. *Medical Teacher* 18, 103–9.
The authors report their experiences with progress testing at the medical faculty of Maastricht University. The testing procedure was found to be effective in preventing test-driven, reproduction-oriented learning behaviour which would interfere with the work in tutorial groups. In addition, the authors point to a number of (partly unforeseen) educational advantages and some drawbacks of the testing method.

Van der Vleuten, C. P. M., Schuwirth, L. W. T., Muijtjens, A. M. M., Thoben, A. J. N. M., Cohen-
   Schotanus, J., and van Boven, C. P. A. (2004). Cross institutional collaboration in assessment: a case on
   progress testing. *Medical Teacher* 26, 719–25.
The paper reports an initiative to jointly construct and administer progress tests by the medical faculties of three universities (Maastricht, Nijmegen, and Groningen) in the Netherlands. The authors provide evidence for the feasibility of the project and the interesting opportunities it offers. It is concluded that the collaboration does indeed improve efficiency, and in addition enables educational improvements that for each individual institute separately would be very hard, if not impossible, to achieve.

Muijtjens, A. M., Schuwirth, L. W., Cohen-Schotanus, J., and van der Vleuten, C. P. (2008). Differences in
   knowledge development exposed by multi-curricular progress test data. *Advances in Health Sciences
   Education* 13, 593–605.

The authors present a method for investigating the between-university differences in the development of medical knowledge in medical students. It is shown that between-university comparison of student performance based on a single test is highly unreliable. These problems can be overcome by using the cumulative data of a jointly constructed and administered progress test. The results indicate that between-curriculum differences in performance can be reliably detected even at the level of a sub–domain of the test.

References

Byrne, G. J., Owen, A., Newble, D., Barton, R., Garden, A., Roberts, T., et al. Sharing resources for UK undergraduate written assessments—one year of UMAP. In: M. B. Maldonado (ed.). *11th International Ottawa Conference on Medical Education. Barcelona: 2004.* P. 192.

Diamond, J., and Evans, W. (1973). The correction for guessing. *Review of Educational Research* **43**, 181–91.

Muijtjens, A. M. M., Hoogenboom, R. J. I., Verwijnen, G. M., and van der Vleuten, C. P. M. (1998). Relative or absolute standards in assessing medical knowledge using progress tests. *Advances in Health Sciences Education* **3**, 81–7.

Muijtjens, A. M., Schuwirth, L. W., Cohen-Schotanus, J., Thoben, A. J., and van der Vleuten, C. P. (2008a). Benchmarking by cross-institutional comparison of student achievement in a progress test. *Medical Education* **42**, 82–8.

Muijtjens, A. M., Schuwirth, L. W., Cohen-Schotanus, J., and van der Vleuten, C. P. (2008b). Differences in knowledge development exposed by multi-curricular progress test data. *Advances in Health Sciences Education* **13**, 593–605.

Muijtjens, A. M. M., Timmermans, I., Cohen-Schotanus, J., Thoben, A. J. N. M., Wenink, A. C. G., and van der Vleuten, C. P. M. (2009). Improving knowledge growth information with progress tests by using the cumulative score. *Conference AMEE 2009, Malaga, Spain, 29 August–2 September.*

Muijtjens, A. M. M., Timmermans, I., Donkers, H. H. L. M.,, Peperkamp, R. P. M., Medema, H., Cohen-Schotanus, J., et al. (2010). Flexible electronic feedback using the virtues of progress testing. *Medical Teacher* (in print).

Norman, G. R., Smith, E. K. M., Powles, A. C., Rooney, P. J., Henry, N. L., and Dodd, P. E. (1987). Factors underlying performance on written tests of knowledge. *Medical Education* **21**, 297–304.

Norman, G. R., Swanson, D., and Case, S. (1996). Conceptual and methodology issues in studies comparing assessment formats, issues in comparing item formats. *Teaching and Learning in Medicine* **8**, 208–16.

Prideaux, D., and Gordon, J. (2002). Can global co-operation enhance quality in medical education? Some lessons from an international assessment consortium. *Medical Education* **36**, 404–5.

Rowley, G. L., and Traub, R. E. (1977). Formula scoring, number-right scoring, and test-taking strategy. *Educational Measurement* **14**, 15–22.

Timmermans, I., Muijtjens, A. M. M., Cohen-Schotanus, J., Thoben, A. J. N. M., Wenink, A. C. G., and van der Vleuten, C. P. M. (2009). ProF; a system for query-based, longitudinal feedback of progress test results. *Conference AMEE 2009, Malaga, Spain, 29 August–2 September.*

Van der Vleuten, C. P. M., Verwijnen, G. M., and Wijnen, W. H. F. W. (1996). Fifteen years of experience with progress testing in a problem-based learning curriculum. *Medical Teacher* **18**, 103–9.

Van der Vleuten, C. P. M., Schuwirth, L. W. T., Muijtjens, A. M. M., Thoben, A. J. N. M., Cohen-Schotanus, J., and van Boven, C. P. A. (2004). Cross institutional collaboration in assessment: a case on progress testing. *Medical Teacher* **26**, 719–25.

Verhoeven, B. H., Verwijnen, G. M., Scherpbier, A. J. J. A., Holdrinet, R. S. G., Oesenburg, B., Bulte, J. A., et al. (1998). An analysis of progress test results of PBL and non-PBL students. *Medical Teacher* **20**, 310–16.

Verhoeven, B. H., Snellen-Balendong, H. A. M., Hay, I. T., Boon, J. M., van der Linde, M. J., Blitz-Lindeque, J. J., et al. (2005). The versatility of progress testing assessed in an international context: a start for benchmarking global standardization? *Medical teacher* **27**, 514–20.

Verwijnen, G. M., Imbos, T. J., Snellen, H., Stalenhoef, B., Sprooten, M., van Leeuwen, Y. D., et al. (1982). The evaluation system at the medical school of Maastricht. *Assessment and Evaluation in Higher Education* **3**, 225–44.

Wainer, H. (2000). *Computerized adaptive testing: a primer*, 2nd edn. Mahwah, NJ: Lawrence Erlbaum.

Wijnen, W. H. F. W. (1971). *Onder of boven de maat*[Below or above par]. Lisse: Swets en Zeitlinger.

Wijnen, W. H. F. W. (1977). Einddoeltoetsen: Waarom en hoe? [Testing the attainment of course objectives: Why and how?]. *Onderzoek van Onderwijs* **6**. 16–9.

Wijnen, W. H. F. W. (1991). The rationale of a school-based centralized examination system. In: A. J. M. Luyten (ed.), *Issues in public examinations*. Utrecht: Lemma. Pp. 149–60.

Chapter 23

Research in education[1]

Cees van der Vleuten, Diana Dolmans, and
Jeroen van Merriënboer

From the time of the foundation of Maastricht University in 1974, educational innovation has
been explicitly incorporated in its mission statement. Indeed educationalists were among the
original pioneering group and have continued to play a prominent role in the university ever
since. During the early years, the educationalists fervently advocated academic status for education and education research. After prolonged and heated debate with opponents who viewed
education as nothing more than a service, academic status was granted to the Department of
Educational Development and Research in 1977. This marked the laying of the first cornerstone
of the education research enterprise in Maastricht. The second cornerstone was put in place by
the decision to recognize education research as one of the few research themes within the Faculty
of Medicine. Dedicated, albeit limited, resources were allocated. More important than the magni-
tude of resource allocation was the official priority given to education research within the medical
school.

In 1982 the education research programme was mandated. The research has supplied evidence
to the educational experiment that the Maastricht programme embodied, especially in the early
years. It has fuelled innovations and innovations have fuelled the research. Over the years, the
research programme has developed into a well-established research strand within the Faculty of
Health, Medicine and Life Sciences (FHML). The two organizational conditions—academic
status for educationalists and a recognized research programme—have been critical for education
research in Maastricht. But other factors have probably been even more crucial for its survival and
success.

Aim and rationale of the research programme

The research programme pursues the following goals:

♦ To investigate the nature of human learning and learning environments;
♦ To collect scientific evidence for health professions education;
♦ To drive educational innovation; and
♦ To educate staff in education research.

The nature of human learning and learning environments

Originally, the research programme was specifically tailored to problem-based learning (PBL).
This was a logical consequence of the radical choice made by Maastricht University to implement

---

[1] A modified version of this chapter was published in *Academic Medicine* (2004): **79(10)**, 990–6.

PBL in all its education programmes, the revolutionary nature of PBL at that time, and the societal need to be accountable for this approach. The research focused strongly on features of PBL, such as issues around the tutor role or the development of assessment instruments for the PBL programme. However, over the years the research has diversified. Currently, the research programme focuses on human learning and the way learning environments can be arranged and evaluated to facilitate learning.

Scientific evidence for health professions education

Building an evidence base to inform educational practice and policies seems quite a logical motivation for education research, but it is not in line with the prevailing way of thinking in educational practice, which is primarily governed by tradition and intuition (Van der Vleuten et al., 2000). Nevertheless, just as medical practice should be supported by evidence, educational practice should be informed by research evidence as much as possible. Although the parallel between evidence-based medicine and best evidence in medical education has been acknowledged (Harden et al., 2000), there is also a wish to emphasize the need for authentic education research, which does not always lend itself to controlled experiments (Berliner, 2002; Dolmans, 2003; Maxwell, 2004; Norman, 2003). The educational research programme at FHML has moved away from broad evaluations of programme effectiveness (Schuwirth et al., 1999) to focus on specific elements within the learning environment (Cook et al., 2008). In addition, both quantitative (e.g., Dolmans et al., 2002) and qualitative research methods (e.g., Prince et al., 2000) or combinations thereof (Schuwirth et al., 2001) are being applied.

Research that drives educational innovation

Education research at FHML is also aimed at innovation in education. This is not only true for the health professions domain in general – by generating and publishing research evidence contributing to health professions education as a scientific discipline - but also, and very importantly so, at the local institutional level. In various national evaluations, the Maastricht undergraduate medical programme is invariably ranked in the top. This attracts many students (national and international) and strengthens the corporate image of the university as an innovative education institution. Education research contributes to this position and thereby legitimizes the allocation of (modest) resources for this research.

Educating staff in education research

Finally, and very importantly, education research has an important role as a faculty development activity. In this view education research is not (exclusively) the domain of educationalists. It is perhaps one of the highest forms of teachers' professional development to engage in critical scrutiny of their own educational work and in education research and thus help expand the scientific field of health professions education. Therefore, it is strongly propagated that FHML staff from all professional domains should undertake education research. Trained educationalist researchers facilitate this professional development process. Also, research carried out by health professionals has inherent credibility for the field and can therefore make a powerful contribution to the implementation of innovations and changes in educational practice within FHML.

Description of the research programme

Research themes

In Table 23.1 the three research themes are given, along with a small sample of ongoing projects.

Table 23.1 The research themes of the Maastricht education research programme with illustrations

Research theme	Sample of ongoing projects
Learning and instruction	◆ Strategies of collaborative learning
	◆ Computer assisted collaborative learning
	◆ Factors influencing self-study in PBL
	◆ Tailored multimodal approaches in Continuing Professional Development
	◆ Real patients as a starting point for learning
	◆ Supervision in practice-based learning
	◆ Clerkship characteristics and quality of learning
	◆ Tutor perceptions and beliefs of group functioning
	◆ Effect of staff training on supervision
	◆ Learning from international clerkships
	◆ Redesigning models for communication skills
Assessment and evaluation of learning and teaching	◆ Transition from theory to practice
	◆ Basic science proficiency of PBL students
	◆ Portfolio assessment for student assessment
	◆ Portfolio use for evaluating teaching competencies
	◆ Feedback effects in progress testing
	◆ In-training assessment in clerkship settings and residency training
	◆ Optimizing final examinations
	◆ Design criteria for programmes of assessment
	◆ Expertise differences in assessment judgements

The logic in these themes is that they range from the basic principles of learning to how learning environments can be arranged to facilitate learning and finally how learning can be evaluated, the process as well as the outcomes. These themes are very broad. Yet, they provide flexibility in meeting the above objectives. The research programme partly follows the research agenda and typically uses the FHML training programmes as field of experimentation. Little research is conducted in lab settings. Research initiatives of staff members within and outside FHML are never discouraged because they appear not to fit well with the thematic priorities. Rather they are reformulated in such a way that they are better aligned with education theory or ongoing issues in the field. Some of the projects are joint collaborative efforts with other research groups within FHML. For example, many insights into learning, teaching, and assessment are transferable to postgraduate training and continuous professional development, and successful projects have been carried out in this area (Gorter et al., 2001; Hobma et al., 2006; Teunissen et al., 2007, 2009).

Organization

There is a more or less fixed volume of internal funding, which is distributed across qualified research staff members who are active and productive in educational research (approximately five full-time equivalents (FTE)). The research is a programmatic activity embedded within the School of Health Professions Education, one of the graduate schools within FHML. Both the Department of Educational Development and Research and several other departments contribute to the research programme. Other internal and external resources are attracted to fund educational research projects. Much of the research is carried out by PhD students. Some of these students are internally funded, but the majority are external candidates pursuing a doctoral degree within the framework of the School of Health Professions Education. Many of the external PhD students are from abroad. They carry out their research in their own working environment and receive supervision at a distance and in scheduled face-to-face meetings. Currently, an approximate number of fifty PhD students take part in the research programme, half of whom are registered doctoral students from abroad.

For a better understanding of these figures some contextual information may be helpful. Within the Department of Educational Development and Research approximately 25 FTEs are available for educational development activities (curriculum construction, faculty development, programme evaluation, assessment, information and communication technology, student counselling) and teaching tasks within the curriculum. Roughly 80% of the educational development activities are more or less structural activities and about 20% are available for educational innovation projects. The acquisition of external research funding is difficult. Most external funding is awarded for education development projects (government and European Union) and additional funding is raised by external consultancies and training programmes for participants outside FHML.

Quality improvement

Every research programme in FHML must meet at least three out of the four following criteria:

◆ At least six international journal publications per FTE internal funding;

◆ Mean impact factor of publications more than 1.5 the average impact factor of the reference group (in this case: Education, Scientific Disciplines);

◆ 0.5 doctoral dissertation per 1 FTE internal funding; and

◆ Equal external matching of internal funding.

So far, the education research programme has managed to comply with these requirements. As far as external funding is concerned the criterion is not (yet) being met and a strategy has been implemented to remedy this. Like any such set of criteria, there is much debate on relevance and strategic consequences. On the other hand the criteria provide an impulse for productivity. They are also applied at the level of individual researchers and more productive researchers are given more formal protected time for research.

In the Netherlands all research is externally audited at regular intervals. The education research programme has always been accredited in these audits. In the last mid-term review the quality, productivity, and viability of the programme were judged as excellent (between four and five on a five-point scale).

Critical success factors

Central to the success of our education research programme is the strong relationship with educational practice in the health domain. All staff members involved in education research also participate in educational development and teaching activities. Actual problems encountered in educational practice are often starting points for research. Because of this strong relationship with educational practice, the research is judged to be highly relevant and contributes to educational innovations both within and outside the FHML programme. Educational relevance also counteracts the frequently mentioned gap between education research and educational practice (Badley, 2003). This does not imply, however, that the research is not theory driven. In many cases practical educational problems are the start of successful research, but in order to be successful research needs to be firmly embedded in the literature and have identifiable added value. And although most research is application oriented, fundamental research is by no means neglected. One of the most successful research programmes in the past—cognitive research on expertise development of medical professionals (Schmidt et al., 1990)—was quite fundamental in nature. But even this fundamental research had a credible and logical relationship with educational practice. In general, education research in Maastricht is not so much deductive and lab-oriented but rather authentic, inductive, and design-based, and as a result highly relevant to educational practice.

Another key aspect of the success of the research programme is its professional alignment. Staff members involved in education research form a mix of trained medical and other health professionals as well as educationalists and psychologists. This mix reflects a deliberate strategy to enhance interdisciplinary synergy between education and the health professions. Since the research programme is carried out partly by health professionals, these professionals gain educational competence, which fosters education mindedness in health professions educational practice, which in turn facilitates the implementation of educational innovations. In this way, the research programme contributes to the strategic institutional mission of excellence in education, thereby creating a self-perpetuating mechanism.

For successful education research a supporting infrastructure is indispensable. This means primarily staff members with sufficient experience in education research, who are also attuned to working in a health profession-oriented manner. Therefore several of our key researchers have a medical background and are pursuing a university career in medical education. Education research rests heavily on research methodology from the social sciences and it requires training and experience to build proficiency in this type of research. The education research is supported by specialists in research methodology and statistics, in qualitative research, in data analysis, and in English language and editorial support.

Risk factors

From the above it is clear that the research programme contributes to innovative education both within and outside Maastricht University. However, with every budget problem and strategic reorganization in the past, education research has been at stake. Whenever priorities had to be set, education research was often considered a frill, a non-essential extra in the organization. Therefore, internal politics will remain the biggest threat to the research programme. It is not illogical in times of hardship for the faculty to prioritize research in health-related sciences over education research. The university and FHML in particular are at a transitory stage from an initially pioneering organization to a large institutionalized one. Research excellence rather than education is generally given greater priority. If this process continues it will eventually go at the expense of the quality of education and the self-perpetuating mechanism may be broken, which might also herald the end of education research. So far, education research in Maastricht has survived to tell the tale of its success because of its contribution to the university's high education quality ratings, the university's corporate image, and satisfaction with educational services, and, finally, the quality of the research itself. These are important arguments in the political debate.

The overall research input into the programme is limited. It is therefore vulnerable in terms of critical mass and personnel changes. A programme of this size would warrant concentration on fewer topics, but this would conflict with the strategy of professional alignment and practice orientation. Nevertheless, programme size and the relatively small number of key researchers make the research programme vulnerable to staff mobility. It is no easy task to recruit and train new young researchers, particularly researchers with a background in medical and health sciences who wish to pursue a career in health professions education. More often than not successful recruitment and follow-up training are rewarded by thankful competitor employers in the job market.

Future challenges

The School of Health Professions Education is a graduate school with multiple training opportunities ranging from short courses to a full Master of Science degree. This international Master Programme in Health Professions Education (MHPE) has an entry of about twenty students or more per year from all over the world (see http://www.she.unimaas.nl). The programme is strongly driven by education research. Quite a few MHPE graduates go on to earn a PhD degree from Maastricht University. A doctoral dissertation is purely research based and typically consists of four to six published research papers in international journals. As was reported earlier, a constant number of international candidates undertake a PhD in education research within the School of Health Professions Education. In all, both activities—the Master programme and the PhD programme—will hopefully provide additional academic anchors for enduring education research.

Another challenge will be to mature the research by embedding it more firmly in educational theory and current issues in the literature. But building a bridge between general education theory and educational practice is quite a challenge. General education research has different scientific platforms and upholding and contributing to both science domains is a tall order indeed.

Finally, over the past thirty years or so there has been an incredible professionalization of the (medical) education community. This has been greatly facilitated by the scientific forums that have been created in this domain. National and international conferences on medical and health professions education are thriving. Workshops, training programmes, and Master programmes are prospering. There is no other profession in higher education that can boast of so many international education journals for disseminating (research) information. These forums are fully targeted at health professionals and characterized by a similar interplay between health professionals and educationalists as FHML education research. This embedding of education research in educational practice and involvement by health professionals is the hallmark of the success of health professions education as a community and therefore of the health professionals being trained by this community. Ultimately this will contribute to the quality of healthcare delivery. It is good to see that a number of other (medical) schools in the Netherlands have started to make similar investments in health education research, following up on the Maastricht model (Ten Cate, 2007). A similar trend can be seen in the international community. Health professions education research is maturing as a scientific discipline. This can help to achieve the final goal of improved education and training of health professionals and, ultimately, better patient care.

References

Badley, G. (2003). The crisis in educational research: a pragmatic approach. *European Educational Research Journal* **2**, 296–308.

Berliner, D. C. (2002). Educational research: The hardest science of all. *Educational Researcher* **31**, 18–20.

Cook, D. A., Bordage, G., and Schmidt, H. G. (2008). Description, justification and clarification: a framework for classifying the purposes of research in medical education. *Medical Education* **42**, 128–33.

Dolmans, D. H. J. M. (2003). The effectiveness of PBL: the debate continues. Some concerns about the BEME-movement. *Medical Education* **37**, 1129–30.

Dolmans, D. H. J. M., Wolfhagen, H. A. P., Essed, G. G. M., Scherpbier, A. J. J. A., and van der Vleuten, C. P. M. (2002). The impacts of supervision, patient mix, and numbers of students on the effectiveness of clinical rotations. *Academic Medicine* **77**, 332–35.

Gorter, S., van der Linden, S., Brauer, J., van der Heijde, D., Houben, H., Rethans, J. J., et al. (2001). Rheumatologists' performance in daily practice. *Arthiritis Care & Research* **45**, 16–27.

Harden, R. M., Grant, J., Buckley, G., & Hart, I. R. (2000). Best evidence medical education. *Advances in Health Sciences Education* **5**, 71–90.

Hobma, S., Ram, P., Muijtjens, A., van der Vleuten, C., and Grol, R. (2006). Effective improvement of doctor-patient communication: a randomised controlled trial. *British Journal General Practitonerst* **56**, 580–6.

Maxwell, J. A. (2004). Causal explanation, qualitative research, and scientific inquiry. *Educational Researcher* **33**, 3–11.

Norman, G. R. (2003). RCT -results confounded and trivial: the perils of grand educational experiments. *Medical Education* **37**, 582–4.

Prince, C. J. A. H., van de Wiel, M. W. J., Scherpbier, A. J. J. A., van der Vleuten, C. P. M., and Boshuizen, H. P. A. (2000). A qualitative analysis of the transition from theory to practice in undergraduate training in a PBL-medical school. *Advances in Health Sciences Education* **5**, 105–10.

Schmidt, H., Norman, G., and Boshuizen, H. (1990). A cognitive perspective on medical expertise: theory and implications. *Academic Medicine* **65**, 611–22.

Schuwirth, L. W., Verheggen, M. M., van der Vleuten, C. P., Boshuizen, H. P., and Dinant, G. J. (2001). Do short cases elicit different thinking processes than factual knowledge questions do? *Medical Education* **35**, 348–56.

Schuwirth, L. W. T., Verhoeven, B. H., Scherpbier, A. J. J. A., Mom, E. M. A., Cohen-Schotanus, J., and Van Rossum, H. (1999). An inter- and intra–university comparison in clinical problem-solving skills. *Advances in Health Sciences Education* **4**, 233–44.

Ten Cate, O. (2007). Medical education in the Netherlands. *Medical Teacher* **29**, 752–7.

Teunissen, P. W., Scheele, F., Scherpbier, A. J., van der Vleuten, C. P., Boor, K., van Luijk, S. J., et al. (2007). How residents learn: qualitative evidence for the pivotal role of clinical activities. *Medical Education* **41**, 763–70.

Teunissen, P. W., Stapel, D. A., Scheele, F., Scherpbier, A. J., Boor, K., van Diemen-Steenvoorde, J. A., et al. (2009). The influence of context on residents' evaluations: effects of priming on clinical judgment and affect. *Advances in Health Sciences Education* **14**, 23–41.

Van der Vleuten, C. P. M., Dolmans, D. H. J. M., and Scherpbier, A. J. J. A. (2000). The need for evidence in education. *Medical Teacher* **22**, 246–50.

Chapter 24

A review of the evidence:
Effects of problem-based learning on students and graduates of Maastricht medical school

Henk Schmidt

There is little doubt that problem-based learning (PBL) is popular as a pedagogical innovation, especially in higher education. For example, the majority of the medical schools in the United States currently include small-group tutorial sessions organized around clinical problems. Most Australian medical schools have adopted PBL as a teaching method, and curricula based on these ideas have also been developed in Germany, Great Britain, Singapore, and Sweden. In addition, PBL has made inroads in K-12 education in the United States and the Netherlands. In fact, PBL is one of the few large-scale educational innovations successfully surviving since the sixties.

Introduction

However, opinions differ as to whether PBL is an *effective* form of education. Some argue that, contrary to expectation, PBL has failed to promote in students higher levels of knowledge (Colliver, 2000). Others maintain that PBL is a form of minimally guided instruction and therefore less effective and less efficient than instructional approaches that place a stronger emphasis on guidance of the student learning process (Kirschner et al., 2006).

This contribution deals with a review of the results of a large number of studies, comparing the performance of medical students and graduates of Maastricht medical school to that of medical students and graduates trained in conventional medical programmes in the same country. This seems a worthwhile endeavour, since roughly one-third of all curriculum comparisons, conducted worldwide since the emergence of PBL in higher education, involve this particular curriculum. However, many of these studies were published only in Dutch or in outlets not easily accessible. In addition, review of *all* studies conducted at one of the major problem-based schools in the world provides an opportunity for sketching an even-handed picture of the problem-based approach. Finally, most studies discussed in this chapter have not been included in previous summaries of research using the curricular comparison paradigm (e.g., Albanese & Mitchell, 1993; Berkson, 1993; Colliver, 2000; Vernon & Blake, 1993).

As stated, this review will concentrate on the results of curricular comparisons, that is: comparisons of the effects of a full curriculum as opposed to the effects of a course or a more limited educational intervention.[1] Generally, comparing the outcomes of different medical curricula is

---

[1] Experimental and process-oriented research on the effects of PBL has been summarized elsewhere (e.g., Hmelo-Silver, 2004; Schmidt & Moust, 2000).

somewhat problematic. Randomization of students over the treatment conditions is almost always impossible, treatments cannot be delivered in a blinded fashion, and, since medical students are highly selected in terms of knowledge and skill required to enter medical school, performance on tests is bound to show ceiling effects, leaving little room for improvement (Norman & Schmidt, 2000). Dutch medical education, however, has features that facilitate comparisons. Admission to Dutch medical schools is organized at the national level by a weighted lottery procedure based on achievement on the same national entrance examination. This procedure (inadvertently) results in groups of students in different schools that are quite similar in terms of past performance, age, gender, and motivation to study medicine (Roeleveld, 1997). Consequently, comparisons between Dutch medical schools in terms of student performance come as close as one can get to controlled field experiments in educational settings. In addition, all schools employ a six-year curriculum and the subject matter taught is largely overlapping. Again, this facilitates comparisons between the curricula.

Unlike previous reviews (e.g., Albanese & Mitchell, 1993; Berkson, 1993; Colliver, 2000; Vernon & Blake, 1993), this chapter will not be confined to the effects of PBL on knowledge acquisition alone. Below, studies will be reviewed on (1) knowledge acquisition, (2) the development of diagnostic competence, (3) interpersonal competencies, and (4) practical medical skills. In addition, (5) student and expert perceptions of the quality of problem-based versus conventional education will be reviewed, and the chapter will pay attention to comparisons in which not individual students or graduates were the focus of study but (6) the relative efficiency of the curricula as a whole. The latter is particularly relevant because a critical analysis of PBL has suggested that such an approach is inevitably less efficient than more guided instruction (Kirschner et al., 2006). The measure of efficiency focused upon here is graduation rate. The characteristics and outcomes of the studies discussed below are summarized in Table 24.1.

Acquisition of medical knowledge

Maastricht medical school developed a medical knowledge test back in the 1970s, which consists of questions about all the subjects covered in the curriculum. This is the so-called progress test (see Chapter 22). In curricular comparison studies, the results of this test lead to curves demonstrating the growth of medical knowledge across the curriculum for each of the schools involved.

The first four comparison studies using the progress test were conducted in the late seventies and early eighties, but not published until later (Verwijnen et al., 1990). These studies involved all students of the problem-based school and large groups of volunteers from three conventional medical schools. The progress tests also included questions submitted by the other universities involved in the comparison study. Although in some of the comparisons, students of one of the conventional schools tended to have higher scores in some curriculum years, these differences disappeared in the sixth year. From these results, the authors concluded that none of the comparisons showed significant differences between the schools involved in students' knowledge at the end of medical training. Verhoeven and colleagues (1998) conducted two comparison studies between all the students of the problem-based school and the majority of the students from the medical school of Nijmegen University. No significant statistical differences emerged in these studies.

A seventh study included all students from four (out of the total of eight) Dutch medical schools, those of Maastricht University, Nijmegen University, University of Groningen, and Leiden University, representing half of the total population of Dutch medical students (Van der Vleuten et al., 2004). As part of an interuniversity collaboration, these medical schools use

Table 24.1 Comparison between the performance of students and graduates of the Maastricht problem-based medical curriculum and conventional medical schools on various outcome measures

First author and publication year	Comparison groups	Statistically significant differences
Medical knowledge		
Answering questions about knowledge		
Verwijnen et al. (1990)	Volunteers from schools A and B, May 1979–September 1980	B better than Maastricht and A
	Volunteers from schools A and B, September–November 1981	B better than Maastricht and A
	Volunteers from schools A and B, non-select sample from C, March–September 1983	No difference
	Random sample from school C, March 1983	No difference
Verhoeven et al. (1998)	Volunteers from the Nijmegen school, December 1994	No difference
	Volunteers from the Nijmegen school, March 1995	No difference
Van der Vleuten et al. (2004)	Populations from the Groningen and Nijmegen school; first 4 years of the Leiden school	Maastricht and Groningen better than Nijmegen and Leiden
Imbos et al. (1984)	Random sample from a non-disclosed medical school	Maastricht better
Prince et al. (2003)	Sample from all 7 other schools	No difference
Self-assessment		
Schmidt et al. (2006)	Volunteer graduates from Rotterdam	Rotterdam better than Maastricht
Diagnostic reasoning skills		
Diagnosing cases		
Schmidt et al. (1996)	Volunteers from Groningen and Amsterdam	Maastricht and Amsterdam better than Groningen
Schuwirth et al. (1999)	Volunteers from Groningen	Maastricht better than Groningen
Processing and recalling cases		
Boshuizen et al. (1994)	Small samples of volunteers from Amsterdam	Maastricht better than Amsterdam
Boshuizen & Claessen (1982)	Small samples of volunteers from Utrecht	Maastricht better than Utrecht on one task; no differences on the other
Interpersonal skills		
Assessment by observers		
Van Dalen et al. (2002)	Volunteers from Leiden	Maastricht better than Leiden
Self-assessment		
Prince et al. (2005)	Volunteer graduates from four unspecified medical schools	Maastricht better than the other 4 schools

(Continued)

Table 24.1 (*continued*) Comparison between the performance of students and graduates of the Maastricht problem-based medical curriculum and conventional medical schools on various outcome measures

First author and publication year	Comparison groups	Statistically significant differences
Schmidt et al. (2006)	Volunteer graduates from Rotterdam	Maastricht better than Rotterdam
Practical medical skills		
Physical examination assessed by observers		
Scherpbier (1997)	Volunteers from Groningen	Maastricht better than Groningen
Answering questions about physical examination		
Remmen et al. (1999)	Volunteers from Ghent and Antwerp	Maastricht better than Ghent and Antwerp
Remmen et al. (2001)	Volunteers from Ghent, Antwerp and Groningen	Maastricht better than Groningen, both better than Ghent and Antwerp
Self-assessment		
Schmidt et al. (2006)	Volunteer graduates from Rotterdam	Maastricht better than Rotterdam
Cognitive skills (problem-solving, seeking information)		
Self-assessment		
Schmidt et al. (2006)	Volunteer graduates from Rotterdam	Maastricht better than Rotterdam
General academic skills (conducting research, writing, presenting papers)		
Self-assessment		
Schmidt et al. (2006)	Volunteer graduates from Rotterdam	No difference
Perception of the quality of the curriculum		
Steenkamp et al. (2004, 2006, 2008)	Samples from all medical schools	Maastricht better than all
Retention rates		
Post et al. (1986)	Graduates from all medical schools, entering 1970	Maastricht better than all
Schmidt et al. (2009a)	Graduates from all medical schools, entering between 1989 and 1998	Maastricht better than all

* The schools compared were anonymized in this study.

identical progress tests, which are administered to the students of all years four times a year. Since this paper focused on the description of this cross-institutional collaboration in assessment, only a graph is provided illustrating the performance of the students from the four schools on the test (Figure 24.1).

The data seem to indicate that differences occurred, slightly favouring Maastricht and Groningen medical school. However, in previous and subsequent administrations, slightly different results emerged, not always favouring these schools (Cees van der Vleuten, written communication, April 2005).

In summary: the comparisons conducted in the Netherlands over the years do not show major differences between the medical schools involved in the studies in terms of the quantity of

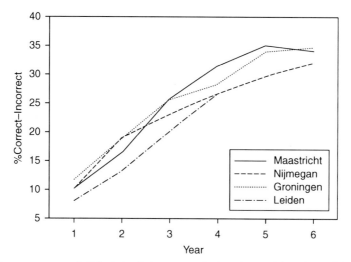

Figure 24.1 Average scores of all first- to sixth-year medical students of four (out of eight) medical schools in the Netherlands on an overall test of medical knowledge called the progress test. The scores are expressed as a percentage of correct minus incorrect answers. Reprinted from C. P. M. van der Vleuten et al. (2004) with permission from Taylor and Francis Group.

medical knowledge gained by students. This conclusion concurs with findings from international reviews (Albanese & Mitchell, 1993; Berkson, 1993; Colliver, 2000; Vernon & Blake, 1993). The results show on the one hand that there is little reason to question the general knowledge of students educated in a problem-based curriculum; their knowledge level appears to be comparable to that of students educated under a more conventional regime. These findings are inconsistent with the prediction by Kirschner et al. (2006) that PBL leads to lower levels of knowledge acquisition, because this is what instruction with less guidance by teachers is expected to do to students. On the other hand, these findings are also inconsistent with results of experimental research on the effects of PBL, demonstrating that students retain more knowledge (De Grave et al., 2001; Schmidt et al., 1989). This issue will be elaborated upon in the Discussion section.

Development of diagnostic reasoning competencies

Relatively little research to investigate whether students attending a problem-based medical school are better at solving diagnostic problems than students attending conventional training has been conducted. (However, see Hmelo (1998b) and Patel et al. (1991).) Several studies were conducted in the Netherlands. In one of these, volunteer students in various years of the Maastricht, Groningen, and Amsterdam medical schools were tested using an assessment instrument intended to evaluate diagnostic reasoning (Schmidt et al., 1996). The instrument consisted of thirty case descriptions that covered all body systems and were epidemiologically representative. Participants produced a differential diagnosis for each of the thirty cases and the number of accurate diagnoses was counted. Students of the Maastricht curriculum and a new patient-focused Amsterdam curriculum achieved better results than did the Groningen students, with statistically significant differences that occurred only in the final years of medical school. In a similar second study, samples of students from Maastricht and Groningen were presented sixty short case descriptions (Schuwirth et al., 1999). In this study, the Maastricht students also achieved significantly higher scores, but, as in the study referred to earlier, the effect seemed to be concentrated in the fifth and sixth years.

Earlier, Boshuizen and her collaborators carried out two comparisons focusing on the relation between knowledge and reasoning. Boshuizen et al. (1994) compared the performances of small samples of students from Maastricht and Amsterdam University. These (preclinical) students were asked to explain how a specific metabolic deficiency and a specific disease could be related, e.g., 'How does a genetic deficiency of pyruvate kinase lead to haemolytic anaemia?' Answering such questions required the application and integration of knowledge about biochemistry and internal medicine. In addition to these student groups, two groups of experts were incorporated in the study: biochemists and internists. Students from the problem-based curriculum and the biochemists took an analytical approach to the problem by first exploring the biochemical aspects of the problem and later linking them to clinical aspects. Students in the conventional curriculum and internists tended towards a more memory-based approach. This latter strategy, however, resulted in significantly fewer accurate answers and more failures by the students from the conventional programme. These results suggest that students in a problem-based curriculum integrate knowledge better than students in a traditional curriculum, resulting in more accurate reasoning. Another study using a clinical case recall paradigm (recall is often seen as a measure of expertise since De Groot's studies in chess) led to mixed results, however: small samples of Maastricht students better recalled an 'atypical' case than did Utrecht students, but recall of a typical case showed no such differences (Boshuizen & Claessen, 1982).

In summary, PBL seemed to have an impact on the diagnostic competencies of students, emerging when students start working with real patients in clinical clerkships. As suggested by the Boshuizen studies, this effect is possibly caused by a better integration of biomedical and clinical knowledge.

Interpersonal skills and other work-related competencies

In a study among a large group of graduates from the medical schools of Maastricht and Rotterdam, participants were asked to assess their own skill levels in eighteen professional competencies (Schmidt et al., 2006). The oldest participants had graduated nineteen years previously and the average time since graduation was slightly over nine years. The competencies concerned interpersonal skills such as the ability to collaborate with others, cognitive skills such as the ability to find relevant information quickly, general academic skills such as the ability to conduct scientific research or write a report, and clinical skills such as performing a physical examination.

The graduates from the problem-based medical school rated themselves more highly, especially on interpersonal competencies. Other research supports the major difference in this area (Prince et al., 2005; Santos Gomez et al., 1990; Van Dalen et al., 2002). It is attributed in part to the fact that students in a problem-based curriculum must work extensively with others in small groups and thus have more opportunities to practise those interpersonal skills. A difference, albeit a smaller one, was also detected with respect to cognitive skills. Hardly any difference was found with respect to general academic competencies (Schmidt et al., 2006).

Finally, graduates from the PBL curriculum felt that they had mastered clinical skills (such as blood-pressure measurement or abdominal examination) at a higher level than their colleagues from the other university. This finding concurs with findings of several other studies (Remmen et al., 1999, 2001; Scherpbier, 1997). One such study compared two groups of Maastricht students with Groningen students in the actual performance of a number of clinical skills (Scherpbier, 1997). The Maastricht students clearly showed better achievement. Two studies tested knowledge about skills (a variable closely related to actual skill level) among volunteer students in the last four years of the medical schools of Maastricht, Groningen, Antwerp, and Ghent—the latter two being Belgian schools (Remmen et al., 1999, 2001). On this test, the Dutch students achieved significantly higher marks than did the Belgian students. Moreover, Maastricht students outperformed Groningen students, especially in the last two years of medical school. Just as in the studies on diagnostic skills, the effects of PBL emerged only in the clerkships. This suggests an incubation effect of what is learned during the first four years; students in a problem-based curriculum apparently seem to reap the benefits of their education only when they begin to interact with patients.

Student and expert judgments of the quality of problem-based instruction

Each year, twenty thousand Dutch students are polled about the quality of their education for the 'Keuzegids hoger onderwijs', a Consumer Reports-type guide to higher education (Steenkamp et al., 2006). In this guide, programmes within a particular domain are compared nationwide to help prospective students make more informed career and education decisions. For each programme, three hundred randomly selected students receive a questionnaire asking them to rate their curriculum on ten dimensions: (1) the quality of the content of the curriculum, (2) electives, (3) coherence of the curriculum, (4) the instructional approach, (5) preparation for professional practice, (6) the quality of the teachers, (7) communication with the students, (8) whether the programme can be completed with the timeframe available, (9) the quality of the classrooms, and (10) student facilities. In the 2006 edition, the problem-based school came out best overall. Students particularly liked the instructional approach; here the difference with the other schools is largest. In addition, the problem-based curriculum received high ratings on contents, coherence, and preparation for the profession. In fact, since the first publication of the report in 1991, the problem-based school has finished first, with only one exemption.

In five-year cycles, an accreditation committee of national experts surveys all medical schools. The resulting reports are used for decision-making at the national level. The findings of these experts, published over the past twenty years, generally concur with the results of the student surveys (e.g., Looijenga, 2004).

Retention rates of Dutch medical schools

The Dutch Association of Universities (VSNU) collects retention rate data of the Dutch medical schools. The retention rate of a programme is expressed as the percentage of entering students that successfully complete the programme. These data have been collected systematically since 1989, but some national data are available from medical schools for previous years. Remember that the first cohorts of Maastricht medical students entered in 1974 and began to graduate in 1980. A study by Post et al. (1986) provides data relevant for this period. It displays the retention rates for all medical students entering the seven medical schools in the Netherlands in 1970 and compares them with the retention rates of the four cohorts entering Maastricht medical school between 1974 and 1978. The comparisons showed that, after six years, 64% of the first Maastricht cohort had earned their medical degree compared to 0% of the cohorts of the other medical schools. Nine years after entering medical school, 96% of the problem-based cohort had graduated, whereas the retention rate for the other schools was 64%.

More recently, a study was conducted on data collected from all students entering Dutch medical education between 1989 and 1998 (Schmidt et al., 2009a). This study demonstrated that, on average, after six years, 73% of the problem-based students had graduated, whereas for the conventional schools the average graduation rate was 48%. After nine years, the difference was still 10% (92 versus 82%) (Figure 24.2). These findings suggest that over the ten-year period surveyed,

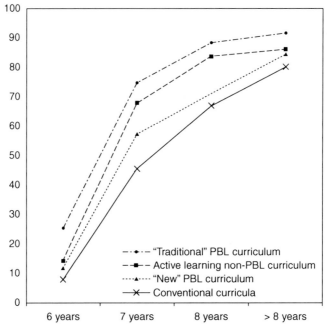

Figure 24.2 Average six- to nine-year graduation rates of all medical students entering medical education in the Netherlands between 1989 and 1998 (Schmidt et al., 2009). The 'traditional' problem-based school is Maastricht medical school. The active learning non-PBL curriculum (Nijmegen) and the 'new' PBL curriculum (Groningen) have many characteristics in common with the Maastricht curriculum. The data of the conventional curricula represent the average graduation rates of all other medical schools over the period mentioned.

the Maastricht problem-based curriculum was consistently more efficient in training medical students than the other schools. Not only does the problem-based school have a considerable lower dropout rate than the other schools, students complete their studies much faster.

Discussion

The review presented here was conducted to provide an overview of the effects of the Maastricht problem-based curriculum on its students and graduates. This curriculum stands out, not only because it is one of the first that began to experiment with PBL and still retains the major characteristics of this approach as originally intended, but also because it is the most extensively studied curriculum in this area (Schmidt et al., 2009b). The results of this review suggest that students and graduates of this curriculum perform better (1) on tests of diagnostic reasoning, and (2) in the area of interpersonal and (3) medical professional competencies. In addition, (4) students in the problem-based school consistently rate the quality of their education more highly than do students in conventional schools. The same applies to national bodies of experts visiting the schools. Furthermore, the problem-based curriculum (5) turned out to be more efficient and effective, as witnessed by lower dropout and less delay. No differences were found with respect to (6) acquired medical knowledge. These findings are generally in agreement with findings from other problem-based schools, when available. Hmelo (1998a), for instance, found similar effects of PBL on diagnostic reasoning tasks in two medical schools. Santos Gomez et al. (1990) and Woodward and McAuley (1983) found graduates from problem-based schools to be better communicators with patients and colleagues than their counterparts from conventional schools. Kiessling et al. (2004) and Kuhnigk and Schauenburg (1999) demonstrated that PBL students felt more supported by this learning environment, and also experienced more social support, less stress, and less alienation. Burch et al. (2006) and Iputo and Kwizera (2005) reported lower dropout rates for students of problem-based curricula. Reviews of comparisons involving the acquisition of knowledge show a pattern similar to that described here: students graduating from problem-based curricula do not acquire more knowledge (Albanese & Mitchell, 1993; Colliver, 2000; Vernon & Blake, 1993).

Taken together, these findings sketch a picture of the effects of PBL that is considerably more positive that that which arises from other contributions to the literature (e.g., Colliver, 2000; Kirschner et al., 2006). Compared to conventional education, the PBL approach to learning and instruction seems to promote, more than conventional education, cognitive skills such as clinical reasoning and information seeking as well as professional skills such as interpersonal competencies and physical examination skills. It does this in a way preferred by students and appreciated by expert judges. In addition, it does this in a more effective and efficient way, as witnessed by higher retention rates and less delay. The latter finding is particularly relevant to note here in the light of suggestions by Kirschner et al. (2006) that PBL, which they classify as minimally guided instruction, is by definition less efficient and effective than conventional education. Schmidt et al. (2009b), Burch et al. (2006), and Iputo and Kwizera (2005) seem to show the reverse. This is the more interesting because, once more as opposed to the expectations of Kirschner et al. (2006), PBL curricula generally show no differences to conventional curricula in terms of the amount of knowledge acquired by students. Combining the lack of difference in knowledge acquired with the higher retention rates of PBL has led Schmidt et al. (2009b) to conclude that differential dropout masks effects of PBL on learning in curriculum comparison studies. They argue that, in curriculum comparison studies such as those reviewed in this paper and elsewhere, sample selection is based on the same performance measures as those used for the actual comparisons (i.e., those who drop out do not contribute to the overall scores). They maintain that this selection method confounds the dependent variable and masks any real differences that may exist between the curricula involved. At the curriculum level, better performance on knowledge tests then translates into higher retention. This may also explain why experimental studies, unlike curriculum comparison studies, find that PBL does in fact have an impact on the knowledge level of students (De Grave et al., 2001).

If PBL works, then a relevant question is *why* does it work? The relevant literature proposes several hypotheses. One line of thought concentrates on the use of *problems as a starting point of learning*. From a cognitive perspective, problems are puzzles that, by their enigmatic nature, evoke epistemic curiosity in students (Inagaki & Hatano, 1977). Curiosity can be interpreted as a form of cognitively induced deprivation that arises from the perception of a gap in knowledge or understanding; learners therefore engage in activities to close that gap (Loewenstein, 1994). Several studies have demonstrated increased levels of curiosity in students after being confronted with a problem in their domain of study. These feelings of curiosity were largely maintained throughout the PBL cycle and were related to subsequent achievement (De Volder et al., 1986; Rotgans, 2009). Second, to the extent that problems can be perceived as pertinent to students' future profession, they contribute to the experience of relevance of the curriculum. It may, therefore, come as no surprise that PBL students report higher levels of perceived relevance of their education in quality-of-instruction surveys (Steenkamp et al., 2004, 2006, 2008).

Others point at the facilitating effects of *small-group instruction*. The cognitive benefits of small-group learning (enabling students to activate prior knowledge, to elaborate upon what is learned, to integrate new knowledge with existing knowledge) have been extensively documented in the literature (e.g., Slavin, 1996; Springer et al., 1999; Webb et al., 1995), and need no further discussion here. There are two other functions of small-group learning. First, the tutorial group is a source of friendships. In addition, the group enables students to develop more personal relationships with teachers than is possible in the larger classroom. Both factors are considered to be protective against premature dropout (Tinto, 1997). Second, regular small-group tutorials in problem-based schools provide peer pressure and natural deadlines for work to be completed and, as a result, encourage students not to postpone self-study. It is suggested here, that this is a reason why students in the PBL curriculum graduate earlier than students from conventional schools.

Self-directed learning is seen as a core element of PBL and much emphasis is put on the developing ability of students to regulate their own learning. It should be noted here that the various instructional activities conducted both in the problem-based and in the conventional context are intended to support self-study of students. However, more emphasis on instructional scaffolding in the curriculum than on direct instruction causes students to spend their time differently. Generally, students in problem-based curricula spend less time in lectures and have more time for self-study. In the problem-based school under study, students received 3 hours of lectures each week and had 27 hours available for self-study, while teachers in the conventional schools lectured on average 14 hours, leaving room for 19 hours of self-study (Schmidt et al., 2009b). As a result of the emphasis on self-directed learning, PBL students were shown to borrow more books and use more learning resources in the library than their counterparts in conventional schools (Blumberg & Michael, 1992; Marshall et al., 1993; Rankin, 1992), suggesting that these students are more self-reliant and feel more responsible for their own learning, a hypothesis corroborated by the quality-of-instruction surveys (Steenkamp et al., 2004, 2006, 2008). A recent study, involving graduation-rate and study-duration data for almost 14,000 graduates from the eight medical schools in the Netherlands, found that time available for self-study in the various curricula was correlated 0.44 with graduation rate and −0.48 with study duration; that is: the more time for self-study was available in these curricula, the more students graduated and the faster they did so (Schmidt et al., 2010). These findings strongly suggest that time available for self-study, as afforded in PBL, leads to better achievement of more students, hence to fewer delays and higher graduation rates. The study also demonstrated that the *more* lectures these students received, the *fewer* students graduated and the longer it took them to graduate. This finding is ironic in the light of the recent emphasis in the literature on the importance of direct instruction, because it demonstrates that this kind of support is not necessarily *good* for students.

The studies reviewed in this chapter involved only one problem-based medical school, the medical school of Maastricht University in the Netherlands. Therefore, the generalizability of the findings presented here can only be claimed to the extent that these findings have been corroborated in studies from other schools, which has happened to some extent. On the other hand, the particular school was established only a few years after PBL was invented at McMaster University in Canada, and has influenced many new schools both within the Netherlands and abroad, particularly in Canada, the UK, Brazil, Thailand, Vietnam, Indonesia, South-Africa, and Egypt. In addition, roughly one-third of all curricular comparisons published in the literature are from this school. Taken together, the findings summarized here indicate that PBL may have several desirable characteristics that seem well worth emulating.

Annoted literature

Albanese, M. A., & Mitchell, S. (1993). Problem-based learning: a review of literature on its outcomes and implementation issues. *Academic Medicine* **68**, 52–81.

This seminal review is among the first summarizing effects of problem-based learning by conducting a meta-analysis-type review of the English-language international literature from 1972 to 1992. Compared with conventional instruction, PBL, as suggested by the findings, is more nurturing and enjoyable; PBL graduates perform as well, and sometimes better, on clinical examinations and faculty evaluations; and they are more likely to enter family medicine. Further, faculty tends to enjoy teaching using PBL. However, PBL students in a few instances scored lower on basic sciences examinations and viewed themselves as less well prepared in the basic sciences than were their conventionally trained counterparts; PBL graduates tended to engage in backward rather than the forward reasoning experts engage in; and there appeared to be gaps in their cognitive knowledge base that could affect practice outcomes. The costs of PBL may slow its implementation in schools with class sizes larger than 100.

Koh, G. C., Khoo, H. E., Wong, M. L., & Koh, D. (2008). The effects of problem-based learning during medical school on physician competency: a systematic review. *Canadian Medical Association Journal* **178**, 34–41.

Rather than reviewing effects on knowledge, these authors conducted a systematic review of evidence of the effects that problem-based learning during medical school has on physician competencies after graduation. They found that, according to self-assessments of students, 8 of the 37 competencies they defined strongly supported PBL. In observed assessments 7 competencies showed strong evidence in favour of PBL. Under both measuring conditions, most of these competencies were in the social and cognitive domain. Four competencies had moderate to strong levels of evidence in support of PBL for both self- and observed assessments: coping with uncertainty (strong), appreciation of legal and ethical aspects of healthcare (strong), communication skills (moderate and strong, respectively), and self-directed continuing learning (moderate).

Schmidt, H. G., Cohen-Schotanus, J., & Arends, L. (2009). Impact of problem-based, active, learning on graduation rates of ten generations of Dutch medical students. *Medical Education* **43**, 211–18.

This study is the first in which graduation rates of populations of medical students up to nine years after admission to medical school are used to study effects of active learning. In addition, duration of study is examined for the first time as a dependent variable in this context. Graduation rates of ten generations of students enrolling in the eight Dutch medical schools between 1989 and 1998 were analysed. In addition, time needed to graduate was recorded. Three of the eight schools had curricula emphasizing active learning, small-group instruction, and limited numbers of lectures; the other five had conventional curricula to varying degrees. Overall, the active-learning curricula graduated on average 8% more students per year, and these students graduated on average 5 months earlier than their colleagues from conventional curricula. Four hypotheses potentially explaining the effect of active learning on graduation rate and study duration were considered: (1) active-learning curricula promote social and academic integration of students; (2) active-learning curricula attract brighter students; (3) active-learning curricula retain more poor students; and (4) students' active engagement with their study required by the active-learning curricula induced better academic performance and, hence, lower dropout. The first three hypotheses had to be rejected. It was concluded that the better-learning hypothesis provides the most parsimonious account for the data.

References

Albanese, M. A., and Mitchell, S. (1993). Problem-based learning: a review of literature on its outcomes and implementation issues. *Academic Medicine* **68**, 52–81.

Berkson, L. (1993). Problem-based learning - have the expectations been met? *Academic Medicine* **68**, S79–S88.

Blumberg, P., and Michael, J. A. (1992). Development of self-directed learning behaviors in a partially teacher-directed problem-based learning curriculum. *Teaching and Learning in Medicine* **4**, 3–8.

Boshuizen, H. P. A., and Claessen, H. F. A. (1982). Cognitieve verwerking en onthouden van patiëntgegevens: een onderzoek bij studenten in Utrecht en Maastricht [Cognitive processing and recall of patient information: a study among Utrecht and Maastricht students]. In: H. G. Schmidt (ed.), *Probleemgestuurd onderwijs [Problem-based learning]*. Harlingen, the Netherlands: Flevodruk. Pp. 83–100.

Boshuizen, H. P. A., Schmidt, H. G., and Wassmer, L. (1994). Curriculum style and the integration of biomedical and clinical knowledge. In: P. A. J. Bouhuijs, H. G. Schmidt, and H. J. M. Van Berkel (eds), *Problem-based learning as an educational strategy*. Maastricht, the Netherlands: Network Publications. Pp. 33–42.

Burch, V. C., Sikakana, C. N. T., Seggie, J. L., and Schmidt, H. G. (2006). Performance of academically-at-risk medical students in a problem-based learning programme. A preliminary report [electronic version]. *Advances in Health Sciences Education*.

Colliver, J. A. (2000). Effectiveness of problem-based learning curricula: Research and theory. *Academic Medicine* **75**, 259–66.

De Grave, W. S., Schmidt, H. G., and Boshuizen, H. P. A. (2001). Effects of problem-based discussion on studying a subsequent text: A randomized trial among first year medical students. *Instructional Science* **29**, 33–44.

De Volder, M. L., Schmidt, H. G., Moust, J. H. C., and de Grave, W. S. (1986). Problem-based-learning and intrinsic motivation. In: J. H. C. van der Berchen, T. C. M. Bergen, and E. E. I. de Bruyn (eds), *Achievement and task motivation*. Berwyn, IL: Swets North America.

Hmelo, C. E. (1998a). Cognitive consequences of problem-based learning for the early development of medical expertise. *Teaching and Learning in Medicine* **10**, 92–100.

Hmelo, C. E. (1998b). Problem-based learning: Effects on the early acquisition of cognitive skill in medicine. *Journal of the Learning Sciences* **7**, 173–208.

Hmelo-Silver, C. E. (2004). Problem-based learning: What and how do students learn? *Educational Psychology Review* **16**, 235–66.

Imbos, T., Drukker, J., Van Mameren, H., and Verwijnen, M. (1984). The growth of knowledge of anatomy in a problem-based curriculum. In: H. G. Schmidt and M. L. de Volder (eds), *Tutorials in problem-based learning: a new direction in teaching the health professions*. Assen/Maastricht, the Netherlands: Van Gorcum.

Inagaki, K., and Hatano, G. (1977). Amplification of cognitive motivation and its effects on epistemic observation. *American Educational Research Journal* **14**, 485–91.

Iputo, J. E., and Kwizera, E. (2005). Problem-based learning improves the academic performance of medical students in South Africa. *Medical Education* **39**, 388–93.

Kiessling, C., Schubert, B., Scheffner, D., and Burger, W. (2004). First year medical students' perceptions of stress and support: a comparison between reformed and traditional track curricula. *Medical Education* **38**, 504–9.

Kirschner, P. A., Sweller, J., and Clark, R. E. (2006). Why minimal guidance during instruction does not work: An analysis of the failure of constructivist, discovery, problem-based, experiential, and inquiry-based teaching. *Educational Psychologist* **41**, 75–86.

Kuhnigk, O., and Schauenburg, H. (1999). Psychological wellbeing, locus of control and personality traits in medical students of a traditional and an alternative curriculum. *Psychotherapie Psychosomatik Medizinische Psychologie* **49**, 29–36.

Loewenstein, G. (1994). The psychology of curiosity: A review and reinterpretation. *Psychological Bulletin* **116**, 75–98.

Looijenga, S. (2004). *Geneeskunde (Medicine)*. Utrecht, the Netherlands: Stichting Quality Assurance Netherlands Universities (QANU).

Marshall, J. G., Fitzgerald, D., Busby, L., and Heaton, G. (1993). A study of library use in problem-based and traditional medical curricula. *Bulletin of the Medical Library Association* **81**, 299–305.

Norman, G. R., and Schmidt, H. G. (2000). Effectiveness of problem-based learning curricula: theory, practice and paper darts. *Medical Education* **34**, 721–8.

Patel, V. L., Groen, G. J., and Norman, G. R. (1991). Effects of conventional and problem-based medical curricula on problem-solving. *Academic Medicine* **66**, 380–9.

Post, G. J., de Graaff, E., and Drop, M. J. (1986). Duur en numeriek rendement van de opleiding tot basisarts in Maastricht (Length and output of medical training in Maastricht). *Nederlands Tijdschrift voor Geneeskunde* **130**, 1903–5.

Prince, K., Van Eijs, P. W. L. J., Boshuizen, H. P. A., van der Vleuten, C. P. M., and Scherpbier, A. J. J. A. (2005). General competencies of problem-based learning (PBL) and non-PBL graduates. *Medical Education* **39**, 394–401.

Prince, K., van Mameren, H., Hylkema, N., Drukker, J., Scherpbier, A. J. J. A., and van der Vleuten, C. P. M. (2003). Does problem-based learning lead to deficiencies in basic science knowledge? An empirical case on anatomy. *Medical Education* **37**, 15–21.

Rankin, J. A. (1992). Problem-based medical education - Effect on library use. *Bulletin of the Medical Library Association* **80**, 36–43.

Remmen, R., Derese, A., Scherpbier, A., Denekens, J., Hermann, I., van der Vleuten, C., et al. (1999). Can medical schools rely on clerkships to train students in basic clinical skills? *Medical Education* **33**, 600–5.

Remmen, R., Scherpbier, A., Van der Vleuten, C., Denekens, J., Derese, A., Hermann, I., et al. (2001). Effectiveness of basic clinical skills training programmes: a cross-sectional comparison of four medical schools. *Medical Education* **35**, 121–8.

Roeleveld, J. (1997). *Lotingscategorieën en studiesucces: Rapportage aan de adviescommissie Toelating Numerus-Fixusopleidingen [Lottery categories and academic achievement: Report to the advisory committee Admissions Numerus-Fixus programs]*. Amsterdam, the Netherlands: University of Amsterdam: SCO/Kohnstamm Instituut.

Rotgans, I. J. (2009). *Motivation, achievement-related behaviours, and educational outcomes*. PhD Thesis, Erasmus University, Rotterdam.

Santos Gomez, L., Kalishman, S., Rezler, A. G., Skipper, B., and Mennin, S. P. (1990). Residency performance of graduates from a problem-based and a conventional curriculum. *Medical Education* **24**, 366–75.

Scherpbier, A. J. J. A. (1997). *De kwaliteit van vaardigheidsonderwijs gemeten [The quality of skills training assessed]*. Maastricht University, Maastricht, the Netherlands.

Schmidt, H. G., and Moust, J. H. C. (2000). Processes that shape small-group tutorial learning: a review of research. In: D. H. Evensen and C. E. Hmelo (eds), *Problem-based learning: a research perspective on learning interactions*. Mahwah, NJ: Lawrence Erlbaum. Pp. 19–52.

Schmidt, H. G., de Grave, W. S., de Volder, M. L., Moust, J. H. C., and Patel, V. L. (1989). Explanatory models in the processing of science text: the role of prior knowledge activation through small-group discussion. *Journal of Educational Psychology* **81**, 610–19.

Schmidt, H. G., Machiels-Bongaerts, M., Hermans, H., Ten Cate, O., Venekamp, R., and Boshuizen, H. P. A. (1996). The development of diagnostic competence: A comparison between a problem-based, an integrated, and a conventional medical curriculum. *Academic Medicine* **71**, 658–64.

Schmidt, H. G., Vermeulen, L., & van der Molen, H. T. (2006). Long-term effects of problem-based learning: a comparison of competencies acquired by graduates of a problem-based and a conventional medical school. *Medical Education* **40**, 562–7.

Schmidt, H. G., Cohen-Schotanus, J., and Arends, L. (2009a). Impact of problem-based, active, learning on graduation rates of ten generations of Dutch medical students. *Medical Education* **43**, 211–18.

Schmidt, H. G., van der Molen, H. T., Te Winkel, W. W. R., and Wijnen, W. H. F.W. (2009b). Constructivist, problem-based, learning does work: a meta-analysis of curricular comparisons involving a single medical school. *Educational Psychologist* **44**, 1–23.

Schmidt, H. G., Cohen-Schotanus, J., van der Molen, H. T., Splinter, T. A. W., Bulte, J. A., Holdrinet, R. S. G., et al. (2010). Learning more by being taught less: a 'time-for-self-study' theory explaining curricular effects on graduation rate and study duration. *Higher Education* accepted for publication.

Schuwirth, L. W., Verhoeven, B. H., Scherpbier, A. J., Mom, E. M., Cohen-Schotanus, J., Van Rossum, H. J., et al. (1999). An inter- and intra-university comparison with short case-based testing. *Advances in Health Sciences Education* **4**, 233–44.

Slavin, R. E. (1996). Research on cooperative learning and achievement: What we know, what we need to know. *Contemporary Educational Psychology* **21**, 43–69.

Springer, L., Stanne, M. E., and Donovan, S. S. (1999). Effects of small-group learning on undergraduates in science, mathematics, engineering, and technology: A meta-analysis. *Review of Educational Research* **69**, 21–51.

Steenkamp, F., de Looper, H., and Bliekendaal, M. (2006). *De keuzegids hoger onderwijs 06/07* [*The higher education guide 06/07*]. Leiden, the Netherlands: Hoger Onderwijs Persbureau.

Steenkamp, F., de Moor, A., and Van Beek, M. (2004). *De keuzegids hoger onderwijs 04/05* [*The higher education guide 04/05*]. Leiden, the Netherlands: Centrum voor Hoger Onderwijs Informatie.

Steenkamp, F., Dobber, L., and Jansen, M. (2008). *Keuzegids hoger onderwijs 2008* [*The higher education guide 2008*]. Leiden, the Netherlands: Hoger Onderwijs Persbureau.

Tinto, V. (1997). Classrooms as communities - Exploring the educational character of student persistence. *Journal of Higher Education* **68**, 599–623.

Van Dalen, J., Kerkhofs, E., van Knippenberg-van Den Berg, B. W., van den Hout, H. A., Scherpbier, A. J., and van der Vleuten, C. P. M. (2002). Longitudinal and concentrated communication skills programmes: two Dutch medical schools compared. *Advances in Health Sciences Education: Theory and Practice* **7**, 29–40.

Van der Vleuten, C. P. M., Schuwirth, L. W. T., Muijtens, A. M. M., Thoben, A. J. N. M., Cohen-Schotanus, J., and van Boven, C. P. A. (2004). Cross institutional collaboration in assessment: a case on progress testing. *Medical Teacher* **26**, 719–25.

Verhoeven, B. H., Verwijnen, G. M., Scherpbier, A. J. J. A., Holdrinet, R. S. G., Oeseburg, B., Bulte, J. A., et al. (1998). An analysis of progress test results of PBL and non-PBL students. *Medical Teacher* **20**, 310–16.

Vernon, D. T. A., and Blake, R. L. (1993). Does Problem-Based Learning Work - a Metaanalysis of Evaluative Research. *Academic Medicine* **68**, 550–63.

Verwijnen, G. M., Van der Vleuten, C., and Imbos, T. (1990). A comparison of an innovative medical school with traditional schools: an analysis in the cognitive domain. In: Z. Nooman, H. G. Schmidt, and E. Ezzat (eds), *Innovation in medical education, an evaluation of its present status*. New York: Springer. Pp. 40–9.

Webb, N. M., Troper, J. D., and Fall, R. (1995). Constructive activity and learning in collaborative small-groups. *Journal of Educational Psychology* **87**, 406–23.

Woodward, C. A., and McAuley, R. G. (1983). Can the academic background of medical graduates be detected during internship? *Canadian Medical Association Journal* **129**, 567–9.

Chapter 25

Internationalization

Gerard Majoor and Susan Niemantsverdriet

As a consequence of progressing globalization, educational institutions, their faculty, and their students must become internationally orientated. Initially Maastricht University's Faculty of Health, Medicine and Life Sciences (FHML) sought international allies to lend support to its educational mission in the Netherlands; later FHML internationally advocated its mission by promoting student mobility, offering short courses on PBL, embarking on development cooperation projects, incepting an international track in medicine, and by hosting the global Network: Towards Unity for Health. These actions have greatly contributed to the international orientation and visibility of FHML.

Introduction

Internationalization has become a dimension of virtually all programmes in higher education worldwide. The intensifying processes of globalization and—in Europe—Europeanization have stimulated institutions of higher education to address international aspects in their curricula and to create opportunities for staff and student exchange. In the early 1970s, the Maastricht Faculty of Medicine adopted the problem-based learning (PBL) approach. Initially, support for this endeavour was sought in the—then few—like-minded institutions dispersed around the globe. In 1979, a Maastricht-based international network was incepted under the auspices of the World Health Organization which now, in 2009, has developed into 'The Network: Towards Unity for Health', an association of 135 institutions with members in 63 countries.

By the end of the twentieth century, Maastricht University had adopted 'international orientation' and 'PBL' as two spearheads for its institutional profile. This emphasis on international orientation coincided with growing attention in Europe for internationalization of higher education, which was boosted by the European Union's (EU) Erasmus programme followed by the Tempus and Socrates programmes and the Bologna declaration (advocating the structuring of academic programmes in a Bachelor and a Master phase). As a consequence the FHML saw an increasing number of its students take study leaves abroad and visiting students participate in educational units presented in English.

The expertise on PBL that has accumulated in Maastricht continues to attract many visitors and (postgraduate) students. Initially, visitors were received throughout the year; later annual summer courses in PBL were offered. The demand for further training in the educational principles and organizational consequences of PBL eventually led to a postgraduate Master programme in Health Professions Education (MHPE). Furthermore, FHML has established cooperation programmes on education with partners in developing countries. The latest initiative was the introduction in 2007 of an English stream of the medical Bachelor curriculum, initially serving Saudi Arabian students.

Definitions of internationalization of education

There is considerable diversity in the definitions of internationalization of education. Definitions by American authors generally emphasize activities, rationales, competencies, and ethics and 'international education' appears to be the preferred term. International education is used in various ways, focusing more on primary and secondary education than on higher education. Authors from Europe, Canada, and Australia refer more often to a process approach and use 'internationalization of higher education'. The most cited process definition of internationalization of higher education is that formulated by Jane Knight. She defined internationalization of higher education as 'The process of integrating an international/intercultural dimension into the research, teaching and services functions of higher education' (Knight, 2008).

Another widely used concept is 'internationalization at home' (Teekens, 2006), which refers to internationalization activities within an educational institution. This definition stresses the importance of international and intercultural content of the curriculum and the role of the international office in promoting internationalization at home in addition to facilitating student and staff mobility (that is, students and staff going abroad and the institution receiving foreign students and faculty for education purposes).

Medical education and internationalization of education

In the field of medicine, participation in internationalization of education has been slow to develop. In November 1991 a European Community conference on 'Erasmus and Mobility in Medical Studies' was organized to discuss why participation in student exchange did not keep pace with the number of individuals involved in medical education and training. At that time medical students represented 15% of all students in the then twelve member states of the European Community but accounted for only 3% of all mobility students. However, at the beginning of the twenty-first century a lively debate about international standardization of medical education commenced at conferences and in medical journals and the first European medical schools adopted Bachelor/Master programmes (FHML started its Bachelor/Master programme in 2006).

Medical education was also pressed to pay attention to internationalization because of health issues related to globalization. Through mobility of people, services, and commodities, globalization affects the health of populations and the delivery of healthcare all over the world. To some extent these issues can be addressed by internationalization of education. This may be done by internationalization of the curriculum and promotion of student and staff mobility. Student mobility has been the most common approach to internationalization in education.

In the medical education literature not much attention has been paid to the effects of student mobility. Some publications have pointed to the potential dangers of international internships, like moral dilemmas and risks of contracting serious infections. Thompson et al. (2003) reviewed all studies from the Medline and ERIC databases for the period 1966–2000 addressing international clinical electives or rotations with evaluation of their educational effects. At that time only eight studies were identified. Thompson et al. concluded that international clinical electives and rotations had positive educational influences on participants' knowledge, skills, and attitudes. In her PhD thesis Susan Niemantsverdriet (2007) has highlighted several positive learning effects of international internships.

Adopting good practices in Maastricht
Internationalization of the curriculum

Internationalization of the regular FHML undergraduate curriculum has been restricted to the inclusion of some English language units (see below) and some clinical cases on imported diseases like malaria. Attempts to introduce intercultural aspects and cross-cultural communication have met little support. On the other hand, for over a decade students of the Maastricht branch of the International Federation of Medical Student Associations (IFMSA) have organized an annual elective on 'Tropical Medicine', which is usually attended by about half of the students of each class. Furthermore, in 2002, the faculty introduced an elective 'International Track in Medicine' for a maximum of twenty students per year. This elective track ran from the second through the sixth year and addressed intercultural communication, international healthcare systems, globalization and health, and health (care) in developing countries. In 2007 this track was converted to a formal honours programme on 'International Medicine', which evolved in 2009 into an honours programme in 'International Health' for medical as well as health sciences students of FHML.

Although in principle taught in Dutch, the medical curriculum features some English language units. The rationale for this is twofold: (a) to enhance the command of (medical) English by medical students (and teachers), and (b) to facilitate the participation of visiting foreign students in the medical programme. Students and staff are offered free courses in medical English to prepare for these units. In the 1988 curriculum a series of three units in the fourth year was exclusively presented in English. With the introduction of the 2001 curriculum English units were only offered in the second year and participation was made optional for Maastricht students. The English language Bachelor programme currently offered to students from Saudi Arabia allows visiting students to participate in any unit of the first two years of the medical Bachelor programme.

Student mobility

Supported by Maastricht University's emphasis on internationalization, FHML has pursued a policy of encouraging medical students to undertake at least one component of their medical education in another country. In order to promote this, FHML allocates substantial resources and staff for internationalization and provides grants to help students cover additional expenses of travelling abroad. FHML has developed a database of some sixty foreign institutions where students can undertake electives and clinical rotations. With a substantial part of these institutions FHML has entered into 'affiliation contracts', while relationships with other institutions have resulted from contacts established on the initiatives of individual students.

Out of the full medical student population of approximately 2000 students, annually about 400 students take a study leave abroad and out of a comparable population of health sciences students between 100 and 125 students do the same. Table 25.1 provides the figures for the academic year 2007/8 and, for comparison, those from five years earlier, 2002/3, just after the curriculum change of 2001. For medicine, the data in Table 25.1 show an increase in clinical rotations in Europe and a decrease in the number of inbound students due to the new curriculum. For health sciences, Table 25.1 demonstrates a growth of student mobility over the same period, especially within Europe.

A laudable initiative by some medical students is 'Maastricht Students Twinning a North Ghanaian Hospital' (MUSTANGH), which aims to support the development of the Damongo Regional Hospital and to create a preferred site in rural Africa for FHML students to undertake clinical rotations and electives.

At the time when FHML was offering three English language units in the fourth year, most of the approximately eighty foreign students who annually visited the school attended these units. When the English units were moved to the second year, the participation of visiting students dropped. This was to some extent compensated by foreign students requesting placements in clinical departments but, obviously, the teaching hospitals can receive only limited numbers of foreign students, because most patients speak only Dutch and hospitals must already accommodate

Table 25.1 Annual student mobility, academic years 2002/3 and 2007/8

FHML programmes	Geography	2002/3		2007/8	
		Outbound	Inbound	Outbound	Inbound
Medicine	Europe	94	61	189	41
	Outside Europe	260	15	273	3
	Total	354	76	462	44
Health sciences	Europe	9	8	72	19
	Outside Europe	62	0	31	0
	Total	71	8	103	19

large numbers of FHML students. The health sciences programme of FHML annually receives 25 visiting students from abroad.

An interesting development was seen with respect to the organization of internationalization at FHML. Initially, a small unit was created, which expanded to an 'international office' staffed by one academic faculty member and about five support staff. At a later stage the tasks of this office were integrated with those of the Institute of Medical Education.

An English international variant of the curriculum

With the consent of the Dutch Ministry for Education, Maastricht and Groningen Universities have entered into contracts with the Ministry of Higher Education in Saudi Arabia to accept Saudi high school graduates for their medical studies. In the course of the academic year 2007/8 the faculty decided to offer these students an English variant of the medical Bachelor curriculum. Candidates enrol in a foundation programme focussing on English language and basic sciences at University College Maastricht (UCM). As of 2009 this English stream will be transformed into an international variant, which is more strongly orientated to 'international health'. Maastricht will use its international contacts to offer the students undertaking this programme clinical clerkships during their Master programmes in English- and Arab-speaking countries.

Programmes on PBL

In order to share Maastricht's experiences with PBL with others, in the early 1980s Dr. Henk Schmidt started a summer course on PBL. This programme has been a continuous success, attracting annually between thirty and fifty participants from around the world. Recently the summer course was included in the programme of the Maastricht School of Health Professions Education (SHE). This programme includes a two-day visitors' workshop, the two-week summer course, a MHPE programme, and a PhD programme. Annually fifteen to twenty international postgraduate students enrol in the MHPE programme and approximately five graduates out of each class of this programme go on to earn a PhD degree.

Development cooperation

Hosting the secretarial office of the Network, offering summer courses, and publishing research on PBL have made Maastricht visible all over the world to those interested in the innovation of medical education. Schools of Medicine and Health Sciences in developing countries have turned to Maastricht for assistance in changing their conventional, 'discipline-based and teacher-centred' medical curricula into 'community-oriented, problem-based, and student-centred' programmes.

Maastricht University's office for development cooperation, 'Mundo', has taken the approach of capacity development in these institutions. Maastricht staff members travel abroad to conduct faculty development workshops in partner institutions and staff members from these schools participate in programmes offered by SHE. Some examples of medical schools in developing countries supported by the Dutch government for cooperation with FHML are Ahfad University for Women, Omdurman, Sudan; Catholic University of Mozambique, Beira, Mozambique; Can Tho and Ho Chi Minh Universities, Vietnam; University for Development Studies, Tamale, Ghana; Gadjah Mada University, Jogjakarta, Indonesia; Hadhramout University, Mukalla, Yemen; Hawassa and Mekelle Universities, Ethiopia; Makerere University, Kampala, Uganda; and Moi University, Eldoret, Kenya.

Discussion

As described above, the intensifying processes of globalization and Europeanization have stimulated FHML to address international aspects in its curricula and to create opportunities for staff and student exchange. The adoption of 'international orientation' and PBL as spearheads for the development of Maastricht University's education profile has generated specific opportunities and challenges with respect to the internationalization of education. FHML has successfully implemented an extensive internationalization programme. For quite some years the faculty has been a role model for the development of internationalization to the other seven Dutch medical schools. Its visibility within the international Network, dedication to educational research, 'organized hospitality' for foreign visitors, and involvement in development cooperation has brought Maastricht world fame in the domain of innovative PBL medical education. Combining the programmes offered by SHE with the Master programmes in Public Health for Professionals and in Global Health offered by the health sciences programme of FHML can further strengthen Maastricht's international position in education in medicine and health sciences.

From the 1990s the faculty has invested considerable manpower and financial resources in the development of internationalization in the medical programme. Initially, the emphasis was on the development of outbound student mobility. However, this affected the organization of education, concentrated in the faculty's Education Office. The Education Office had streamlined the organization of the medical education programme, during the clinical phase in particular, which gave students the possibility of completing their studies within the nominal six years of the curriculum. By contrast, internationalization required the organization to be flexible to allow students to undertake clerkships abroad, to skip progress tests when studying abroad, etc. It took quite some years before the Education Office accepted internationalization as an integral component of the medical programme. As mentioned earlier, eventually the organization of internationalization was fully integrated in the tasks of the Institute for Education.

Two issues that have caused the progress of the internationalization of medical education to be somewhat slow should be mentioned. Firstly, there is still reluctance to include aspects of international health in the curriculum. International aspects of health, such as globalization, public health, healthcare systems, and intercultural communication are not included in the regular medical programme but are covered by electives like 'Tropical Medicine' offered by IFMSA and an honours programme on 'International Medicine'. Secondly, some staff members remain very sceptical about the quality of clinical clerkships abroad, in developing countries in particular. Nevertheless, the extended responsibilities often given to medical students in hospitals in developing countries can provide strong learning opportunities (Niemantsverdriet, 2007). Moreover, the experience of practising medicine outside our 'technology-driven' clinical settings teaches students to rely on their basic clinical skills in diagnosing patients. Apart from all the positive results the deviant construct of PBL curricula initially posed a barrier to international student exchange. The lack of programmes that were in line with the PBL approach hampered outbound student mobility and students from conventional schools were usually not rewarded by their home institutions for attending theme-oriented, multidisciplinary units at a PBL school like Maastricht. However, over the course of time more medical schools all over the world have adopted integrated and PBL programmes, which has mitigated this problem.

Annotated literature

Knight, J. (2008). *Higher education in turmoil: the changing world of internationalization.* Rotterdam: Sense. This book offers a critical perspective on the rationales, benefits, risks, strategies, and outcomes of internationalization. A look at the diversity of approaches to internationalization across institutions and countries around the world emphasizes that 'one size does not fit all' when it comes to integrating international and intercultural dimensions into the teaching, learning, research, and service functions of higher education. This book extensively addresses the definition of concepts used in internationalization, provides tools for quality assurance in internationalization, and demonstrates the interplay between internationalization and globalization through the impact of the General Agreement on Trade in Services (GATS) on higher education.

Niemantsverdriet, S. (2007). *Learning from international internships: A reconstruction in the medical domain.* PhD thesis, Maastricht: Datawyse.
In this PhD thesis the educational effects of learning in international internships were investigated. The study was set up according to the principles of grounded theory. Data were gathered through surveys of coordinators of internationalization programmes, interviews with students at Dutch medical schools and with supervisors at the sites of students' international internships, and a questionnaire administered to an international panel of experts on student mobility. In the resulting grounded theory of learning in international internships the emerging core category was 'sense of belonging'. Together with the 'central categories' of supervision, learning processes, and learning outcomes the theory provides an explanation for students' differing learning outcomes. Experiential (unstructured) learning processes predominated. Students' learning was fostered by a 'sense of belonging' and hampered when this 'sense of belonging' was weak, e.g., due to an unfavourable social climate. Results suggest that active learning processes (either self-directed or guided) can improve the effectiveness of international internships.

Teekens, H. (ed.) (2006). *Internationalization at home: a global perspective.* Den Haag: Nuffic, 2006.
The concept of internationalization at home was the central topic of a 2005 conference organized by the Netherlands' Organization for International Cooperation in Higher Education (Nuffic). The book is meant for practitioners in the field of international and intercultural education, academics, and higher education policy-makers. The following themes are dealt with: approaches to structural internationalization beyond mobility, areas for improvement, and new strategies for preparing students to live and work in an international and intercultural environment. Part I of this book presents more philosophical and theoretical contributions; in part II case studies show how diversity is considered and handled in practice.

Thompson, M. J., Huntington, M. K., Hunt, D. D., Pinsky, I. E., and Brodie, J. J. (2003). Educational effects of international health electives on US and Canadian medical students and residents: a literature review. *Academic Medicine* **78**, 342–7.
This paper presents a meta-analysis of eight independent reports on the educational effect of electives abroad ('international health electives', IHE) taken by US and Canadian medical students and residents. In seven of these studies educational effects of IHE were assessed using self-reported questionnaires; one study used an objective measurement of knowledge. Taking IHE was found to be associated with career choices in underserved or primary care settings and recruitment to residency programmes. Positive effects on participants in IHE included their clinical skills, certain attitudes, and knowledge of tropical medicine. An important aspect of this paper is the set of inclusion criteria for reports in this meta-analysis, as defined by the authors.

These criteria can be useful to any investigator in the domain of internationalization of education considering reporting on electives and internships of medical and health sciences students taken abroad. The meta-analysis may be somewhat outdated by now. The most recent study included was published in 2000.

De Wit, H. (2002). *Internationalization of higher education in the United States of America and Europe: A historical, comparative, and conceptual analysis.* London: Greenwood Press.

This comprehensive book describes and compares the historical development of the internationalization of higher education in the United States and Europe and provides a comparative and conceptual analysis. First, de Wit describes and compares the historical development of internationalization in higher education in the United States and Europe. In part two, the political, economic, social/cultural, and academic rationales for the internationalization of higher education are described and a critical analysis of the different meanings and definitions as well as organization models and strategies is provided. In the last section, internationalization of higher education is placed in the context of recent globalization. The book may serve those in search of a thorough introduction to internationalization of higher education.

References

Knight, J. (2008). *Higher education in turmoil: the changing world of internationalization.* Rotterdam: Sense.

Niemantsverdriet, S. (2007). *Learning from international internships: A reconstruction in the medical domain.* PhD thesis, Maastricht: Datawyse.

Teekens, H. (ed.) (2006). *Internationalization at home: a global perspective.* Den Haag: Nuffic, 2006.

Thompson, M. J., Huntington, M. K., Hunt, D. D., Pinsky, I. E., and Brodie, J. J. (2003). Educational effects of international health electives on US and Canadian medical students and residents: a literature review. *Academic Medicine* **78**, 342–7.

Chapter 26

A role for problem-based learning in higher education in the developing world

Gerard Majoor and Han Aarts

Higher education in the developing world is facing many challenges. Problem-based learning (PBL) may help to overcome some of these. Interest from the developing world in PBL as applied at the Faculty of Health, Medicine and Life Sciences (FHML) of Maastricht University has elicited many cooperation projects between FHML and medical and health sciences schools in the developing world. To initiate and manage these projects Maastricht University created an office for academic development cooperation: Mundo.

A global need to expand higher education

The world of today is increasingly dependent on knowledge and therefore on people who are capable of generating and applying knowledge. Thus, the potential of a society to develop is critically related to the comprehensiveness and quality of its educational system and the rate of participation of the population in that system. This is especially true for higher education which provides society with academic professionals (World Bank, 2002).

The biggest challenges to higher education are seen in developing countries. Most of the world's 120 developing countries are located in Africa, Asia, and Latin America. Some 80% of the world population lives in those developing countries, which face the world's major development problems like poverty, poor health, poor education, environmental degradation, and the impact of climate change. In the emerging 'global knowledge society' one of the keys to 'development for all' lies in how effectively knowledge can be applied to promote development in a local context. Well-educated people are needed to attain that aim. Consequently a huge expansion of higher education capacity in the developing world is needed (see, e.g., World Bank, 2008).

However, higher education in the developing world is confronted by both a quantitative and a qualitative challenge. The quantitative problem arises from the recent explosion of demand for higher education as seen almost everywhere in the developing world. This demand has not been met by an adequate expansion of capacity to absorb students. In fact, public funding for higher education often decreased, even in absolute terms. Most universities have increased student enrolment but not sufficiently to meet the growing demand. Also many new universities have been established, often with private funding, but the quality of education in these new universities remains to be proven. The qualitative problem has its roots in the traditional lecture-based didactic tradition, which continues to dominate education in many developing countries. Higher education in the established universities has not been adjusted to the changing needs of society. Graduates usually have acquired a static and often outdated knowledge base. As students they were taught neither how to locate, retrieve, and critically assess new information, nor how to apply relevant information to problems encountered. Taken together, 'the overall quality of higher education has declined in much of the developing world as a result of overcrowding and inadequate resources' (Altbach, 2008).

In conclusion, in higher education in the developing world, quantitative capacity must be expanded and the quality of education needs to be improved. It is of the utmost urgency that these changes take place.

The need for a different paradigm in higher education

The qualitative challenge described above calls for redefinition of the aims of higher education, particularly in developing countries. Graduates and academic professionals can no longer work *from* a static knowledge base, but they must be able to work intelligently *with* knowledge resources. To that end, students need to learn to analyse the problems prevailing in their country and to define the relevant sub-problems contained therein. Next, they should be able to determine what knowledge is needed to solve these particular problems, how to retrieve relevant information, and how to assess its reliability; in other words how to distinguish evidence-based information from opinions and ideas. Lastly, students need to learn how to apply the knowledge acquired to the issue or problem to be addressed. In brief, there should be a shift in higher education from 'teaching' and 'instruction' towards training in 'retrieval and critical appraisal of information' and 'application of knowledge to current problems'. As stated in a 2008 policy paper by the World Bank on tertiary education in Sub-Saharan Africa:

> Perhaps the most difficult task facing tertiary institutions (in Africa) as they transition to a culture favouring innovation is to change their traditional pedagogy. The changes are well known: *interdisciplinary rather than disciplinary perspectives; flexibility in learning; group work instead of lectures; problem solving rather than memorization of facts; practical learning as a complement to theory; learning assessment through project work that demonstrates competence instead of multiple choice examinations; communication skills; and computer literacy.*

> (World Bank, 2008; italics by the authors)

The desired features of higher education mentioned in this quotation are almost identical to the guiding principles of PBL as applied at Maastricht University, especially by the FHML. This may explain why, since the inception of the Maastricht PBL medical curriculum, many institutions for higher education in the developing world have shown an interest in PBL as practised in Maastricht University.

PBL: a panacea for higher education in developing countries?

PBL challenges the paradigm of teaching in which knowledge is transferred from teacher to students. PBL is a form of 'student-centred learning', which implies that students are encouraged to take responsibility for their own learning. This may require a big effort of higher education institutions in developing countries, because pre-university education is almost exclusively based on classroom teaching. But if students accept the student-centred format, the usually inefficient classroom teaching may be substituted by more rewarding learning formats. Students could meet in small groups to jointly analyse problems carefully selected and described by their teachers, then individually consult resources (in the library or in the local internet café) and, again in their small groups exchange newly acquired knowledge and apply that to the problem initially analysed. There may be additional advantages of this 'teacher-independent learning' approach. First, the problems presented to the students to rouse their curiosity (or, in other words, to trigger their intrinsic motivation) may confront them with current problems of their own country, region, city, or community. In that way any information acquired by the students will be relevant to solving local problems. Second, information gathered by the students may be more up-to-date than that provided by teachers. Particularly if students have access to the Internet and an electronic library, they can easily obtain the latest information. To that aim, availability of some recent textbooks and computers with Internet access is more helpful than a library with outdated journal issues. Third, this format teaches students to search for and retrieve recent and relevant information, a skill most helpful for their future professional career. Fourth, working together in small groups develops collaborative and communication skills: like chairing a session, keeping notes, phrasing their own contribution and—above all—listening to others. All in all, there may be many important reasons that favour a change to student-centred and problem-oriented educational approaches in higher education in developing countries. For the domain of medicine and health sciences such changes were already proposed for example in 1987 in a WHO report on 'community-based education of health personnel' (WHO Study Group, 1987).

If your PBL car is so posh, why does it run this slow?

The barriers to the introduction of new educational approaches like PBL are many, and some may be hidden or even go unrecognized. Lack of financial resources to restructure lecture halls into tutorial rooms and to equip the library is often explicitly put forward. The next is an insufficient number of staff to run all tutorial group sessions—while alternatives like using advanced students as tutors for freshmen are overlooked. (National) culture may be mentioned as incompatible with collaborative learning, although examples of PBL schools in countries dispersed all over the world contradict this view. Most importantly, strong resistance to change may reside in the faculty. Usually staff members were educated in the traditional format and it may be very difficult for them to accept the advantages of an education paradigm so fundamentally different from the one by which they were trained. Furthermore, national culture and derived organizational structures may influence the propensity to adopt an integrated curriculum (e.g., a PBL curriculum). Integrated programmes require a multidisciplinary, centralized organization of a school but in many cases academic departments are still rather monodisciplinary, highly autonomous, and strictly hierarchically organized. And finally it may be difficult for faculty in developing countries to adopt new academic roles in addition to their other jobs which they need to earn a decent income. However, the world has changed and therefore it may be worthwhile to (re)consider the essential features of PBL as a new paradigm for higher education in developing countries.

Assisting schools of medicine and health sciences in the developing world

In the 1990s the number of requests from universities in the developing world to the former Faculties of Medicine and Health Sciences of the then 'Rijksuniversiteit Limburg' for assistance with educational change increased rapidly. After a successful cooperation with Suez Canal University in Egypt, subsequent partnerships were established with universities in El Salvador (University of El Salvador), Sudan (Ahfad University for Women), and Kenya (Moi University). With these partners, projects were developed for which substantial external funding was obtained, in most cases from the Dutch development aid budget. This prompted the need for an organizational unit to manage these projects and to administer the budgets involved. In 1993 the initiative was taken by both faculties together with Maastricht University's central international office to establish a 'University of Limburg International Centre for Educational development' (Ulice). When the Rijksuniversiteit Limburg was renamed Maastricht University, 'Ulice' changed to 'Mundo': Maastricht University centre for international cooperation in academic development.

From the 1990s up to mid-2009, over twenty projects in the domain of medicine and health were executed in close cooperation between FHML and Mundo (Table 26.1). Below a general outline of such projects with some guiding principles for this type of cooperation is described and one case example is presented.

Generic project setup

The common overall aim of a typical project is to improve an existing education programme (for instance, part of a medical curriculum) with a partner university in Africa or Asia. Sometimes the

Table 26.1 Cooperation projects with partner universities in the developing world implemented by FHML with the support of Mundo.

I. Projects in progress (in October 2009)

Partner institution	Project objectives	Running time
Catholic University of Mozambique (UCM), Beira, Mozambique	Establishment and development of a new medical school (among other objectives)	2000–4 (initial and first phase); 2005–10 (second phase)
Ho Chi Minh City University of Medicine and Pharmacy, HCMC, Vietnam	Development of medical skills training at the major public medical schools of Vietnam	2004–9
Hanoi Medical University and other medical schools, Vietnam	Development of a curriculum for general physicians for rural areas in Vietnam	2008–12
Gadjah Mada University, Yokyakarta, Indonesia	Development and introduction of PBL, skills training and community-based internships in the medical curriculum	2004–6 (first phase) 2006–10 (second phase)
University for Development Studies, Tamale, Ghana	Development and implementation of a PBL curriculum in medicine	2005–9
Makerere University, Kampala, Uganda	Various improvements in the medical curriculum as offered by Makerere	2004–9
Ministry of Education, Science and Technology (MESCT), Mozambique	Development of educational modules on HIV-AIDS; training and research by educational staff on HIV-AIDS issues	2005–8 (extended until 2009)
Mekelle and Hawassa Universities, Ethiopia	Various improvements in medical education at two Ethiopian universities	2006–10
Hadhramout University, Mukalla, Yemen	Various improvements in medical education at Hadhramout University, Mukalla, Yemen	2003–7 (first phase); 2008–11 (second phase)
Ege University, Izmir, Turkey	Educational development and primary care research at the medical faculty of Ege University	2004–9
University of Venda for Science and Technology, Thohoyandou, South Africa	Development and implementation of PBL in health sciences education at Venda University (among others)	2005–9
Faculty of Health Sciences, Moi University, Eldoret, Kenya	Development of the first Master programme in Family Medicine in East Africa	2006–9
National University of Kyiv Mohyla Academy, Ukraine	Development of the first MBA in Health Management in Ukrain	2007–10

Table 26.1 (*continued*) Cooperation projects with partner universities in the developing world implemented by FHML with the support of Mundo.

II. Track record of completed projects

University of Syiah Kuala, Faculty of Medicine, Banda-Aceh, Indonesia	Support to the faculty in recovering from the consequences of the tsunami and to introduce innovations in the medical curriculum, specifically medical skills training	2006–8
Atma Jaya University, Jakarta, Indonesia	Support for the development of a medical undergraduate curriculum using problem-based learning methodology	2007–8
School of Medical Sciences, Kathmandu University, Dhulikhel, Kathmandu, Nepal	Training in strengthening problem-based learning approaches	2007–8
Universidad de El Salvador (UES), San Salvador, El Salvador	Intervention mapping applied to health promotion	2007–8
Faculty of Medicine, University of Cairo, Egypt	Development of an electronic learning environment for medical students	2005–7
Thamassat University, Bangkok	'Higher and continuing family medicine curriculum development for rural physicians'	2004–6
Centroamericana University (UCA), Managua, Nicaragua	'Educación de la sexualidad'. A train-the-trainers programme in health education and promotion	2004–5
Can Tho University, Can Tho, Vietnam	'Strengthening medical education', phases I and II	1996–9 (phase I); 2000–4 (phase II)
Moi University, Eldoret, Kenya	'Strengthening community-based medical education', phases I and II	1995–2000 (phase I); 2000–4 (phase II)
Technikon Northern Gauteng, Pretoria, South Africa	'Academic staff development health', phase I	2000–4
University of El Salvador (UES), San Salvador, El Salvador CA	'Strengthening public health education at the University of El Salvador', phase I, I, and III	since 1989; final phase 1997–2000; finalized 2002
Ministry of Health, Gujarat State, India	'Gujarat Netherlands demand-driven health care project'	1998–2001
Ahfad University for Women, Omdurman, Sudan	'Strengthening community-based medical education'	1994–9; finalized 2000
Ministry of Health, Egypt	'Training programme in primary health care for PHC physicians'	1998–2000
Suez Canal University, Ismailia, Egypt	Developing a community-based curriculum in medicine	1984–6

aim is to develop an entire new curriculum. A project spans a certain period, usually three or four years, but may be extended to double that time and more. Funding is usually provided by an external party, such as the Dutch government or an international development donor. The main activity is often to train the faculty how to develop or change (part of) the education programme in accord with the PBL approach. Also there is a great demand for development of systematic skills training programmes—another feature of Maastricht University's educational approach that has drawn widespread attention. Sometimes these components have been complemented by strengthening community-based education and clinical training.

Projects usually target local staff—the people expected to manage and deliver the new programme. They are trained according to their learning needs. This may include tailor-made individual training or graduate training abroad, at Maastricht University or elsewhere. Training may be at Bachelor, Master, and even PhD level. Staff may also be trained on the job in their own institution, for instance through workshops or seminars. Such courses are usually facilitated by Maastricht faculty. Workshops focus on components of the new education programme to be developed. Common topics are defining the desired profile of a graduate in consultation with local stakeholders; curriculum design based on such graduate profile; design of problem scripts suited to trigger students' learning; tutor training; student assessment; quality assurance in PBL; and development of skills training programmes.

Next to this generic outline of a project there are several principles to which all projects should adhere and which, in combination, make up what internally is referred to as 'the Mundo approach'.

The 'Mundo approach'

Cooperation projects must be initiated by a university in the South. Often these universities are already familiar with Maastricht University and its educational approach, for instance through the 'Network: Towards Unity for Health' or through workshops on PBL offered by FHML's School of Health Professions Education (SHE). Because FHML and Mundo in principle work only in a responsive way, it may be presumed that educational innovation is really wanted by the applying institution and therefore 'need driven'.

A second leading principle is that FHML and Mundo through these cooperation projects try to make a significant contribution to development. This implies that projects always relate to generic development aims—including the Millennium Development Goals. Targeted groups may include mothers and their young children, pregnant women, poor people, etc. Consequently, for instance, a project to assist in the design of a postgraduate training programme for family physicians would receive priority over a project to develop an organ transplantation programme.

The third principle is to build educational capacity in the partner university in a sustainable way. This means that changes introduced through the project can be sustained after its expiration. By training local staff how to manage and maintain the curriculum and to generate funds to sustain it, a basis is laid for successful continuation of the programme after the project has stopped.

Case presentation: promoting community-oriented and problem-based learning at Moi University, Eldoret, Kenya

In the early 1990s, the first Dean of the Faculty of Health Sciences at Moi University (MU-FHS) in Eldoret, Kenya, was a psychiatrist. He met Maastricht's Professor of Social Psychiatry and through him sought assistance from the Maastricht medical school to develop PBL at MU-FHS. In 1994, a Maastricht team visited Eldoret to assist MU-FHS in drawing up a project proposal for funding by the Dutch government. The final project plan focused on faculty development in PBL (e.g., tutor training, exam construction), in medical skills training, and in research (through training for

Master's and PhD degrees). For the latter purpose the school was advised to concentrate on 'nutrition' as a central research theme. To assist the school with project implementation many FHML staff visited Kenya. In addition, twice a Maastricht 'long-term expert' was fielded to Eldoret. PBL continues to be maintained successfully at MU-FHS, despite its resource-scarce environment. Supported by the Dutch project a research laboratory and a learning resources centre were also built and equipped. Eight members of MU-FHS staff obtained Master's degrees abroad and three PhD degrees at, or in cooperation with Maastricht University. Finally, a fund was created to support female medical students who had insufficient income to cover their studies.

For political reasons, Dutch government support for projects in Kenya was phased out after 2000. Nevertheless, a new initiative for the development of a postgraduate Master programme in Family Medicine, the first of its kind in East Africa, was started. The initiative was supported with funds from various private donors. The first students enrolled in 2005 and graduated in 2007. Also thanks to this project 'family physicians' are now formally recognized as medical specialists in Kenya.

In parallel to its first contact with Maastricht, MU-FHS had also established a link with the Faculty of Health Sciences at Linköping University in Sweden, another Network member practising PBL. This institution had secured funds from the Swedish government to support the undergraduate 'Community-Based Education and Service' programme at MU-FHS. This effective and successful triangle of collaborating institutions has expanded to include a few more universities (e.g., Indiana University, USA) and formalized for the purpose of mutual donor adjustment as the 'Friends of MU-FHS' (Oman et al., 2007).

Conclusion

There is growing agreement about the need to urgently and significantly increase the quantitative capacity of higher education institutions in developing countries. At the same time education delivered by those institutions must become more relevant to the problems faced by the developing world. This chapter advocates student-centred PBL as an approach to learning that may be instrumental in addressing the latter challenge. The educational approach for health professions education as practised and investigated by FHML over many years may have great potential for higher education in all kinds of domains in the developing world. This seems to be confirmed by the observation that many education institutions in the developing world have shown interest in the Maastricht PBL approach to education. Since the 1980s, FHML and its predecessors have entered into partnerships with institutions in developing countries with the aim of assisting them with the introduction of new approaches to education. And since 1993, Mundo has been instrumental in the design, management, and administration of projects to facilitate these collaborations. Key characteristics of these projects are that they are need driven; that 'content' is delivered by FHML experts; that they contribute not only to educational innovation but also to generic development goals; and that the achievements of cooperation are sustainable in the long term.

Development cooperation projects are not only beneficial to partner institutions in the developing world but also to FHML. These projects contribute to a broader perspective on health and healthcare than a view based on just the Maastricht region or the Dutch context. Collaboration with partners in the developing world has played a significant role in the development and design of education programmes for professionals, like the international Master of Public Health for Professionals (MPHP) and the international Master of Health Profession Education (MHPE). In addition, significant numbers of graduates from these programmes are based in the developing world and have obtained their PhD degree at, or in close collaboration with Maastricht University. Members of FHML staff have participated enthusiastically as consultants and content experts in development cooperation projects, or supervised Master and PhD students from developing countries. Their experiences impact on their work for FHML. All in all, development cooperation has significantly added to FHML's international reputation in innovative medical and health sciences education.

Annotated literature

Altbach, P.G. (2008). The complex roles of universities in the period of globalization. In: *Higher education in the world 3—Higher education: new challenges and emerging roles for human and social development.* GUNI Series on the Social Commitment of Universities 3. Pp. 5–14.

In this era universities are called on to be entrepreneurial and market-relevant, in addition to their traditional core functions of education and research. These core functions may be negatively affected by the new challenges. Altman first describes the central academic roles of universities, i.e., preservation and dissemination of knowledge; acting as intellectual and international centres; guarding access and equity; functioning as engines of economic development; and providing general education. After a sketch of the historical perspectives the implications of massification of higher education are discussed. Firstly in relation to the emergence of private educational institutions next to public institutions, and secondly in relation to the special challenges faced by developing countries. In the chapter's conclusion it is stated with respect to universities in general that 'there seems to be neither the time nor the resources to consider new approaches to educating students or serving society'. With respect to the developing world this statement forms the linchpin of Altbach's chapter and the one above.

World Bank (2002). *Constructing knowledge societies—new challenges for tertiary education.* Washington, DC: World Bank; and

World Bank (2008). *Accelerating catch-up—tertiary education for growth in sub-Saharan Africa.* Washington, DC: World Bank.

During the 1990s the World Bank emphasized the importance of primary education for development. For many years the consequence was political neglect of the higher education sector, which was in particular severely felt in African higher education. It was only at the turn of the century that the World Bank—on the wave of the emerging global knowledge society—'rediscovered' the crucial role of higher education for development. The 2002 World Bank policy paper *Constructing Knowledge Societies* is probably the most obvious reflection of the Bank's mind shift. Specifically for Sub-Saharan Africa, this change of mind was taken a few steps further in the 2008 report *Accelerating Catch-Up–Tertiary Education for Growth in Sub-Saharan Africa.* This paper not only (re)emphasizes the importance of higher education for development, but also analyses what kind of higher education is needed. In the view of the World Bank current higher education does not deliver well. In the Bank's view, drastic changes are needed to make higher education effective for fostering development. The report was well received because of its support for the higher education sector in Africa in general and for pushing badly needed change. However, the report also met with criticism, predominantly for assigning an almost exclusive instrumental role to higher education in support of economic development. Critics prefer to see higher education also perform more generic functions, such as developing critical intellectual mass and contributing to culture and society.

References

Altbach, P.G. (2008). The complex roles of universities in the period of globalization. In: *Higher education in the world 3—Higher education: new challenges and emerging roles for human and social development.* GUNI Series on the Social Commitment of Universities 3. Pp. 5–14.

Oman, K., Khwa-Otsyula, B., Majoor, G., Einterz, R., and Wasteson, A. (2007). Working collaboratively to support medical education in developing countries: the case of the Friends of Moi University Faculty of Health Sciences. *Education for Health* **20**, 1–9.

WHO Study Group (1987). *Community-oriented education of health personnel.* Technical Report Series 746. Geneva: World Health Organization.

World Bank (2002). *Constructing knowledge societies—new challenges for tertiary education.* Washington, DC: World Bank.

World Bank (2008). *Accelerating catch-up—tertiary education for growth in sub-Saharan Africa.* Washington, DC: World Bank.

Index